Sexual Health

For Baillière Tindall:

Senior Commissioning Editor: Jacqueline Curthoys
Project Manager: Gail Murray
Project Development Manager: Karen Gilmour
Designer: George Ajayi

Sexual Health
Foundations for Practice

Edited by

Heather Wilson BEd(Hons) RGN RHV
Education Officer, English National Board for Nursing,
Midwifery and Health Visiting, York, UK

Sue McAndrew MSc BSc (Hons) Marital & Sex
Therapist CPN Cert RMN
Nursing Lecturer, University of Leeds, Leeds, UK

Foreword by

Ben Thomas BSc(Hons) MSc RGN RMN DipN RNT FRCN
Director of Nursing, Somerset Partnership NHS and Social Care Trust,
Bridgewater; Principal Lecturer
Mental Health, University of Plymouth, Plymouth, UK

Introduction by

Robert J. Pratt BA MSc RN RNT DN(Lond)
Centre for Sexual Health and HIV Studies,
School of Health and Science,
Thames Valley University, London, UK

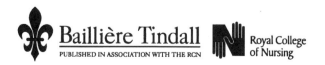

Baillière Tindall
PUBLISHED IN ASSOCIATION WITH THE RCN

Royal College
of Nursing

EDINBURGH LONDON NEW YORK PHILADELPHIA ST LOUIS SYDNEY TORONTO 2000

BAILLIÈRE TINDALL
An imprint of Harcourt Publishers Limited

© Harcourt Publishers Limited 2000

is a registered trademark of Harcourt Publishers Limited

First published 2000

ISBN 0 7020 2269 1

British Library Cataloguing in Publication Data
A catalogue record for this book is available from the British Library

Library of Congress Cataloging in Publication Data
A catalog record for this book is available from the Library of Congress

Note
Medical knowledge is constantly changing. As new information
becomes available, changes in treatment, procedures, equipment and
the use of drugs become necessary. The editors, contributors and the
publishers have, as far as it is possible, taken care to ensure that the
information given in this text is accurate and up to date. However,
readers are strongly advised to confirm that the information, especially
with regard to drug usage, complies with the latest legislation and
standards of practice.

The
publisher's
policy is to use
**paper manufactured
from sustainable forests**

Printed in China

Contents

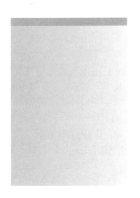

Contributors

Jo Adams
Manager, Sheffield Centre for HIV and Sexual
Health, Sheffield, UK

Kevin P. Corbett BA(Hons) MSc RN PGCE
Senior Lecturer Primary Care, Faculty of
Health and Social Care Sciences,
Kingston University & St George's Hospital
Medical School, London, UK

David T. Evans BA(Hons) PGDip Psychol Couns PGCE
(Health Professions) MPhil (Wales) RN
Freelance Educational Consultant in Sexual
Health, London, UK

Gordon Evans MSc RGN RMN RNT
Pathway Leader, Department of
Health Studies, University of York,
Scarborough Hospital,
Scarborough, UK

Jackie Green MB BS MSc
Senior Lecturer, School of Health and
Community Care, Leeds Metropolitan
University, Leeds, UK

Ian Hicken RGN RMN CPN (Cert)
Formerly Lecturer,
University of Manchester,
Manchester, UK

John C. Hooker BSc RGN RMN DN Cert
Primary Care Manager (Service Development),
Central and East Gateshead Primary
Care Group, Gateshead, UK

Steve Jamieson MSc BSc(Hons) RMN RGN DipCPN
Advisor in Sexual Health,
Royal College of Nursing, London, UK

Damon D. Lab BSc DClinPsy
Clinical Psychologist, Department of
Psychology, Institute of Psychiatry,
London, UK

Sue McAndrew MSc BSc(Hons) Marital & Sex
Therapist CPN Cert RMN
Nursing Lecturer, University of Leeds,
Leeds, UK

Anne McNall BA(Hons) RGN RM CertEd
Senior Lecturer, Faculty of Health, Social
Work and Education, University of
Northumbria at Newcastle,
Newcastle, UK

Hugh Palmer BSc(Hons) CertEd RGN RMN
Nursing Lecturer, Division of Nursing,
School of Healthcare Studies,
University of Leeds, Leeds, UK

Robert J. Pratt BA MSc RN RNT DN(Lond)
Professor of Nursing, Centre for Sexual
Health and HIV Studies, Thames Valley
University, London, UK

Gerald Anthony Samociuk MEd RMN DN(Lon)
Adv Dip Guidance & Counselling CertEd FETC
Lecturer in Mental Health Nursing, School of
Healthcare Studies, University of Leeds,
Leeds, UK

Keith Tones MA MSc PhD Hon MFPHM
Emeritus Professor of Health Education,
Leeds Metropolitan University, Leeds, UK

Robert Tunmore BSc(Hons) PG Dip(Ed) MA RMN RGN
IPD Cert
Principal Lecturer/Academic Co-ordinator,
Institute of Health Studies, Faculty of Human
Sciences, University of Plymouth, Plymouth, UK

Barbara Wallace MPH
Child Care Co-ordinator, Jersey Child
Care Trust, St Helier, Jersey, UK

Heather Wilson BEd(Hons) RGN RHV
Education Officer, English National Board for
Nursing, Midwifery and Health Visiting,
York, UK

Foreword

Sexual health promotion is rarely out of the news these days. At the time of writing this foreword, news is coming through that the incidence of HIV amongst heterosexuals is rising faster than amongst the homosexual population. The controversy about repealing Section 28 of the Local Government Act (which restricts the promotion in schools of the acceptability of homosexuality) rages on, with prominent religious leaders entering the debate and questioning whether there is a moral difference between gay and straight relationships. The Government, while firmly promoting marriage and traditional family values, also acknowledges that various aspects of sexual health promotion have not received the attention they deserve. New draft guidance to schools on the teaching of sex education is due to be sent out for consultation. The Department of Health is on the verge of launching a national sexual health strategy which is intended to incorporate the main thrust of the HIV/AIDS strategy and the key messages of the Social Exclusion Unit's report on teenage pregnancy. The report reveals, for example, that in England and Wales the conception rate for teenagers has risen to nearly 90 000 a year. The report also highlights how poorly informed many British children are about sex and parenthood, contraception and sexually transmitted diseases.

Many of us have long thought that nurses have a special distinct contribution to make in sexual health promotion on a number of levels. A cursory look at the Social Exclusion Unit's report on teenage pregnancy supports this claim. The report shows the enormous potential for nurses to become involved in sexual health promotion in various ways. These include not only preventative work to reduce the rate of teenage parenthood through education about sex, relationships and contraception but also the promotion of a positive sexual identity, personal growth and increased self-esteem.

Sexual Health: Foundations for Practice contains examples of both these approaches. Jackie Green and Keith Tones remind us that to focus exclusively on the problems caused by sexual activity would deny the more positive, life-enhancing aspects of sexuality. In case nurses are still unconvinced of the enormous role they have to play in sexual health promotion, then delving into the first part of the book should change their minds. This part addresses the question of why sexual health is an issue for health carers. It includes exploration of the complex relationships between sexual health, sexuality, culture, government involvement, and a concern with the ways power has shaped our ideas and opinions about sexuality. This theme continues with the more troublesome aspects of sexuality or, more precisely, the darker side of sexual behaviour, highlighting particular groups of people who are vulnerable to the physical and emotional effects of sexual activity. Damon Lab provides a sober account of research which shows the lack of awareness of male sexual abuse and the paucity of training in this area for all health professionals.

Ideas and approaches to the inclusion of sexual health promotion in practice form the main thrust of this book. Included are examples of models and innovations in service delivery in primary care, and the acute and continuing care settings. Whatever the setting or perspective, the authors all share the same commitment, enthusiasm and values relating to sexual health promotion. The authors recognize that the planning and delivery of nursing care is incomplete without an understanding of sexuality and an informed proactive approach to sexual health promotion. Such an understanding begins with exploring our own values, attitudes and beliefs.

Of course, nurses do not practise in a vacuum and our willingness to act as change agents in the delivery of sexual health promotion depends not only on personal initiative, strengths and weaknesses but also on our professional regulation and the organizations in which we work. Heather Wilson provides a review of professional regulation as prescribed by the statutory bodies and asks some searching questions relating to practising safely in the area of sexual health, being properly prepared and demonstrating accountability. If the assessment of sexual well-being is to become part of mainstream practice, as suggested by Kevin Corbett, rather than the preserve of specialists, then a strategic approach is required. Such an approach must involve the development of policy and practice guidelines. Organizations must support staff and ensure that appropriate supervision, education and training are provided. Unfortunately, organizations often hinder or limit nurses' abilities and

militate against their promoting sexual health. Robert Tunmore explores the impact of organizational culture and behaviour on the development of sexual health related policies. Like the other chapters within the book, his takes a refreshing journey into those grey areas of sexual health, highlighting how the process of social exclusion has its roots in seemingly innocuous everyday behaviours. Sexual harassment and bullying are examples used to draw out the process of social exclusion in the context of organizational culture. Again the analysis is enriched by an emphasis on promotional proactive measures rather than merely pointing out the shortcomings and telling us what we already know.

Sexual Health: Foundations for Practice is a timely introduction to and reference book for this important area of health care. Through its learning activities and reflection points it tackles uncomfortable topics and seeks to open up lines of debate rather than foreclosing discussion. In the lively arguments and informative pages that follow, nurses will find no better framework to take forward practice developments in the area of sexual health and to ensure that sexual health promotion has a much higher priority.

Ben Thomas

Preface

Sexual health is not a single-topic subject – it covers numerous aspects of care. In high-quality health-care provision sexual health should be integrated with all aspects of patient or client care and should hold equal status with physical, spiritual, social and emotional care.

Sexual health is a right for any individual or group, irrespective of their age, gender, race, religion, sexual orientation, economic or social status, political affiliation or existing medical condition. Sexual health encompasses a number of rights, which include the right to be a sexual being; access appropriate information and resources to enable sexual safety; access appropriate services; not be at the mercy of other individuals' sexual attitudes; not be sexually harassed, exploited or assaulted; and, confidentiality and sensitive information gathering (Adapted from Royal College of Nursing 1996 Sexual health: key issues within mental health services. A position statement. RCN London).

In order to provide good-quality, effective health care which embraces this philosophy, health-care workers need to be sure of their personal and professional role in sexual health related practice, wherever it is delivered. This book aims to help clarify those roles and assist in defining boundaries for practice.

The editors and contributing authors believe that in order to meet the sexual health needs of consumers of health services, there is a natural order and priority for a learning set. The book therefore takes a 'view global, think local' approach, working from the macro level of health care through the professional and political issues of personal health care.

Following an introduction by Professor Robert J. Pratt from the Centre for Sexual Health and HIV Studies, Thames Valley University, which looks at the global challenge of acknowledging and providing appropriate sexual health care, the book is divided into three main parts. Part 1 addresses why sexual health is an issue for health-care delivery and practice. It sets into context sexual health, sexual ill health and sexual abuse by highlighting cultural, political and legal issues and the implications for both clients and health-care professionals. Chapter 1, 'Sex and the world', looks at sexual health and sexual health promotion on a global scale and emphasizes a need on the part of health-care workers to become more vigilant with regard to sexual health in their everyday practice.

Chapter 2, 'Sex and politics', defines the legal and moralistic aspects of sex and sexual health from a personal as well as a political point of view, as well as raising awareness of power, powerlessness, discrimination and prejudice.

Chapter 3, 'Sexual health abused', focuses on the sensitive issue of sexual abuse. Although this considers a national study, it reminds us of the global problem of childhood sexual abuse and its devastating effects on the adults of the future.

Part 2 considers the influences on professional practice related to sexual health. It explores the way in which society, professionals and organizations work towards meeting the sexual health-care needs of clients as individuals, groups and communities.

Chapter 4, 'Sexual health and professional practice', focuses on nursing clients in a community setting and looks at ways in which health and local authority services combine resources to meet their clients' needs.

Chapter 5, 'Sexual health for sale', describes the context of purchasing services for sexual health provision and the influence that nurses and other health-care professionals can have on strategic development.

Chapter 6, 'Sexual health: sense and sensibility', discusses the influence of culture on organizations that have a responsibility for sexual health-care delivery, and issues that can arise from sexual harassment in the workplace.

Chapter 7, 'Sex and the statutory bodies', refers to the legislation that affects sex, sexuality and sexual health and professional accountability in practice.

Part 3 focuses on service users, the skills and knowledge of health-care professionals and the context in which care is delivered.

Chapter 8, 'Sexual health and the service user', explores what users of health-care services want in order to have their sexual health-care needs met.

Chapter 9, 'Sexual health and you', describes the challenges facing health-care professionals.

Chapter 10, 'Skills for sensitivity', enables readers to develop their professional practice by enhancing the skills necessary when dealing with sensitive issues. This chapter also acknowledges the difficulties faced by professionals and provides a framework for integrating coping strategies into practice.

Chapter 11, 'Sexual health, the process: primary care', looks at those working at the interface and how they respond to the sexual health needs of communities.

Chapter 12, 'The process: acute care', identifies the ways in which acute illness can impinge on sexual health, putting forward a model for sexual history taking and also addressing some of the skills pertinent to this activity.

Chapter 13, 'Sexual health in the continuing care setting', deals with the stigmatization and fear of dealing with sexual health in continuing care settings.

Chapter 14, 'Sexual health: support and supervision', describes ways in which structured clinical supervision can enhance professional practice and improve the delivery of sexual health care.

Although this book is aimed primarily at pre-registration nursing students, it is anticipated that other health- and social-care students undertaking specific programmes, either pre- or post-registration, will find it invaluable for supporting their sexual health-related practice.

How to use this book

In order to maximize the learning experience we hope that readers will use a workshop approach to the subject of sexual health. Individual chapters will give an overview of what is to follow, with guidance on background reading. In order to help readers relate the subject to their own area of practice or study, *reflection points* will be highlighted throughout the text. It is anticipated that these will facilitate personal and professional growth and development relating to sexual health. The editors recommend that a reflective journal is kept for this purpose.

In addition, structured *learning activities* and *case studies* (some of which offer feedback) have been designed to deepen understanding and aid the application of new knowledge in practice. In some cases the learning activities can be undertaken in groups. At the end of each chapter identified resources and annotated reading will enable the reader to access further information relating to specific areas of sexual health.

Each chapter will summarize key points and contain clear signposting to other sections that address related topics.

Heather Wilson
London and Leeds 2000
Sue McAndrew

Acknowledgements

To Ian Hicken, without whom this book would never have got started, and for offering us the opportunity to experience the agony and ecstasy of book editing!

To Malcolm Wilson, without whom this book would never have got finished.

And to Peter, for being there.

Introduction

Sexual health and disease: an international perspective

Robert J. Pratt

Understanding human sexuality is a prerequisite to the promotion of sexual health, and yet all over the world sexuality remains one of the most problematic and dangerous aspects of personhood.

In this introduction, this personal impression of sexuality describes how, worldwide, traditional well organized and powerful forces have historically colluded and conspired to deprive humankind in many parts of the world of their right to express their sexuality positively and to achieve and maintain some degree of sexual health. These impressions have been formed from more than 20 years of practice in the arena of one of the most serious threats to public health within our lifetime, a pandemic daily fired by a lack of any real comprehension of sexuality, and a resulting deprivation of individual sexual health which is politically, socially and culturally premeditated.

WHAT IS SEXUALITY?

Professor Catherine Ingram Fogel (1990), of the School of Nursing at the University of North Carolina at Chapel Hill, has defined the elements of sexuality perhaps more succinctly than most authors in this field. She describes sexuality as 'an important dimension of the human personality' and sees it as being 'inextricably woven into the fabric of human existence'.

Expressing their own sexuality is important to most people at some time or another in their lives. Sexuality is an essential component of personhood; it is 'a powerful and purposeful aspect of human nature and it is an important dimension of our humanness' (Fonseca 1970). It is 'the way we individually and uniquely express and project our identity and interrelate our physiological and psychosocial processes which are inherent in the way we sexually develop and sexually respond, both to ourselves and to others' (Fogel 1990, Fonseca 1970).

Sexuality is more than just overt sexual behaviour: it spans and underlies the complete range of human experience and contributes to our lives, and to the lives of our families, friends, neighbours, colleagues and clients, in many ways.

In positively expressing sexuality, 'we are able to build our unique identity, to communicate subtle, gentle or intense feelings, to realize sexual pleasure and physical release, to emotionally bond with others, to achieve a sense of self-worth and, for many, to link with the future through their children' (Fogel 1990). Being able to positively express sexuality is one of the most joyful and enriching aspects of the human experience, which for many people in socially and economically deprived communities and countries helps compensate for many of the less positive aspects of life today. It is one aspect of life to which all persons are entitled and, for many, makes waking up in the morning worthwhile, purposeful and exciting.

Sexuality is, of course, socially and culturally constructed, and concepts of sexuality have changed over time and remain dynamic today.

Nurses, attempting to define a meaningful, relevant and applicable concept of sexual health, will remain impressed with the challenge of working towards promoting this elusive goal.

An important aspect of the art of nursing is concerned with helping clients to strive for and to achieve their maximum human potential.

Being able positively to express sexuality is an essential component of the drive to realize our ultimate potential as a person. True potential cannot be achieved unless we can positively express our sexuality and enjoy a basic level of sexual health.

The vast majority of people throughout the world today are prevented from expressing a positive sexuality, and as a consequence any concepts of sexual health that nurses in Europe subscribe to will be, to them, unachievable, irrelevant and provocative.

On a global scale there are several issues that prevent individuals from positively expressing their sexuality. These are not by any means all inclusive but they are not being addressed by nurses or anyone else: issues that are 'fixable', for which a remedy could be applied if the will existed. They include:

◆ illiteracy and poverty
◆ the taboo against discussing sexuality openly and honestly
◆ sexually transmitted infections
◆ reproductive health and family planning
◆ female genital mutilation
◆ a variety of other issues.

Finally, there is a need to reflect on those greatest of all impediments, male power, poverty and illiteracy. In 1999 there were almost 6 billion people (5716.4 million) inhabiting our planet, 80% (4549.8 million) of them living in the less developed regions, where even access to safe water and adequate food are daily challenges. Within less than 20 years the world's population will increase by a further 2 billion, principally in the developing regions. Along with great poverty, almost 1 billion (960 million) people today cannot read or write, and two-thirds of these are women. Some 130 million children, including over 90 million girls, are denied access to primary schooling (UNFPA 1995).

Being able to positively express sexuality and to acquire an acceptable level of sexual health is part of a wider agenda in which population growth, poverty and illiteracy are adequately addressed. There is no detectable will or commitment in the world to share the resources of the north with those in the south, just as in the author's field of clinical practice there is no real effort being made to provide appropriate and effective antiretroviral drugs to the 90% of individuals infected with HIV and who, by an accident of birth, live in the southern part of the world. The remedy for this is political, and a legitimate target with which professional nurses, acting within the philosophy of the International Council of Nurses, must engage.

SEXUALITY AS A TABOO

All over the world there are powerful constraints to being able openly and explicitly to discuss sexuality and sexual behaviour. Consequently, even the most superficial models of sexual health cannot be enabled and the effective promotion of primary prevention measures for sexually transmitted infections, including HIV, cannot be engaged.

Our Centre for Sexual Health Studies is currently engaged in a 5-year project in southern Asia. In India, as in many other countries in this region, the open discussion of sexuality is difficult and the acknowledgement and exploration of sexual diversity is at times impossible, if not outright dangerous. For example, India is the second most populated country in the world, with a population of almost 1 billion; this is over 16% of the world's population: more than that of South America, Africa and Australia combined. By the year 2025 India's population will have increased to 1.4 billion, and shortly thereafter will overtake China as the world's most populous nation. India is impoverished and crowded, and almost half of all Indians cannot read or write.

Along with the increase in population India will also become home to the largest number of HIV-infected people in the world, with the greatest number of new cases each year. How can this have happened? How could India jump from a practically 0% HIV prevalence rate in the mid-1980s to being engulfed by this epidemic within less than 8 years?

Many factors have conspired to position India as the developing AIDS capital of the world, not least the cultural inability of Indians to discuss sexual behaviour openly. There is little public discussion of sexuality in India and sex education is virtually non-existent. Along with high rates of illiteracy, poverty and a massive commercial sex industry, this clearly leaves Indians vulnerable to all forms of sexually transmitted infection, including HIV.

It was not always thus. Hindu culture in India has a long and rich tradition of erotic expression and discourse. The temples at Khajuraho, situated in the hot, dry plains of northern India, were built by the Chandela kings over 1000 years ago. Since their rediscovery in 1838, the erotic temple sculptures have facilitated an insight into how sexuality might have been constructed, at least by one aspect of Indian culture, at that time. Among other things, these sculptures seem to celebrate sensuality, freedom of sexual expression and a society at ease with sexual gratification.

A thousand years before the building of Khajuraho temples the great Hindu sage Vatsyayana wrote and illustrated the *Kama Sutra*, one of the most important works in a long tradition of Indian erotic literature and art. Vatsyayana's work, and that of others, celebrated sexual expression without shame, sexual diversity, and a positive joy in living.

Although the Indian epidemic is dominated by heterosexual transmission, men who have sex with other men are also part of the epidemiological equation. Today, male sexual behaviour remains diverse and men having sex with men have been recorded in Indian literature and erotic art for centuries.

The world, of course, changes, and Indian sexuality and sexual behaviour have been reshaped by many forces throughout the ages. The centuries of Muslim and then Imperial British rule, with the imposition of Islamic and British Victorian values and inhibitions, probably ended forever in India what was left of an earlier, more open, healthier and joyful approach to expressing human sexuality.

The challenge in exploring sexuality and promoting the primary prevention of sexually transmitted infections in India, as in other parts of the world, is to devise culturally sensitive and appropriate methods that allow public discussion to take place, such as the use of puppet shows, classical Hindu dance and street theatre.

The taboo against discussing sexual behaviour can also be identified in the nursing profession and in many of the cultures that make Europe. Many British nurses (and nurse teachers) are uncomfortable with their sexuality and remain embarrassed and reluctant to engage in any seemingly appropriate discussions about the sexuality of either themselves or their clients. Any strategy to promote sexual health must take into account the need to facilitate nurses – the largest group of health-care providers in the world – gaining confidence and competence in discussing sexuality and sexual behaviours.

SEXUALLY TRANSMITTED INFECTIONS

Although it is clear that any definition of sexual health means more than just simply the absence of sexual dysfunction or disease, no definition can ignore the fact that the pandemic of all forms of sexually transmitted diseases, including HIV and hepatitis B virus (HBV) infection, precludes many people throughout the world from enjoying sexual health. Over one-third of a billion people become infected with a preventable, sexually transmitted disease every year, and the number becoming infected with HIV each day (currently well over 16 000) is increasing. The remedy in part lies within the solution of the first two issues under discussion, i.e. poverty and illiteracy, and an ability to skilfully engage in communications that promote primary prevention.

REPRODUCTIVE SEXUAL HEALTH AND FAMILY PLANNING

Health issues related to reproduction and sexuality affect women and men of all ages worldwide. Individuals who have good reproductive health can enjoy healthy sexual relations: they have the ability to reproduce, and the freedom to decide if, when and how often to do so.

Several factors determine the possibility or quality of reproductive health, including social and economic development levels, lifestyles, women's position in society and their power and ability to make choices, and the quality and availability of health services.

Millions of women worldwide do not enjoy reproductive health or safe motherhood because of premature and excessive childbearing. Women are also more vulnerable to reproductive tract infections (RTIs), as well as sexually transmitted infections (STIs), including HIV. Finally, hundreds of thousands of women are at daily risk of domestic violence, rape and genital mutilation.

Understanding sexuality and promoting sexual health will lead to improvements in both reproductive health and health generally. Good reproductive health is the basis for the empowerment of women and the critical foundation in all countries for meaningful social and economic development focused on protecting women, and their children, from ill health subsequent to HIV infection.

FEMALE GENITAL MUTILATION

The United Nations (UN) estimates that between 85 and 114 million women and girls worldwide have undergone one form or another of female genital mutilation (FGM), and each year another 2 million will be subjected to these procedures. Although this is principally an Islamic practice, it is a cross-cultural and cross-religious ritual. The phenomenon is not restricted to Africa, Asia and the Middle East: it also takes place in Europe and in North America, where it is estimated that thousands of girls are at risk each year. Various forms of FGM are practised and, beyond the obvious initial pain and shock of the procedure, the long-term physiological, sexual and psychological effects are dreadful. FGM is the antithesis of sexual health, an obscene assault in which women often collude with men in its perpetuation.

OTHER GLOBAL ISSUES ASSOCIATED WITH SEXUALITY AND THE PROMOTION OF SEXUAL HEALTH

There are other equally important issues within the arena of sexual health that must be considered by health-care providers, who often deal with these issues or their consequences. The continuing global acceleration of HIV infection and AIDS is occurring in a socially constructed arena of poverty, ignorance, illiteracy, inequity, inequality and unsustainable population growth. These factors conspire to deprive people of their ability to express their sexuality safely and appropriately and to attain a basic level of sexual health. This in turn leaves them unfilled and vulnerable to sexually transmitted infections, and further intensifies the increasing epidemics of HIV infection and AIDS.

The author's centre has been active in promoting sexual health as part of an international schedule of HIV-related research and educational programmes in disparate parts of the world, including Africa, south and southeast Asia, the Middle East and eastern Europe. The work of the centre is currently focused on major AIDS-related research and education projects in south Asia and in the Arabian Gulf States, and it is true to say that the risk behaviours associated with sexually transmitted infections are the most complex area of work.

The author's impression is that in Europe, as in many other regions of the world, nurses frequently fail to relate to many of these issues. Consequently, their influence is negligible in initiating and contributing to a much-needed global discourse among health-care workers, focused on developing appropriate culture-sensitive solutions which can facilitate people's aspirations for sexual health.

Sexual diversity remains problematic even in the more liberal and enlightened countries of Europe. However, in some European states, and in general in most nations throughout the world, expressing a different sexual orientation (i.e. other than an exclusively heterosexual) remains dangerous. Even among the caring professions there is ample evidence that homophobia is common and that clients suffer as a result of subtle expressions of this attitude. Other global issues include the sexual exploitation of children, male rape and commercial sex. There is a need to highlight the recent expansion in the commercial sex industry with child sex workers, both boys and girls. This increase in demand is related to many factors, including a perception in some cultures that having sexual intercourse with a young child reduces the risk of being exposed to HIV or, even more sinister, the myth that sexual intercourse with a young boy or girl will effect a cure for a sexually transmitted disease, including HIV infection.

Another ill-discussed issue surrounds the fact of male rape, which is underreported, poorly understood and not uncommon. Male rape occurs in the community and is in many cultures a not-infrequent occurrence in many institutions, including prisons and the military.

MALE POWER

To conclude, attention should be drawn to the very heart of all the issues surrounding sexuality. It has previously been stated that sexuality is socially and culturally constructed, but it would have been more accurate to say that sexuality is socially and culturally constructed by the dominant male group in any society, which is always heterosexual and often explicitly or subliminally misogynistic. Men control all of the critical institutions in any society and determine the cultural mores of sexuality. What is more, women often collude with this domination, continuing to accept a female role constructed by men.

Throughout the world women are often economically dependent on men, their status is lower than that of men, and they have fewer opportunities for education and to acquire financial independence and personal freedom. This often means that they have little power or control over decisions relating to their sexuality and the sexual behaviour of their partner, and of accessing information on sexuality and safer sexual behaviour. Women are vulnerable to coerced sex, including marital and non-marital rape, sexual abuse within and outside the family, and/or being forced into the sex industry. In most cultures women are expected to be passive and submissive in their sexual relationships, which are invariably controlled by men. They lack the skills and confidence to discuss sexual behaviour with their partners, and have little bargaining power within their sexual relationships.

This sexual subordination makes it impossible for women to protect themselves from sexually transmitted infections or to realize their true human potential as sexual beings.

All over the world, a more open and healthy expression of human sexuality is literally being daily beaten into the ground by massive male power. Until men stop discriminating against women, and fight to empower them as equals in all aspects of life, including sexuality, women and their children, and all of our futures, will be at risk. Nurses can be positioned to influence the growth and development of sexuality, both in individuals and in societies, and can change our world.

REFERENCES

Fogel C I 1990 Human sexuality and health care. In: Fogel C I, Lauver D (eds) Sexual health promotion. WB Saunders Philadelphia

Fonseca J D 1970 Sexuality – a quality of being human. Nursing Outlook 18: 25

UNFPA 1995 The state of the world population. New Internationalist Publications, Oxford

1

Part One
Why is sexual health an issue for health care?

1

Sex and the world

Jackie Green   Keith Tones

> '*Sexual intercourse is a grossly overrated pastime; the position is undignified, the pleasure momentary and the consequences utterly damnable.*' (Lord Chesterfield)

KEY ISSUES/CONCEPTS

- ◆ Interpretations of health
- ◆ Definitions of sexual and reproductive health
- ◆ Sex, sexuality and the social construction of sexual health
- ◆ Assessing the sexual health of communities
- ◆ The promotion of sexual health
- ◆ Health education and health promotion
- ◆ Healthy sexuality: a global perspective

OVERVIEW

Chapter 1, *Sex and the world*, explores the notion of sexual health and methods of measuring it. It identifies the major influences on an individual's sexual health and the way they combine to make up what might be termed a 'sexual health career'. It also looks at strategies for promoting sexual health and how they relate to national and international initiatives, such as the Health For All movement.

INTRODUCTION

National and international concern about HIV and AIDS, unwanted pregnancies and the increasing size of the world's population has focused attention on sexual activity as a contemporary public health issue. However, to focus exclusively on the problems would deny the more positive, life-enhancing aspects of sexual experience. Furthermore, at the personal level, individuals' sexuality is integral to their sense of identity and self-esteem. It is generally accepted that there is no single objective definition of health. This applies equally to sexual health, and a number of interpretations exist. How sexual health is defined will inevitably be influenced by the values and attitudes acquired through personal experience and the process of socialization. For those working to promote sexual health, the way in which it is conceptualized has important implications for practice. It will determine:

- ◆ the acceptability of various possible indicators as measures of sexual health
- ◆ the identification and prioritization of goals
- ◆ the selection of methods to achieve those goals
- ◆ what constitutes success and how it can be evaluated.

Insight into our own understanding of sexual health and development of a sound conceptualization provides a secure basis for working with others.

There is widespread recognition of the influence of culture in shaping sexual attitudes, activities and orientation (Porter 1994). Value systems have a major direct impact on sexual health. They also have an indirect effect by imposing restrictions about what can and cannot be expressed openly, what kind of sex education can legitimately be provided, and the way sex and sexuality are treated by society in general, and in particular by health and social services.

INTERPRETATIONS OF HEALTH

Views about sexual health will inevitably be influenced by more general interpretations of what it is to be 'healthy'. Both professional and lay understandings of health exist (Aggleton and Homans 1987). Alternative interpretations of health and sexual health can be the source of misunderstanding and raise barriers to effective communication between professionals and clients, between different professionals, and indeed more generally. It is therefore important to recognize and acknowledge the range of different lay and professional perspectives. Furthermore, lay and professional beliefs do not necessarily exist completely independently of each other. Biomedical explanations may be incorporated into lay beliefs, and conversely, professionals may be influenced by the lay views acquired during their early socialization (Helman 1978, Frankel et al. 1991).

Professional interpretations of health

Health is frequently interpreted as the absence of disease. This view is central to the biomedical interpretation of health, which is based on the premise that disease and dysfunctional states can be objectively diagnosed, thereby providing a rational basis for defining health, albeit in a negative sense. This *biomedical model* has, however, been subjected to criticism because of its mechanistic, disease-orientated focus. Moreover, it tends to objectify human experience and to place authority and control in the hands of professionals.

Beattie (1993) comments on different modes of thought in describing health, and contrasts the mechanistic approach of biomedicine with humanistic approaches that focus on the meaning of health within everyday life. Aggleton and Homans (1987) identify social and holistic models

of health in addition to the biomedical model. Rather than being concerned with disease, the *social model* recognizes the importance of the subjective experience of illness and the way people respond to it. Factors such as age, gender, class and poverty may have an effect on the way individuals both interpret and react to the experience of discomfort, pain and disability. The subjectivity and relativism that are integral to the model have also been the focus of criticism. This model would in addition take a broader view of the causes of health and ill health, and acknowledge their social and environmental determinants.

The *holistic model* of health is encapsulated by the definition offered in the constitution of the World Health Organization (1946):

'. . . *a state of complete physical, mental and social well-being and not merely the absence of disease or infirmity.*'

This introduces the notion of wellbeing as distinct from freedom from disease, and draws attention to the mental and social aspects of health. Although this definition has been criticized for being unrealistic and even utopian, it extends the area of interest to include a positive dimension.

Lay interpretations of health

Lay interpretations of health include the absence of disease, but also incorporate the more subjectively defined states of illness. Exploration of these interpretations by, for example, Herzlich (1973), Blaxter and Patterson (1982), Williams (1983) and Cornwell (1984), show health to be a more complex concept incorporating a number of dimensions:

◆ The absence of disease, illness, pain, and any deviation from expected norms
◆ A reserve for coping with stress and illness
◆ Functional ability to allow tasks to be performed
◆ An ideal state including positive wellbeing.

Cornwell (1984) noted that people hold both public and private accounts of health and illness. The public accounts conform with prevailing socially accepted values, and tend to be used in communication with professionals. Although this applies to health in general, there are particular implications for communicating about sexual health. People may even use different language to talk about sex or sexual parts in public from that used in private. Indeed, many people feel uncomfortable using 'popular' words with their partner and those close to them, let alone professionals. Without a precise vocabulary that they feel able to use, people often resort to vague euphemisms, such as 'doing it'; 'private parts'; 'down below'; and so on. Communication couched in such terms is clearly open to misinterpretation.

Explanations for the occurrence of disease are also incorporated into lay beliefs. Again, these explanations often include biomedical interpretations, which however may be overlaid by notions of personal responsibility for ill health. Indeed, ill health in general is often associated with moral wrong-doing (Blaxter 1990) and this must apply particularly to sexual ill health. In the context of HIV and AIDS there has been the distinction of the 'innocent victim' from those who are judged to have brought it on themselves by going against conventional moral or social norms (Aggleton and Homans 1987). Taken to its most extreme, illness may even be seen as retribution for past misdemeanours.

The British survey of social attitudes (Social and Community Planning Research 1994) found that in 1993, 49% of people agreed that most people with AIDS had only themselves to blame (in contrast to 57% in 1989); and also in 1993, 20% thought that AIDS was a way of punishing the world for its decline in moral standards (compared to 29% in 1987 and 27% in 1989).

Overall, then, it can be seen that in defining health a number of different perspectives emerge. These are summarized below:

Professional - - - - - - - - Lay
Positive - - - - - - - - - - - Negative
Subjective- - - - - - - - - - Objective
Biomedical - - - - - - - - Holistic
Public - - - - - - - - - - - - Private

Reflection point 1.1

Consider what implications these perspectives have for you when trying to define sexual health.

DEFINITIONS OF SEXUAL AND REPRODUCTIVE HEALTH

Reproductive health

Reproductive health was defined by the International Conference on Population and Development and endorsed in Resolution 49/128 of the United Nations General Assembly as:

'. . . a state of complete physical, mental and social well-being and not merely the absence of disease or infirmity, in all matters relating to the reproductive system and its functions and processes. Reproductive health therefore implies that people are able to have a safe and satisfying sex life and that they have the capacity to reproduce and the freedom to decide if, when and how often to do so.' (Rice 1996)

Reflection point 1.2

To what extent can this definition be used to describe sexual health or reproductive health?

On the positive side

◆ It includes wellbeing and sexual satisfaction.

◆ It includes safety and freedom from disease.

◆ It refers to choice about the number of children, or not having any.

On the negative side

◆ It locates sex in the context of reproduction.

◆ It omits sex as part of emotional relationships.

◆ It may imply a heterosexual norm.

Reflection point 1.3

Brainstorm the various groups of people who come into contact with health services who may have health-care needs related to reproductive health.

Feedback on Reflection point 1.3

Did you include in your response the following groups:

◆ Pregnant women of all ages, where the pregnancy was planned, unexpected, wanted or unwanted?

◆ Infertile men and women?

◆ Women undergoing hysterectomy?

◆ Partners and families of pregnant women?

◆ Clients experiencing altered body image?

◆ Clients experiencing long-term health problems and their effects on future fertility and parenthood?

◆ Widows and widowers considering artificial reproduction?

◆ Clients with sexually transmitted diseases?

◆ Parents suffering loss after stillbirth, abortion or the death of child?

◆ Homosexual parents?

Sexual health

There are many areas of overlap between sexual health and reproductive health; however, there are also clearly important distinctions, and for some the two may be entirely unrelated.

Self-identity, emotional wellbeing and the ability to develop mutually satisfying relationships would be included in holistic definitions of sexual health. The World Health Organization (1975) defined sexual health as:

'. . . *the integration of the somatic, emotional, intellectual and social aspects of sexual being,*

in ways that are positively enriching and that enhance personality, communication and love.'

Hendriks (1992, p. 155) proposes that:

'Sexual health is an integral part of overall health, not restricted to the avoidance of STDs and HIV/AIDS. Sexual health contributes to the fulfilment of individual sexuality, enabling a person to share this with consenting others, without jeopardising the health and well-being of other persons. Sexual health requires the enjoyment of free choice, expression and responsibility, with particular regard to the prevention of transmission of STDs/HIV. The sexual health of an individual contributes to the health and well-being of the individual involved, his/her sexual partner(s), and the ultimate community as a whole.'

This definition draws attention to the right of self-determination, but not if this conflicts with the right of others.

Goldsmith (1992, p. 121) acknowledges the range of interpretations of sexual health, and suggests that they include three components:

◆ *'Absence and avoidance of STDs and disorders which affect reproduction*

◆ *Control of fertility and avoidance of unwanted pregnancy*

◆ *Sexual expression and enjoyment without exploitation, oppression or abuse.'*

These definitions of sexual health derive essentially from a professional perspective. It is important not to lose sight of the fact that sexual health is interpreted and experienced by individuals in the context of their lives.

Reflection point 1.4

In your reflective journal, create your own definition of sexual health.

How might sexual health be interpreted by the following people, and what do think might be the implications for them, given their personal circumstances?

◆ **John**, a 25-year-old man with Down's syndrome.

◆ **Margaret**, a 69-year-old widow living in a residential home.

◆ **Rani**, a 21-year-old woman living in Bihar in India who has three girls under 5 years old.

◆ **David**, a 15-year-old who knows he is homosexual.

◆ **Mary**, lives in Uganda and her husband is a long-distance lorry driver.

Feedback on Learning activity 1.1

Did you consider any of the following issues in your response?

The importance of avoiding stereotyping should always be recognized and any issue related to sexual health may be relevant to **John**, **Margaret**, **Rani**, **David** or **Mary**. **John** faces the additional problems of living in a society which often ignores the sexuality and sexual needs of those with learning disability. **Margaret** may also face discrimination because of her age and gender, and the practical difficulties of sexual relationships for those in residential care. **Rani** may feel under pressure to produce a son, even though a fourth pregnancy may carry risks for her health. **David** will most likely feel more insecure than most adolescents in a predominantly heterosexual society, and be less able to share his concerns with others. **Mary** will face not only separation from her partner but also uncertainty about her absent husband's behaviour and the possible risk of HIV infection.

SEX, SEXUALITY AND THE SOCIAL CONSTRUCTION OF SEXUAL HEALTH

The term sex, in addition to distinguishing between male and female, is generally used to describe physical acts and experiences and the feelings aroused. Again, there is no common understanding of what this involves: it may involve penetration and orgasm, or alternatively be used for a much wider range of activities, such as kissing and cuddling. Sexuality is a broader concept including gender, sexual orientation, sexual preferences, desires and sexual expression. As already noted, it is likely that individuals' feelings about their sexuality will affect their self-esteem. Awareness and a positive acceptance of one's sexuality is also integral to the development of sexual health. In stark contrast to this is the view of sexuality as a weakness which should be controlled, and sex as being acceptable only within marriage for the purpose of procreation. Fustukian et al. (1994, p. 2) emphasize the point that:

> *'Working on sexual health requires a knowledge and understanding of human sexuality. We cannot promote behaviour change without promoting sexuality awareness.'*

Many cultures attempt to define what is natural or 'normal' in relation to both sex and sexuality, labelling anything that deviates from this as promiscuous, pornographic, abnormal, deviant or even perverted. These normative views would include:

◆ who may be sexually active (e.g. generally considered to be able-bodied adults over the age of consent)

◆ with whom (usually a partner of the opposite sex)

◆ the kind of sexual activity they can engage in (ordinarily penetrative vaginal sex)

◆ how often (heavily influenced by age and gender)

◆ under what conditions (within marriage and in private).

Within society there are frequently powerful forces to encourage (or even dictate) conformity to these norms. Both the law and medicine have been used to this effect. For example, in Britain homosexuality was a criminal offence until 1967, and was on the American Psychiatric Association's list of disorders until 1974 (Field et al. 1994). In some parts of the world adultery can still incur a death sentence, and in Britain earlier this century there were instances of women being admitted to mental hospitals after giving birth to illegitimate babies. Indeed, the term illegitimate itself implies the legal sanctioning of some births and not others, and until recently carried a considerable stigma. The definitions of sexual health offered earlier attached a central importance to the element of personal choice and self-actualization and established sexual health as a basic human right. Like many other human rights it is 'often denied or abused through social, political, economic, cultural or psychological forces' (Hughes 1994, p. 4).

Comparisons between different cultures and over time show that there is no universal consensus about normal sexual behaviour. The work of Kinsey et al. (1948, 1953) in the United States revealed considerable differences between private accounts of sexual experience and notional public norms. It also challenged assumptions about what is 'normal' by revealing substantial variations in sexual behaviour, and that homosexuality and homosexual experience were much more common than had been supposed.

The survey of sexual behaviour in Britain (Wellings et al. 1994) acknowledged that people's sexual preferences and practices cannot be neatly categorized as heterosexual or homosexual, but that a continuum exists. It also distinguished between sexual experience ('any kind of contact with another person that you felt was sexual') and sexual attraction. In face-to-face interviews 90.2% of men and 92.4% of women said that their attraction and experience were exclusively heterosexual. It is noteworthy that in anonymous written answers to a different set of questions both men and women admitted to more homosexual experience than in the interviews. The difference was greatest for men, and increased with age (Field et al. 1994). Even with the liberalization of

Reflection point 1.5

Think of the ways in which sexual activity may be regulated; identify examples from your personal and professional experience from the following:

◆ Peer pressure

◆ By law

◆ By religious and moral codes

◆ By the existence of social sanctions

◆ Through the use of fear

◆ Creating myths about sexual activity.

attitudes towards homosexuality, reluctance to acknowledge it publicly clearly still exists.

Public accounts of health tend to conform with perceived norms. This is particularly so in relation to sexual activity and sexuality, where these norms may be overlaid by moral imperatives. The survey of sexual attitudes and lifestyle of almost 19 000 people in Britain (Wellings et al. 1994) revealed that:

◆ three-quarters of the sample considered sex before marriage not wrong at all

◆ 8.2% of men and 10.8% of women believed it to be always or mostly wrong

◆ nearly 80% (78.7% men and 84.3% women) considered sex outside marriage to be always or mostly wrong. In addition, two-thirds of men and more than three-quarters of women disapproved of sexual relationships outside a live-in relationship

◆ 70.2% of men and 57.9% of women believed that sex between two men was always or mostly wrong, and there was only marginally less condemnation of sex between two women (64.5% of men and 58.8% of women saw this as always or mostly wrong).

The fact that within cultures some forms of sexual expression are valued more highly than others (Aggleton et al. 1989) has important implications for individual sexual health. First, it affects how people see themselves and their self-esteem. Having high self-esteem may be considered healthy in its own right, and it will be shown later that it is a key component in both making and implementing health-related decisions. Secondly, it influences whether people are able to speak openly to others about their sexuality, sexual preferences and practices. This applies to communication with partners, the wider social circle and professionals.

Cultures may also value one gender more highly than the other. Prejudice against women and girls may show itself in a number of ways. In its most extreme form it may lead to the death of female babies and children, either directly by infanticide and selective abortion or indirectly as a result of neglect, inadequate nutrition and a poorer quality of care (including medical care) than that given to their more highly valued brothers. It has been estimated that some 60 million females globally are 'missing' for these reasons (Coale 1991).

Anthropological studies in the Pacific Islands and the United States led Mead (1962, p. 215) to conclude that 'Most societies persistently emphasise the child-rearing aspects of femininity as the significant ones'. For women who have internalized this view there is pressure to conceive, and repercussions as to how they see their femininity for those who either cannot or choose not to do so. In some parts of the world marriage and motherhood (particularly of sons) is the only way for women to achieve fulfilment and social status (Armstrong 1990). However, there are also expectations in virtually all societies that women will control both their fertility and their sexuality.

Within sexual relationships the role of women may be seen as giving pleasure to their partners, rather than experiencing it themselves. The ultimate manifestation of this attitude is female genital mutilation. Although somewhat trivial in comparison, the absence of non-medical words for the clitoris could be seen as a linguistic equivalent. Even in countries that pride themselves on gender equality, it may still be less acceptable for women to be assertive in sexual relationships and insist on protection against pregnancy and sexually transmitted disease.

Reflection point 1.6

Consider a situation where your cultural background has differed from that of your client. To what extent does the awareness of a cultural difference affect your health-care practice in this situation? Try to identify practical examples related to the delivery of sexual health care.

SEXUAL HEALTH: A CONTINUUM

It is possible to think of sexual health as a continuum ranging from negative to positive (Box 1.1). At the negative end would be disease states, unwanted pregnancy and a range of factors affecting wellbeing, such as ignorance, embarrassment, frustration, fear, and access to appropriate services.

Downie et al. (1990) reject this simple continuum as a basis for describing health in general. They suggest that it is possible for wellbeing to exist independently of states of disease or ill health, and represent this by using two intersecting axes (Fig. 1.1)

If this interpretation is applied to sexual health, it is perfectly possible for someone with gonorrhoea, who would be located towards the negative end of the health/ill-health axis, to be sexually active and experience high levels of personal wellbeing as a result. In complete contrast, an individual may have no problems in terms of their disease status, but not experience sexual wellbeing.

Box 1.1

Negative	Positive
STDs	Freedom from disease
HIV	Planned pregnancy
Unwanted pregnancy	Mutually satisfying
Abortion	relationships
Frustration	Respect for self
Exploitation	Respect for others
Embarrassment	Pleasure
No self-respect	

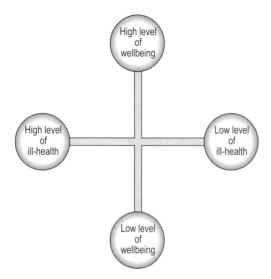

Fig. 1.1 Ill health and wellbeing (derived from Downie et al. 1990). Reproduced with permission of Oxford University Press.

ASSESSING THE SEXUAL HEALTH OF COMMUNITIES

Although sexual health is experienced by individuals, assessment of the sexual health status of communities and populations is an essential basis for:

◆ identifying and prioritizing need
◆ planning services
◆ exploring determinants of sexual health and ill health
◆ evaluating interventions.

Which measures we choose to accept as indicators of sexual health will be determined in part by the concept of health to which we adhere. The validity of each measure must therefore be judged in relation to the concept it is describing. It is also useful to reflect on whether proposed indicators are:

◆ **necessary** for describing sexual health (is it possible to describe sexual health without including them?)
◆ **sufficient** to describe sexual health (do they include all the variables required or is anything else needed?).

Epidemiological measures

The traditional 'tools' of epidemiology are morbidity and mortality data, which are used to measure disease and death, respectively. It will be clear that these are negative indicators and assess health by the absence of disease. However, data of this nature are often collected routinely and are therefore readily available.

Learning activity 1.2

Identify two sources of morbidity data and mortality data related to sexual health.

HIV/AIDS and sexually transmitted diseases

Most countries have systems to monitor the number of AIDS cases, which are frequently presented as the cumulative total since the disease was first recognized (Table 1.1).

The Public Health Laboratory Service estimates that there is about 13% underreporting of AIDS in England and Wales (Health Education Authority 1994), but worldwide this may be much greater. By December 1996 1.5 million cases of

Reflection point 1.7

What are the advantages and disadvantages of using cumulative totals of AIDS?

Advantage

It represents the total disease burden that a country has experienced.

Disadvantages

◆ It does not distinguish between those living with AIDS and those who have died.

◆ It does not reflect the fact that the size of the populations of different countries may differ widely; the use of **rates** would compensate for this.

Table 1.1   European AIDS figures (cumulative tables to 30 June 1996)

Country	Cases	Country	Cases
Austria	1 609	Norway	533
Belgium	2 203	Portugal	3 575
Czech Republic	85	Romania	4 198
Denmark	1 957	Russian Federation	245
France	43 451	Spain	41 598
Germany	15 308	Sweden	1 445
Greece	1 422	Switzerland	5 397
Israel	403	Turkey	214
Italy	35 949	United Kingdom	13 394
Netherlands	4 199		

Learning activity 1.3

List the factors that might influence the number of cases of AIDS in a country.

Feedback on Learning activity 1.3

You might have considered the following:

◆ The extent of 'unsafe' sexual practices.

◆ The sharing of drug injecting equipment.

◆ The safety of donor blood supplies and blood products.

◆ The accuracy of diagnosis and reporting.

◆ The stage in the development of the 'epidemic' – countries that AIDS has only recently reached are unlikely to have as many cases as those in which it has been present for much longer.

AIDS had been officially reported to the World Health Organization, but it is estimated that more than 8.4 million cases have actually occurred since the beginning of the epidemic (UNAIDS 1996).

The long interval between infection with HIV and the development of symptoms of AIDS also means that the data may reflect what was happening in terms of transmission some years ago. This period tends to be longer in developed countries than in developing ones, where the progression

of the disease is usually more rapid. Data on HIV-positive status would give a much more up-to-the-minute picture on current trends. However, some countries do not have the resources to fund extensive testing facilities. Furthermore, HIV-positive reports need to be interpreted with caution as they only apply to those who have actually been tested and omit two important groups, i.e. those who are unaware that they have been at risk but may in fact be HIV positive; and those who are aware that they have been at risk but who have decided not to be tested, possibly because of the fear of prejudice against those who are HIV positive, or indeed the negative consequences of taking the test itself.

To compensate for this problem some countries have set up surveillance surveys. In the United Kingdom, for example, a programme of unlinked anonymous testing of blood samples obtained primarily for other purposes was set up in 1990.

A distinction also needs to be made between the number of *new* cases (i.e. the incidence) and *all* the cases, which would include existing cases and new ones for the period in question (i.e. the prevalence). **Incidence** gives a clearer picture of the trend in the spread of the virus; **prevalence** is more useful in planning services.

Data on HIV and AIDS are often broken down according to the probable source of exposure (Table 1.2).

UNAIDS (1996) estimates that throughout the world there are about 22.6 million people living with HIV and AIDS, and that each day a further 8500 become infected. The total number of deaths

Table 1.2   UK AIDS and HIV infections (1996). Derived from AVERT 1997

Probable route of infection	HIV	AIDS
Sexual intercourse between men	1634	1165
Sexual intercourse between men and women	779	440
Injecting drug use	173	135
Blood factor (e.g. haemophilia)	5	48
Blood and tissue transfer	20	15
Mother to child	28	31
Other	257	28
Total	2896	1862

Learning activity 1.4

Describe the advantages and disadvantages of using the categories of transmission from Table 1.2.

Feedback on Learning activity 1.4

You might have considered the following:

◆ It allows the spread of the virus through different routes to be tracked.

◆ It might lead to stereotyping of different groups.

◆ HIV is transmitted by what people do, not which groups they belong to.

from AIDS is expected to exceed 8 million by the year 2000 (WHO 1995). Although there is much current concern about HIV and AIDS, it is important not to lose sight of other sexually transmitted diseases. WHO (1996) estimates that worldwide, not including AIDS and other viral STDs, there is an annual incidence of 333 million cases of curable STDs. The four most common are:

◆ trichomoniasis: 170 million cases per year
◆ chlamydia: 89 million cases per year
◆ gonorrhoea: 62 million cases per year
◆ syphilis: 12 million cases per year.

It is also thought that trichomonas vaginal infection makes women more vulnerable to infection with HIV.

Some indication of the incidence of STDs in the United Kingdom may be gained from new cases reported to STD or genitourinary medicine clinics (Table 1.3). However, it must be acknowledged that not everyone with an STD will come forward for diagnosis and treatment. The discrepancy will clearly be greatest for those conditions without obvious symptoms, such as chlamydia, where there may be considerable underreporting. Chlamydia has been identified as a major cause of infertility, and lack of public awareness of the condition (Sheldon 1996) may have contributed to its current high prevalence.

The decline in the incidence of STDs such as gonorrhoea, which have a much shorter incubation period than AIDS, has been attributed to safer sexual practices. Indeed, the Health of the Nation strategy for England (Department of Health 1992) has set targets for reducing the incidence of gonorrhoea as a proxy indicator for HIV. WHO (1995) notes that the use of condoms contributed to the 77% decline in STDs in Thailand between 1986 and 1993, and the 66% decline in Harare (Zimbabwe) between 1990 and 1993.

Overall, then, it can seen that a range of data is available to describe trends in sexually transmitted diseases and to make international comparisons. Mortality data exist on AIDS, but are less usual for other sexually transmitted diseases which are

Table 1.3 Incidence of sexually transmitted diseases: new cases seen at STD/GUM clinics in the United Kingdom (thousands). (Derived from CSO, 1996.) Crown copyright is reproduced with the permission of the controller of HMSO

| | Males | | | Females | | |
STD	1986	1991	1994	1986	1991	1994
Wart virus	46	55	55	30	39	42
Non-specific urethritis	–	58	53	–	19	18
Chlamydia	–	19	19	–	22	21
Herpes	11	12	13	9	12	16
Candidiasis	13	11	11	56	54	60
Gonorrhoea	28	12	8	18	8	4
Syphilis	2	1	1	1	–	1
Trichomoniasis	1	–	–	14	6	5

not a major cause of death. Morbidity data provide information on incidence or prevalence. Because it has been possible to monitor the spread of the disease since its emergence in the early 1980s, cumulative totals for AIDS and HIV are available.

Learning activity 1.5

Using the information from Learning activity

1.2, check the availability of data on sexually transmitted disease in your local area. How does your local information compare with national and global trends?

Control of fertility and avoidance of unwanted pregnancy

Reliable estimates of the number of unwanted pregnancies are not readily available. Although data on births are routinely collected, there is limited information as to whether the pregnancy was planned or not. There is also a point of distinction in that being unplanned is not necessarily the same as being unwanted. It has been suggested that in England and Wales between one-third and a half of conceptions may be unintended (HEA 1994). Women with an unplanned pregnancy may choose to continue with it; alternatively, they may attempt to terminate the pregnancy, either legally (in countries where such abortions are possible) or illegally. Although they may represent only the tip of the iceberg, abortion rates can be used as indicators of unwanted pregnancy. However, they need to be interpreted with caution as only very approximate estimates can be made for the numbers of illegal abortions. Throughout the world there are thought to be about 20 million abortions per year, accounting for the death of 70 000 women. It has also been estimated that in 1990 there were 140 unsafe abortions for every 1000 live births (World Health Organization 1995).

Teenage pregnancies are of particular concern because of the greater risk of negative health,

Table 1.4 Teenage conceptions in England and Wales by age and outcome, 1993 (thousands) (Derived from CSO, 1996). Crown copyright is reproduced with the permission of the controller of HMSO

Age at conception	Leading to maternities	Leading to abortion
13 and under	0.2	0.2
14	0.7	1.1
15	2.6	2.5
16	6.5	4.4
17	11.3	6.2
18	15.8	7.6
19	19.5	8.3
All under 20	56.5	30.2

social, educational and economic consequences than in women over 20 (NHS Centre for Reviews and Dissemination 1997). Between 50% and 90% of teenage pregnancies in England and Wales are unintended (HEA 1994). The proportion of pregnancies leading to abortion is much greater for young women under the age of 16, and tends to decline with age, as shown in Table 1.4.

For women aged 16–19 in England protection from pregnancy is a more important consideration than protection against HIV and AIDS (HEA/MORI 1990). The General Household Survey (OPCS 1995) shows that in Great Britain 72% of women aged 16–49 use some form of contraception:

◆ pill 25%
◆ condom 17%
◆ sterilization 12% women and 12% partners.

Women's reports of condom use by their partners increased from 13% in 1986 to 17% in 1991, and remained reasonably stable until 1993.

Reproductive health

The absence of unwanted pregnancy is integral to the notion of reproductive health. The safety of mothers during pregnancy and childbirth is also a key component. Maternal mortality rates (expressed as deaths per number of live births) provide some indication of this. WHO (1995) reports that maternal mortality in Europe is 50 per 100 000 live births, whereas in Africa it is 13.5 times greater at 675 per 100 000 live births. Many women, particularly in developing countries, also suffer long-term ill health and disability as a consequence of giving birth. Although it is difficult to quantify this exactly, WHO estimates that it may be in the region of 18 million women.

Sexual attitudes and behaviour

The absence of disease and unwanted pregnancies are important components of sexual health. The epidemiological and demographic data referred to above provide some insight into this dimension, and in many countries data of this nature are routinely collected and readily accessed. There has been a more general call for epidemiology to address positive measures of health (Kemm 1993). The type of data required from this may need to be gathered by specific surveys. On the one hand this means that data may not be so readily available, and on the other that there may be problems with comparison between countries and over time because of methodological differences between different surveys. Within the United Kingdom national surveys which address aspects of sexual health include the following:

◆ British Social Attitudes 1989 and 1993 (Social and Community Planning Research)
◆ Contraceptive Services and Recent Mothers (Department of Health)
◆ Emergency Contraception (Health Education Authority)
◆ Health Education Monitoring Survey (Health Education Authority/Office for National Statistics)
◆ Admonitor (Health Education Authority)
◆ AIDS Research in Gay Bars (Health Education Authority)
◆ Health and Lifestyles – General Population (Health Education Authority)
◆ Health and Lifestyles – Black and Minority Ethnic Groups (Health Education Authority)
◆ Young Travellers and HIV Prevention (Health Education Authority)

◆ Today's Young Adults (Health Education Authority)
◆ Project Sigma (Medical Research Council/ Department of Health)
◆ Omnibus (Office for National Statistics)
◆ General Household Survey (1989) (1991) (1993) (Office for National Statistics)
◆ Sexual Attitudes and Lifestyle (Wellcome Trust).

The Wellcome Trust's survey of almost 19 000 people in Britain provides a comprehensive view of contemporary sexual behaviour (Wellings et al. 1994). The median age of first sexual intercourse (i.e. the age at which half the population will have had sexual intercourse and half not) appears to be falling with successive generations. Over the last 40 years it has declined from 21 years to 17 for women, and from 20 years to 17 for men. Currently about 19% of young women report having had sex before the age of 16 (the legal age of consent), in contrast to less than 1% of women who are now aged 55 or over. More than half those who had sex before the age of 16 felt that they had done so too early, although overall only 1 in 4 women and 1 in 8 men thought so. There was found to be a widespread acceptance of sex before marriage, which may indicate more liberal attitudes. However, in contrast to many media representations of a permissive society, the survey also showed:

◆ relatively few people reporting more than one sexual partner in the last year
◆ negative attitudes towards sex outside marriage or cohabitation
◆ disapproval of casual sex
◆ positive attitudes towards monogamy.

Indirect indicators

In addition to attempting to measure sexual health directly, other factors might be included which support the development of sexual health. The health field concept (Lalonde 1974) identified four key areas of influence on health in general, but these might equally be applied to the area of sexual health (Fig. 1.2).

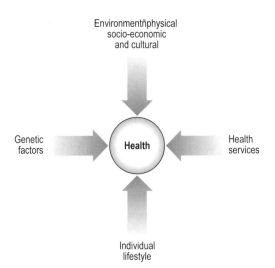

Fig. 1.2 The health field concept (Lalonde 1974).

Individual lifestyle is clearly a key factor already noted in some sources of information. Although genetic counselling and advances in genetic engineering may herald changes for the future, this area is perhaps not of major current significance. In contrast, the health service and environment are both important factors.

Service Provision and Utilization

As will be apparent from Figure 1.2, health services are one of the key areas that influence sexual health. The provision of high-quality care antenatally, postnatally and during delivery is clearly important to maternal and reproductive health. In developed countries many women are concerned about the overmedicalization of childbirth. In stark contrast to this, mothers of half the babies born in the least-developed countries have no access to antenatal care (WHO 1995). A range of services may contribute to the broader notion of sexual health in one way or another.

The uptake of services may be influenced by a number of factors, including:

◆ availability (are services provided in the area?)
◆ awareness (do people know about them?)
◆ accessibility (can people get to them at reasonable times and with minimal inconvenience?)

◆ acceptability (is it socially acceptable to use the service?).

Clearly these need to be borne in mind when interpreting service utilization data. For example, the 1989 Demographic and Health Survey in Kenya found that 14.1% of women were not using contraception because of a lack of access (cited in Pritchett 1994).

Reflection point 1.8

Consider the specific health services you feel are relevant to your concept of sexual health.

Feedback on Reflection point 1.8

You might have considered:

◆ Family planning services
◆ Counselling
◆ Screening for breast cancer and cervical cancer
◆ Genitourinary medicine clinics
◆ Antenatal and postnatal clinics

Environmental factors

Social and cultural factors within the environment will determine the ease with which people can talk about sex and sexuality and their ability to access services openly. Developing an overall objective measure of this is fraught with difficulty. The influential study of teenage pregnancy in developed countries conducted by the Alan Guttmacher Institute (Jones et al. 1985) assessed openness about sex on the basis of four items:

◆ media presentation of female nudity
◆ the extent of nudity on public beaches
◆ sales of sexually explicit literature
◆ media advertising of condoms.

It found lower birth rates (which were used as an acceptable proxy for pregnancy rates) in teenagers in those countries with more liberal views and adequate availability of contraception and sex education. In contrast, those countries characterized by 'religiosity' had higher rates.

The ability of parents to tell their children about sex is also a useful indicator. Many parents feel uncomfortable talking to their children about sex. An English study of young women's experience of menstruation (Prendergast 1992) found that one-third of girls had not been told about it by their parents before their periods started, and 12% had not been told by anyone at all. This reluctance was also noted by Allen (1987), who found that 43% of teenagers had never spoken to their mother and 72% to their father on any of 14 sex education topics.

Having accurate information and the opportun-

Reflection point 1.9

'Parents, and people in general are very peculiar when it comes to sex. Instead of telling their sons and daughters everything at the age of 12, they send their children out of the room the moment the subject arises and leave them to find out everything on their own.'

Anne Frank, 18 March 1944
(Frank and Pressler 1997)

Why do you think parents find it difficult to talk to their children about sex?

---

ity to discuss views about sex and sexuality is important to the development of sexual health. Schools are often charged with the task of educating young people about sex. As agencies of secondary socialization they reflect dominant values and social norms and provide a useful mirror of the way different countries respond to the issue of sexual development. Do they ignore it completely, respond reluctantly and at a minimalist level, or deal with it as a natural part of growing up?

Studies into sources of information about sex have consistently identified friends as the main source (Allen 1987, HEA/MORI 1990, Balding 1994, Wellings et al. 1995), but there are no guar-

antees that information passed on from friend to friend is accurate! A somewhat sad indication of the failure of friends, families and schools to respond to young people's needs for information about sex is to be found in the letters to problem pages in magazines (McFadyean 1986).

Sexual imagery can be used to sell anything from cars to newspapers. Clearly, a large number of factors in the environment will have an influence on sexual health, as succinctly summarized by Jones et al. (1985).

> '. . . Movies, music, radio and TV tell
> [teenagers] that sex is romantic, exciting,
> titillating; premarital sex and co-habitation are
> visible ways of life . . . Yet at the same time,
> young people get the message good girls
> should say no.'

Furthermore, the actual experience of discrimination on the basis of gender or sexuality will inevitably affect sexual health. A whole range of indicators could therefore be developed, ranging from the existence of antidiscriminatory legislation to personal reports of prejudice and harassment.

It has only been possible here to refer to selected examples of environmental influences, which have a clear and obvious link to sexual health. However, it is important not to forget that general environmental factors may also have an effect. It is well recognized that the more economically prosperous nations tend to have lower birth rates. The study of teenage pregnancy referred to above (Jones et al. 1985) found that factors associated with low teenage pregnancy rates included a high gross national product, an equitable distribution of wealth within countries, and a smaller proportion of the population being engaged in agriculture (indicative of a higher level of industrial and economic development).

Listening to people: the lay perspective

Assessing the sexual health and health needs of communities is clearly a complex task. We have proposed a number of possible indicators, but these tend to provide a fragmented view of individual experience. They also tend to stem from a 'professional' perspective, leading to a 'top-down' or professionally led process of describing health. In contrast, 'bottom-up' processes consciously attempt to involve individuals in describing sexual health as they experience it, and in identifying their needs. A range of participatory techniques is available (Gordon and Gordon 1994), including constructing a sexuality lifeline. Facilitating this kind of approach is a skilled task which requires confidentiality and a high level of trust from participants, but it allows a more holistic view to emerge.

The sexual health of communities reviewed

Previous definitions of sexual health have established it as a multidimensional concept. It follows that there cannot be a single indicator of sexual health, but that we need to draw on a number of indicators to assess the sexual health of communities or populations. The types of data and information we can draw on can be summarized as follows:

◆ positive or negative measures
◆ direct or indirect measures
◆ routinely collected (official) data, or data collected by specific surveys
◆ professionally led or client-led descriptions.

Clearly, the type of indicator selected must be consistent with the concept of sexual health and the specific purpose for which it is required. The ultimate constraint will of course be data availability. Each indicator can be thought of as a piece of a mosaic. Which pieces are used will determine both the type and the completeness of the picture that emerges.

THE PROMOTION OF SEXUAL HEALTH

We have discussed the nature of sexual health and noted how a wide variety of factors influence it, both directly and indirectly. Before turning our attention to the promotion of sexual health, we need to consider in greater detail the ways in which some of these psychological, social and environmental factors contribute to individuals' choices and actions in the context of their sexual health.

A sexual health career

The health career concept is especially useful for those engaged in planning health promotion programmes. Whereas a sexuality lifeline provides a personal interpretation of highs and lows and perceptions of major influences to date, the health career provides a more comprehensive view. Because it looks at the way a whole social system influences individuals, it can be used to make generalizations and predictions about future circumstances. It may thus be used to attempt to explain present behaviours in terms of past influences, or to predict future behaviours. For example, if we understand the effects of child-rearing practices on attitudes to gender and sexuality later in life, we can take account of this in developing more sensitive and appropriate health promotion. It is a device which helps the planner identify the many and various factors that influence the development of health and illness-related behaviours during the whole of the individual's lifespan. Moreover, by mapping out key stages, transitions and 'life events' in the health career, it is possible to identify strategic points at which agencies and settings might intervene, and to maximize effective collaboration between those agencies.

The influences on a health career are best explained in terms of socialization, i.e. the direct or indirect effect of social norms on individuals' beliefs, values, attitudes, knowledge and behaviours. The family plays a major part in this process, and is joined later in the health career by other agencies, notably the school and the health service (Fig. 1.3).

Influences on individual sexual health: the Health Action Model

The Health Action Model provides a useful framework for identifying the ways in which psycho-

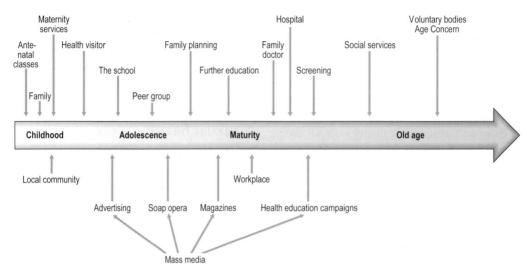

Fig. 1.3 The sexual health career.

logical, social and environmental factors combine to influence health-related decisions (Tones and Tilford 1994). Figure 1.4 shows how an intention to undertake a given health action is the product of three interacting systems. In the discussion that follows the model will be applied, by way of example, to the appropriate use of a condom, but could equally be applied to any other behaviour.

The belief system

A belief is the extent to which someone accepts that something is true or not. A number of beliefs may have to be considered. For instance, the 'Health Belief Model' (Becker 1984) states that people will not take preventive action unless they believe that:

Learning activity 1.6

Create your own sexuality life map identifying the direct and indirect external influences that may have had an effect on your sexual health.

Suggest how each of the organizations or groups in Figure 1.3 could have a positive or negative influence on your sexual health.

◆ they are susceptible to a particular disease
◆ the disease is serious
◆ preventive action will be effective and beneficial
◆ preventive action will not involve too many disadvantages.

Although people will certainly see AIDS as a serious condition, they may well refuse to accept that they are personally at risk. Even if they consider that condoms are effective in preventing disease or pregnancy, they may still refuse to use them because they believe that they interfere with sexual pleasure and are messy or just inconvenient.

The beliefs mentioned above, in turn, depend to some extent on certain subordinate beliefs and understanding – for instance about the nature of AIDS and HIV infection. If, for example, people believed that the virus was so minuscule that it could pass through any barrier, they would not accept the effectiveness of condoms in protecting them from disease.

Beliefs about one's ability to carry out actions are especially important. These are known as self-efficacy beliefs. In short, if people did not believe they would be capable of negotiating condom use with their partners, they would have no intention of using or even buying them.

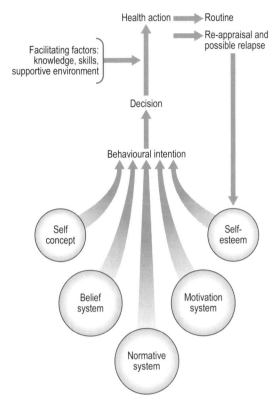

Fig. 1.4 The Health Action Model.

The motivation system

This complex of motives comprises a mixture of emotional 'pushes and pulls'. A number of funda-

Learning activity 1.7

Catherine, aged 20, met Michael (aged 25) in a nightclub last week. They are both keen to engage in sexual activity with each other. What might (a) influence and (b) deter Catherine and Michael to/from use/using condoms? Consider the application of the Health Belief Model in your answer.

Feedback on Learning activity 1.7

Did you consider the potential of sexually transmitted diseases, unwanted pregnancies, cost implications, pleasure, etc?

mental values can influence attitudes and reduce the likelihood of action. In the context of sexuality there are powerful, culturally rooted moral values which can generate negative attitudes towards the use of condoms. Values, however, often compete with even more fundamental motivational pressures, which psychologists have traditionally called 'drives'. The sex drive is manifestly one of the more significant of these. Other motivational states, such as fear, anxiety and embarrassment, can influence the intention to act. Again, these negative states may compete with a range of positive gratifications and pleasures, including addictions of one sort or another. Indeed, it has been suggested that one of the more important strategies for promoting condom use is the eroticization of safer sex. To complicate matters there is typically a constant interaction between the belief system and the motivation system: not only may beliefs influence attitudes, but conversely values and feelings may control beliefs. It is a universal human characteristic to believe only what it is comfortable to believe, and to take defensive action to avoid exposure to threat and to information that challenges values.

In relation to condom use, a worst-case scenario can illustrate the ways in which a mix of motivations can militate against condom use. Imagine a young woman whose socialization has inculcated a strong moral sense which proscribes a number of sexual activities. It is, therefore, not merely embarrassing: it is virtually impossible for her to contemplate sex outside marriage. The very thought triggers anticipatory shame and anxiety. Clearly it would be impossible for her to follow recommendations to carry a condom in her handbag as a prophylactic measure in anticipation of a sexual encounter. None the less, it could well happen that she finds herself faced with a very close

Reflection point 1.10

Identify the values, attitudes and emotional states that influence decisions about the use of condoms. List separately those that make use *more* likely and those that make use *less* likely.

sexual encounter in which the power of the sex drive outweighs the dictates of morality – or indeed common sense!

The normative system

The normative system should need little explanation. Many decisions are substantially influenced by expectations of what other people do and how they might react to proposed activities. Social pressures vary from the general 'norm-sending' function of mass media to the more powerful and intimate pressures of close acquaintances and peers. Mass media convey conflicting norms about sex; communities will offer examples of 'normal behaviours'; friends will inevitably convey views not only about the acceptability of condom use, but perhaps more importantly, about gender roles.

Translating intention into practice

It is self-evident that many a good (or bad) intention is never translated into action. The Health Action Model acknowledges the importance of describing the major factors that either facilitate or inhibit this translation of behavioural intention into routine practice. Two distinct kinds of influence operate. The first refers to whether or not people have the necessary skills and knowledge needed to carry out what they want to do. This is especially important in determining the likelihood of condoms being used on the first 'risky' encounter and being routinely adopted thereafter. It involves:

◆ knowing where to obtain condoms
◆ the psychomotor skill of proper use and disposal
◆ the social interaction skills needed to communicate intimately but assertively with a partner.

The second influence is arguably even more important, and is concerned with the degree of support offered by the environment. Key features include:

◆ ready availability of condoms in relation to cost and access
◆ the kinds of social support available

◆ the general barriers associated with poverty and disadvantage.

The problem of 'relapse'

As with most health actions, the use of a condom on one occasion offers no guarantee of future use. Accordingly, the provision of anticipatory guidance and associated skills is one of the more important health promotion functions identified by the Health Action Model. Effectively, this involves providing a realistic expectation of what is involved, together with the skills needed to manage the aftermath of the sexual encounter.

The empowerment dimension

The notion of empowerment is central to the promotion of sexual health, and its psychosocial and environmental dimensions may be seen in the health action model. Empowerment has two aspects:

1. The extent to which the environment actually limits or enhances individuals' power and capacity to act.
2. Individuals' beliefs about their capacity to exert control over their lives, together with the various competences they need to do so.

Accordingly, the self-concept – i.e. the sum total of individuals' beliefs about themselves – features prominently within the belief system. It includes self-efficacy beliefs (i.e. level of confidence about ability to achieve specific goals and perform particular actions) together with more general capability beliefs such as 'perceived locus of control'. This latter concept is based on the assumption that people differ in the extent to which they attribute success or failure to their individual efforts ('internal locus of control') or to the generalized effect of uncertainty, chance, fate or powerful others ('external locus of control'). Self-efficacy and internality will typically increase the likelihood of individuals undertaking any health-protective behaviours.

Again, the motivation system incorporates people's overall attitudes to self, i.e. the extent to which they respect and value themselves as people. The most commonly used term for this phenomenon is self-esteem. Exercising control is one of the factors that enhance self-esteem. Self-esteem exerts an independent influence both on wellbeing and on the adoption of health-enhancing behaviours.

Within the framework of the Health Action Model, those environmental and personal factors that facilitate the adoption and maintenance of healthy choices might just as well be labelled empowering influences.

Health Education and Health Promotion

It will be clear that sexual health is the product of both personal and environmental factors. It follows, then, that the promotion of sexual health involves two main strands of activity:

◆ Encouraging healthy lifestyles
◆ Providing supportive environments.

Health education has been seen as a means of influencing individual lifestyles. A healthy public policy can contribute to the development of environments that support healthy choices and lifestyles, as encapsulated in the familiar phrase 'making the healthy choice the easy choice'. This can be simply summarized as:

$$\text{Health promotion} = \text{Health education} \times \text{Healthy public policy.}$$

Learning activity 1.8

Healthy public policy is concerned with creating supportive environments for health. Consider the following and try to identify which factors in the environment would support sexual health:

◆ learning about sex
◆ seeking advice about symptoms of a sexually transmitted disease
◆ using contraception
◆ obtaining advice about sexual difficulties.

Remember that the environment is not only the physical environment but also includes social circumstances; economic factors such as poverty and unemployment; cultural beliefs, etc.

Health education

Health education and healthy public policy operate in such a way that the one reinforces the impact of the other – that is to say, synergistically. The following definition of health education, derived from the Health Action Model, indicates its key features:

'Health education is any intentional activity that is designed to achieve health or illness-related learning, i.e. some relatively permanent change in an individual's capability or disposition. Thus, effective health education may produce changes in knowledge and understanding or ways of thinking; it may influence or clarify values; it may bring about some shift in belief or attitude; it may facilitate the acquisition of skills; and it may even effect changes in behaviour or lifestyle.' (Tones 1997, p. 786)

Traditionally, health education has been primarily concerned with persuading individuals to adopt appropriate lifestyles in order to prevent disease. The social and environmental determinants of health and ill health were effectively ignored. In contrast, the approach described here is concerned to support and empower individual choice. Health education therefore has a key role in raising awareness of factors that adversely affect sexual health – for instance in reducing oppression and prejudice. Individual empowerment, coupled with raising public awareness and concern about the effects of the environment on sexual health, may lead to individual or community action to improve the environment. This might, for instance, generate a groundswell of public opinion supporting (or even lobbying for) policy change. The legalization of homosexuality and abortion in the United Kingdom and the recent reduction in the age of homosexual consent from 21 to 18 are perhaps examples of this. Some HIV/AIDS programmes have also specifically challenged prejudice against people who are HIV positive or living with AIDS, and the wider issue of homophobia.

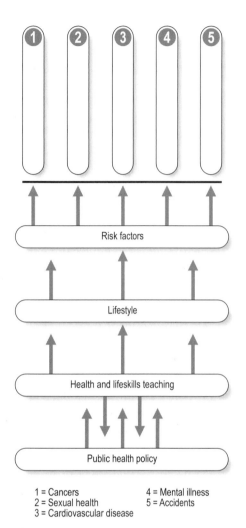

1 = Cancers   4 = Mental illness
2 = Sexual health   5 = Accidents
3 = Cardiovascular disease

Fig. 1.5 The relationship between horizontal and vertical programmes.

Horizontal or vertical programmes?

Clearly there are a number of different strategies that might be used to achieve sexual health promotion goals, and a variety of different settings through which they might be delivered. Within these settings, an equally varied repertoire of specific methods and initiatives can be mobilized. Further exploration of these is beyond the scope of this chapter, but it is important to distinguish between two broad approaches: horizontal and vertical.

Vertical programmes are those interventions that adopt a narrow focus on specific topics or diseases.

For instance, the English Health of the Nation strategy (Department of Health 1992) identified five specific 'key areas', including sexual health. However, there are a number of broader and more significant factors that underpin a whole range of health-related behaviours. Figure 1.5 includes the most important of these, and shows how general lifestyle may contribute to a variety of risk factors which in turn exert an influence on a number of different diseases. Similarly, individuals' lifestyles are determined by the extent to which they are in possession of empowering 'action competencies'; all of these are to a greater or lesser extent determined by the nature of social, economic, cultural and physical environmental influences. Accordingly, **horizontal programmes**, which involve building healthy public policy and the provision of various 'all-purpose' life skills, will be both more effective, more ethical and more economic than a narrow concern with vertical programmes.

HEALTHY SEXUALITY: A GLOBAL PERSPECTIVE

Health promotion strategies in general are shaped by ideological imperatives. For instance, the English strategy outlined in *Health of the Nation* is essentially derived from a quite narrow biomedical model. The specific targets for 'sexual health' are listed below:

◆ To reduce the incidence of gonorrhoea among men and women aged 15–64 by at least 20% by 1995 (from 61 new cases per 100 000 population in 1990 to no more than 49 new cases per 100 000)

◆ To reduce the rate of conceptions among the under-16s by at least 50% by the year 2000 (from 9.5 per 1000 girls aged 13–15 in 1989 to no more than 4.8)

◆ To reduce the percentage of injecting drug users who report sharing injecting equipment in the previous 4 weeks by at least 50% by 1997, and by at least a further 50% by the year 2000 (from 20% in 1990 to no more than 10% by 1997, and no more than 5% by the year 2000). (Department of Health 1992)

It is apparent that the fundamental concern is with the prevention of disease, although more holistic and even radical approaches may well be introduced by practitioners at the implementation stage.

In contrast, since its inception WHO has steadfastly adopted a more holistic and positive approach to health issues. This approach was given further impetus in 1977 at the World Health Assembly with the emergence of the Health for All movement. A series of conferences, publications and radical declarations followed, in which health promotion featured prominently. The following major ideological principles permeated these productions:

◆ An emphasis on equity and a determination to tackle inequalities in health
◆ The centrality of empowerment and community participation
◆ the building of healthy public policy and supportive environments
◆ the importance of primary health care and the reorientation of health services, involving a shift in emphasis from hospital to community and an exhortation that services should be accessible and relevant to consumer needs.

Various agencies concerned with sexual health, both national and international, have either explicitly adopted these principles or work in accordance with a philosophy that is entirely congruent with a positive and radical empowerment perspective.

CONCLUSION

This chapter has explored a variety of interpretations of sexual health. It further has identified ways of assessing the sexual health of communities together with those factors which impinge on it. Some key dimensions of health promotion and health education have been discussed and contextualized with WHO's current ideology and strategic purpose.

Sexual health is clearly a right; a right which is frequently marginalized or even abused. Commitment to promoting sexual health should be a central concern for all those involved in health care, health promotion and health education.

We conclude with the example of The International Planned Parenthood Federation (IPPF) Charter on

Reflection point 1.11

Using each of the rights listed, reflect on the ways in which you can contribute to upholding those rights.

Sexual and Reproductive Rights (1995), which provides an ethical framework for work on sexual health and lists rights as:

1. The right to life (to protect women whose lives are currently endangered by pregnancy)
2. The right to liberty and security of the person
3. The right to equality and to be free from all forms of discrimination
4. The right to privacy
5. The right to freedom of thought
6. The right to information and education
7. The right to choose whether or not to marry and to found and plan a family
8. The right to decide whether or when to have children
9. The right to health care and health protection
10. The right to the benefits of scientific progress
11. The right to freedom of assembly and political participation
12. The right to be free from torture and ill treatment.

ANNOTATED FURTHER READING AND RESOURCES

If you have access to the Internet try to obtain information from sites such as:

AVERT at http://www.avert.org
Department of Health at http://www.open.gov.uk/doh/dhhome.htm
World Health Organization at http://www.who.ch/
WHO (Europe) at http://www.who.dk/

Aggleton P, Homans H 1987 Educating about AIDS. National Health Service Training Authority. Chapter 2 Explaining health and disease, and Chapter 3 Explaining AIDS

These chapters provide a comprehensive overview of models of health and how they relate to HIV and AIDS.

Health Education Authority 1997 Health update: sexual health. HEA, London

This provides an authoritative and detailed account of sexual health and contains a wealth of data on different dimensions of sexual health.

Wellings K, Field J, Johnson A M, Wadsworth J 1994 Sexual behaviour in Britain. Penguin, London

A fascinating insight into sexual attitudes and behaviour in Britain.

REFERENCES

Aggleton P, Homans H 1987 Educating about AIDS. NHS Training Authority, London

Aggleton P, Homans H, Mojsa J, Watson S, Watney S 1989 AIDS: scientific and social issues. Churchill Livingstone, London

Allen I 1987 Education in sex and personal relations. Policy Studies Institute, London

Armstrong S 1990 Labour of death. New Scientist 31/3/90

AVERT 1997 United Kingdom HIV and AIDS Statistics. http://www.oneworld.org/avert/stats. htm

Balding J 1994 Young people in 1993. Schools Health Education Unit, University of Exeter

Beattie A 1993 The changing boundaries of health. In: Health and well being: a reader. Open University Press, Milton Keynes, pp 260–271

Becker M H (ed) 1984 The health belief model and personal health behaviour. Charles B. Slack, Thorofare, New Jersey

Blaxter M, Patterson E 1982 Mothers and daughters: a three-generational study of health attitudes and behaviour. Heinemann Educational Books, London

Blaxter M 1990 Health and lifestyles. Tavistock/Routledge, London

Coale 1991, quoted in Daugherty H G, Kammeyer C W 1995 An introduction to population. Guilford Press, New York

Cornwell J 1984 Hard earned lives. Tavistock, London

CSO 1996 Social trends 26. HMSO, London

Department of Health 1992 Health of the nation. HMSO, London

Downie R S, Fyfe C, Tannahill A 1990 Health promotion models and values. Oxford University Press, Oxford

European Centre for the Epidemiological Monitoring of AIDS 1996 HIV/AIDS surveillance in Europe No. 51. September 1996

Field J, Johnson A, Wadsworth J, Wellings K 1994 The sex survey: part two. The Independent on Sunday 23/1/94

Frank O H, Pressler M 1997 The diary of a young girl: the definitive edition. Viking Press, London

Frankel S, Davison C, Davey Smith G 1991 Lay epidemiology and the rationality of responses to health education. British Journal of General Practice 41: 428–430

Fustukian S, Macdonald J, Hughes H, Klouda T 1994 More than just a health issue. Health Action 10: AHRTAG, London

Goldsmith M 1992 Family planning and reproductive health issues. In: Curtis H (ed)

Promoting sexual health. British Medical Association Foundation for AIDS, London, pp 121–128

Gordon G 1994 Learning to listen. Health Action 10: 6–7 Health Education Authority/MORI 1990 Young adults' health and lifestyle: sexual behaviour. HEA, london

Health Education Authority 1994 Health update 4: sexual health. HEA, London

Helman C G 1978 'Feed a cold and starve a fever': folk models of infection in an English suburban community and their relation to medical treatment. Culture, Medicine and Psychiatry 2: 107–137

Hendriks A 1992 The political and legislative framework in which sexual health promotion takes place. In: Curtis H (ed) Promoting sexual health. British Medical Association Foundation for AIDS, London, pp 155–166

Herzlich C 1973 Health and illness: a social psychological analysis. Academic Press, London

Hughes H 1994 Understanding sexual health. Health Action 10: 4–5

International Planned Parenthood Federation 1995 The IPPF charter on sexual and reproductive rights. http://www.oneworld.org/ippf/charter_rep.html

Jones E F, Forrest J D, Goldman N et al. 1985 Teenage pregnancy in developed countries: determinants and policy implications. Family Planning Perspectives 17(2): 53–63

Kemm J R 1993 Towards an epidemiology of positive health. Health Promotion International 8(2): 129–134

Kinsey A C, Pomeroy W B, Martin C E 1948 Sexual behaviour in the human male. WB Saunders, Philadelphia

Kinsey A C, Pomeroy W B, Martin C E, Gerhard P H 1953 Sexual behaviour in the human female. WB Saunders, Philadelphia

Lalonde M 1974 A New perspective on the health of Canadians. Government of Canada, Ottawa

McFadyean M 1986 Youth in distress – letters to *Just Seventeen*. Health Education Journal 45(1): 49–51

Mead M 1962 Male and female. Penguin, Harmondsworth

NHS Centre for Reviews and Dissemination 1997 Effective health care: preventing and reducing the adverse effects of unintended teenage pregnancies. NHS Centre for Reviews and Dissemination, University of York

OPCS 1995 General household survey 1993. HMSO, London

Porter R 1994 The literature of sexual advice before 1800. In: Porter R, Teich M (eds) Sexual knowledge, sexual science. The history of attitudes to sexuality. Cambridge University Press, Cambridge, pp 134–157

Prendergast S 1992 This is the time to grow up: girls' experiences of menstruation in school. Health Promotion Research Trust, Cambridge

Pritchett L H 1994 Desired fertility and the impact of population policies. Population and Development Review 20(1): 1–55

Rice M 1996 A framework for developing health promotion and education initiatives in reproductive health. Promotion Education III(3): 7–10

Sheldon T 1996 Dutch catch the love line. Healthlines 37: 6

Social and Community Planning Research 1994 British social attitudes: the 11th report. Social and Community Planning Research, Aldershot

Tones K, Tilford S 1994 Health education: effectiveness, efficiency and equity. Chapman & Hall, London

Tones K 1997 Health education, behaviour change and the public health. In: Oxford textbook of public health, 3rd edn, Vol. 2: Public health sciences. Oxford University Press, Oxford

UNAIDS 1996 HIV/AIDS: the global epidemic. http://www.unaids.org/highband/document/epidemio/situa96.html

Wellings K, Field J, Johnson A M, Wadsworth J 1994 Sexual behaviour in Britain. Penguin, London

Wellings K, Wadsworth J, Johnson A M, Field J, Whitaker L, Field B 1995 Provision of sex education and early sexual experience: the relation examined. British Medical Journal 311: 417–420

Williams R 1983 Concepts of health: an analysis of lay logic. Sociology 17: 185–205

World Health Organization 1946 Constitution. WHO, Geneva

World Health Organization 1975 Education and treatment in human sexuality: the training of health professionals. Technical Report series 572. WHO, Geneva (also quoted in AIDS Action 13, AHRTAG, London)

World Health Organization 1978 Primary health care: report of the conference on primary health care. WHO, Geneva

World Health Organization 1995 The world health report 1995. WHO, Geneva

World Health Organization 1996 Sexually transmitted diseases (STDs) factsheet. http://www.who.ch/programmes/asd/facsheet.htm

2

Sex and politics

Jo Adams

> *'Personally, I want the Government out of my underwear.'*
> (Palac 1995)

KEY ISSUES/CONCEPTS

◆ Definitions of legality and morality
◆ Criteria for definitions
◆ Social and political factors
◆ Influence of power, powerlessness, discrimination and prejudice

OVERVIEW

Chapter 2, *Sex and politics*, explores the complex relationships between sexual health, sexuality and politics. It looks at who defines and decides what is and is not morally and legally acceptable in relation to sex and sexuality, in order to establish a framework against which to consider the social and political and other factors that shape sexual relationships and a sense of the sexual self. It also looks at the influence of power, powerlessness, discrimination and prejudice in the construction of common understandings of sex and sexuality.

INTRODUCTION

The relationship between sex, sexual health and politics, both past and current, is vexed, contentious and much contested. The boundaries and separations between what appropriately constitutes the private and the public have been drawn and redrawn by politicians and moralists, theologians and sociologists, by community activists and the judicial system, by journalists and philosophers, and still there is no consensus to be found.

The territory of sexual health and sexual politics is strewn with legislative and ethical issues, from rape in marriage to the law on the age of consent: from purchasing arrangements that privilege the rights of some women above others to receive fertility treatment to sex education; from the policing of 'victimless crime' (e.g. prostitution or gay men cruising) to abortion laws. What is common to all of these scenarios is that there is some conflict, if only in the perceptions of some people, some of the time, between the rights of the individual and either the actual law or common wisdom about the common good.

SOCIAL INFLUENCES

Religion

Originally sexual activity was seen as the appropriate domain of theology and religion. Sex was only sin-free if it consisted of limited, prescribed sexual activity, namely in relation to the procreation of children, as stipulated in the Christian marriage service. Women's sexuality was perceived by theologians (unquestionably male) as powerful, destructive and to be feared. An 11th-century manuscript for monks asserts that 'There is no plague which monks should dread more than woman: the soul's death' (de Caen, quoted in O'Faolain and Martines 1973). The polar opposites of Eve tempting Adam with her nakedness, and the virginal Mary, offer a clear choice to women about where spiritual damnation or salvation lay in terms of their experience of sexuality. Although in the Pauline doctrine it was better to marry than to burn, the implication is 'only just' (1 *Corinthians* 7: 8–9).

Religion and theology dictated sexual morals, including divorce laws, the taboo on masturbation, the moral outlawing of adultery or 'fornication', and imputations of 'uncleanness' in menstruating women that exist in many societies. One example comes from ancient Persia, where any woman menstruating for longer than the statutory 4 days allowed would receive 100 lashes, and women in the Orthodox Jewish communities were excluded from the synagogue while menstruating (Crawford, quoted in Weideger 1978). Such proscriptions did not prevent such activities occurring, but simply caused enormous emotional and psychological distress to those whose activities and religious faith were dissonant. It also caused great social suffering to those such as unmarried mothers, whose situation damned them to ruin and poverty and, more recently, to incarceration in mental hospitals and asylums for their sin of 'deviance'.

Science

A 19th-century shift from the predominance of theology to the 'new religion' of science was accompanied by a similar reframing of the sexual, which was thought to be an appropriate field for scientific study. This saw biological determinism becoming the new imperative and the rise of sexology as a quasi-science. With this emerging conceptual model, women were constructed as bodies of reproduction, prey to hormonal vicissitudes that rendered them irrational vessels of nature (Segal 1994).

Prisoners of their reproductive organs and their biology, women were again rendered inappropriate for positions of responsibility and power, as they had been within the religious construct. In the 'sexuality as a science' model women were perceived as being at the mercy of irrational tides of nature, rather than because of their 'sinful' sexual drives. So, between them, religion and science neatly justified women's social, political and economic subjugation, albeit in the name of two entirely separate and often opposing dogmas. Not for nothing did the Women's Liberation Movement badge in the 1970s read 'Eve Was Framed'!

Politics

The final shift, during the 20th century, has been the social construct of sexuality, which in turn has led to sexuality and sexual health being seen as fit subjects for both psychological and political study. Here the body politic has been transformed into the body political. In this paradigm shift, key issues such as gender and age, race and class, (dis)ability and sexual preference are all seen to have a bearing on sexuality, and in turn to be affected by sex, sexual health and sociosexual relationships.

Critical awareness has grown out of the link between how a person's sexuality is constructed, how it is expressed, and how it is reflected back to them by the wider society. There is an increasing consciousness that sexual health is not a fixed commodity to be aspired to, achieved, and then settled down with for a long and happy life: it is, rather, of a shifting and liquid nature. The nature of someone's sexual identity, whether this is legally and morally proscribed or prescribed; whether the law forbids it or church services bless it; whether it has financial or legal impact, such as tax allowances for married couples or the blight of a prison sentence for men involved in under-age gay relationships; does not exist in a vacuum: it is not a freely made choice, and is seen as being appropriate territory for policing.

'The person is political' was a popular tenet of 1970s feminism, capturing the sense that everything that happened to a person – their education, childhood, family experience, friendships, domestic and paid work, their relationship with their own body and with those of others – is part of the mosaic of experience that builds the lived and quotidian politics of ordinary lives in ordinary towns. It is in fact the collective politics formed from the experience of all individuals, not the politics that is simply the preserve of professional politicians.

However, this radical definition can be reversed into something much more reactionary. A perhaps more sinister interpretation could be that whatever goes on between two or more individuals sexually, with total consensus and no coercion involved, is open to public moral censure, and to intrusion and intervention by the state, the judiciary and the penal system. It is perhaps understandable, then, for Lisa Palac, writing on cybersex in an article in the *Observer* on developments in sexual politics, to protest that 'Personally, I want the government out of my underwear'! (Palac 1995).

This chapter will go on to explore further the particular way in which social/political identities, such as age or gender, affect and interact with sexual identities and experience, and whether the level at which the government is involved is appropriate or inappropriate.

Reflection point 2.1

In your reflective journal, consider the social factors that have influenced your views of morality in relation to sexual activity.

All too often the tabloids and the media present sex and sexuality in a hermetically sealed compartment, a sort of 'Carry on' world of 'three in a bed' sex romps and 'five times a night' orgies, but clearly things are more complex and subtle than that. Sex and sexuality reside at a nexus of other relationships, influences and factors, and are profoundly affected by influences as various as race, age, economic status, physical and mental abilities, childhood experiences and mental and emo-

tional health. Most particularly they are shaped by gender and sexuality, and this theme has been well explored by gender theorists over the centuries (for a review of these see Spender 1982).

Learning activity 2.1

Using your knowledge of any major political sexual scandal, consider the impact that it made on the general public. Write a list of the factors that influenced the public views and opinions at the time. Categorize these and compare them with your opinion of what should have happened.

Feedback on Learning activity 2.1

Did you consider any of the following issues in your response?

◆ The person's role in politics, as a family member, in society

◆ Legal, moral and ethical issues

◆ Views held by church groups and other political groups

◆ Other people involved

◆ General media coverage

◆ The range of public opinion

◆ What was your view of the event, and did you describe how it was influenced and formed?

GENDER AND SEXUAL HEALTH

The argument that if sexual partners are of different genders there is likely to be a crucial difference in power between them in a society which is still constructed along patriarchal lines, has been well rehearsed. Within society men maintain institutional power and are still in the overwhelming majority as lawmakers and sculptors of the culture, as it is men who hold the senior positions in central and local government, in churches and other faith groups, in the judiciary and in the media. Even if there are individual factors within a heterosexual relationship that confer a particular power on a woman – for example she may have a higher income, the privilege of a better education, or she may be white and he black – the socialized imbalance of power between the sexes may very possibly mean that she will feel less powerful about her ability to negotiate whether they have sex and, if so, on whose terms and how. (Painter 1994). These issues raise great concerns for those working in sexual health, and often this is felt particularly strongly about young women who come into contact with services and are particularly vulnerable. Women have historically and contradictorily been seen as both a threat to the nation's sexual health and guardians of it, stuck in the cleft stick of 'vamp or virgin'.

Folk history, myths and legends

Folk history and lay beliefs about STDs and HIV include the 19th-century bogeywoman 'Typhoid Mary', who was supposed to have profligately spread STD among the ranks of sailors in Portsmouth (Davenport-Hines 1990). More recently, part of the oral history accumulating about HIV is the story told with absolute certainty of the woman who went home with a man after meeting him at a nightclub, had sex with him all night and then left. When he woke the next morning he found the words 'Welcome to the wonderful world of AIDS' written in lipstick on the bathroom mirror.

This is a folk devil story familiar to those working in the field of HIV prevention, told the length and breadth of the country by participants on training days as categorically true (and usually having occurred to a 'friend of a friend'), and recounted with a shiver of horror and sympathy for the man. What both these stories highlight is that women's sexuality is dangerous, perhaps even fatal, and that they will inveigle unsuspecting men into their clutches, trap them and destroy them. No matter how counter this may run to the norm of where power resides in mixed-gender relationships, this myth continues to run and run.

For centuries the corollary to this great fear of women's sexuality has been the framing of laws,

religious codes and cultural conditions to contain women and tame sex so that it does not threaten the order of society. These can be as geographically separate and far-flung as the hunting down and burning of single women as witches in 16th-century Europe, to the genital mutilation of girl children in parts of Africa, the epidemic of hysterectomies in the USA in the 1960s, and the foot-binding in China a century ago. What they have in common in their subtext, if not their main message, is the subjugation of women's free expression of self and sexuality (Daly 1978). However, this sense of women as dangerous and primitive coexists, albeit uneasily, with an image of them as the guardians of the nation's sexual health, the partner who is expected to carry and insist on using condoms, to negotiate and provide contraception. This portrays a new reworking of the 'vamp or virgin' polarity, updated to suit the millennium.

Contemporary views

In the early 1980s the Health Education Authority ran an advertisement in its HIV prevention campaigns which showed an image of a rather depressed-looking young woman: the caption underneath read: 'She doesn't carry condoms because people will think she's easy. What's your excuse?' This is a classic piece of double-think about women and their sexuality, and many messages can be teased out of it. Three of these are:

1. that she is being irresponsible by not carrying condoms: therefore, the implicit message is that she should take the responsibility for safer sex

2. that she has the prerequisite power in any relationship to negotiate the kind of sex she has, and, in particular, to insist that it is protected sex. At the very least this can be called a moot point

3. that she is 'using excuses' for not carrying condoms, rather than responding to very real pressure on her. Yet surely it is patently true that she may well be called 'easy' if she were to do so. This is not an unusual experience for young women, who know how easily the term 'slag' is applied and how tenaciously it sticks. No wonder she is looking hopeless and confused (Painter 1996).

From the man's point of view the pressures are very different. Men in sexual health training and group work testify again and again to the excruciating pressures they came under when growing up, and from which they are by no means exempt as adults, in relation to their sexuality: they must be constantly 'horny' and ever-ready for sex; they must never have anxieties or insecurities, e.g. about their sexual performance, or the size of their penis; they must always be able to have an erection and satisfy a woman (and of course it *will* always be a woman that they want to satisfy); they must not admit to shyness or inexperience, or anything less than absolute prowess (Metcalf and Humphries 1985); they must be willing to brag about sexual conquests and must never feel anything remotely like passion or desire or intimacy for another man, unless of course it is on the football field, when they might be allowed the luxury of a triumphal hug.

So, while women are contending with the vamp-or-virgin, Madonna-or-whore polarities, men are doing battle with the stud-or-wimp, stallion-or-'poofter' polarities. What is certain from both these sets of social images is that they are tragically limiting: they force everyone into stereotypes that constrain and circumscribe humanity. Too often the only response that appears to be available is to acquiesce to the image and conform in the hope of gaining social approval. The challenge of much of sexual health work today is to find another way that leaves those stereotypes behind and refuses to be moulded by them any longer, that forges new ways of being sexual and alive that do not forswear the female gender but that no longer collude with it as being determinist and rigid.

SEXUALITIES AND SEXUAL HEALTH

If gender can be seen to be constructed within society as determining the way in which people should behave, with the threat of social castigation if they stray from this path, then sexuality does the same thing, with greater tenacity. The choice of words and labels adopted by a society says much about what that society expects of its citizens in terms of their sexuality, and how fierce the judgement is if those expectations are not met. Not only are the malefactors labelled abnormal, deviant, criminal, sinful and sick, they are also seen as posing a danger to the common good. Most particularly they are typified as being predatory and abusive, paedophiles and child-molesters, with a mission to corrupt and pervert the morals and behaviour of others.

Learning activity 2.2

Take four sheets of paper with a heading on each:

◆ Heterosexual

◆ Homosexual

◆ Bisexual

◆ Lesbian.

Brainstorm with colleagues all the words associated with each sexual preference.

Now consider:

◆ The derivations of these words?

◆ Where have you heard or read them?

◆ Do they hold positive or negative connotations?

◆ What percentage on each paper is positive or negative?

◆ What are the differences and similarities between the groups and genders?

◆ What do the results of this learning activity tell you about yourself and/or the group you have worked with?

Reflection point 2.2

◆ Think about your personal relationships.

◆ What has influenced your decision to engage in or restrain from sexual activity?

◆ How easy was it for you to make that decision?

◆ What are the external pressures that challenge or support your decision?

It seems that contemporary British society finds it hard to tolerate, let alone celebrate, diversity, perceiving it as a threat to order rather than an opportunity. This struggle with difference takes many forms, such as fears and phobias that are projected on to people from non-white races, and non-Anglo-Saxon ethnicities and cultures. Probably the most crude expression of this is reserved for people who are not heterosexual. Homophobia is prevalent in the press, in Parliament, in Christian churches and in other faiths, bearing witness to the fact that mainstream modern Britain is, in equal measure, obsessed, horrified and fascinated by gay and lesbian sexuality.

Society and sexualities: psychological implications

Much has been written about the psychological aspects of such strong reactions, about the potentially closet gay sexuality of the most ardent and evangelical homophobics. Whatever the deeper wellsprings of such attitudes, however, the effect is to isolate and blame homosexual men and lesbian women, to treat them as social pariahs and exile them from the warmth and approval of society to some twilight zone. The adverse effects of such treatment are profound and can lead not least to a sense of hopelessness and disempowerment, and at worse to mental health problems of depression, despair and suicide (Trenchard and Warren 1984).

In terms of sexual health, being offered such consistently negative and demonized images of oneself and being denied access to good information and support often has catastrophic consequences, for example in a health needs assessment of gay and bisexual men in Sheffield in 1996, 98% of the men surveyed had received no sex education at school that mentioned gay sexuality or safer sex.

If the wider culture has always asserted that what you are is deviant and contemptible, then it is difficult to develop any positive sense of self-esteem. For both gay men and lesbians this is likely to lead to a very negative self-image being internalized, believed in and acted upon. When this happens it can pose real health issues, as low self-esteem clearly leads to taking less than the best possible care of oneself. For many gay men this may mean risking unsafe sex, and for both gay men and lesbians it may result in the use of alcohol or drugs to numb the emotional pain, putting up with abusive sexual relationships, or seeking oblivion through casual relationships (Hillin and Bremner 1993).

All of this behaviour may be an understandable, though self-destructive, compulsive response to messages of low self-worth and feeling that one deserves nothing better. However, all too often the effect is to reinforce and compound the negative societal stereotypes that caused these feelings and this behaviour in the first place, thereby completing the vicious circle.

The changing social and political culture

In much of the work that has been carried out over the past 10 years in response to the HIV epidemic, there has been an opportunity for professionals and other staff to review their attitudes and understandings about sexuality. This has resulted in some impressive pieces of practice, although it has also revealed some startling and shocking things. An article in the *Nursing Times* reports on a survey which revealed that 10% of nurses believe that gay men with AIDS deserve it: that 30% of nurses automatically suspect that gay men have AIDS; and that a very worrying 43% of nurses questioned 'will not condone homosexual practices' (Roberts and Taylor 1994). Although there is no concrete evidence in the article of such attitudes translating into less than supportive and respectful behaviour towards gay men and lesbians, it would be dangerous and naive to assume that this might not happen.

In recent years, particularly with the growth of HIV prevention and AIDS support work, a new category and experience of sexuality has been named. It has become apparent to many of those working with men who have sex with other men that by no means all of these self-identify as gay: many are married or living in heterosexual partnerships, and many are from black or ethnic minority communities in which the very concept of being gay may not be entertained, let alone its lived reality.

To target HIV prevention programmes and materials at men who identify as gay or bisexual may therefore risk excluding many whose sexual practices may also put them at risk (Doyal 1994). The term 'men who have sex with men' has therefore emerged from this work and the understanding gained from it, while discussion continues about whether it is what you do, who you perceive yourself to be or how you describe yourself that is the key element in sexual identity.

In addition there are 'twilight zones' of sexuality, such as bisexuality, transsexuality and transgendered sexuality. Whereas at least some greater acceptance and consciousness may be developing in relation to gay and lesbian sexuality, in the case of these more 'Cinderella' subjects there is still taboo and mystery, and inaccurate assumptions and prejudices abound. Bisexuality is all too often characterized as greedy ('wanting your cake and eating it'), indecisive (as in 'Betty Both-Ways'), or lacking the courage fully to come out as gay or lesbian (Harvey Fierstein's character in the film 'Torch Song Trilogy' memorably said that he had yet to meet a bisexual man who lived with his boyfriend and secretly snuck out at night to meet his girl . . .).

In the case of transgendered people debate continues about whether this is predominately a gender or a sexuality issue: however, their inclusion in the 1997 Pride celebration in London to make it 'Lesbian, Gay, Bisexual and Transgendered Pride', marks a movement into a more centrally acknowledged position.

Reflection point 2.3

Think back over your life and try to focus on a time when you found out something that challenged a strongly held belief (e.g. discovering for the first time that your parents had sexual intercourse, or that a friend was gay). Write down your thoughts and feelings at that time, noting in particular how comfortable you felt immediately after the discovery, and whether and how your behaviour changed towards them.

AGE AND SEXUAL HEALTH

At either end of the age spectrum sexual activity and sexual expression are either formally or informally policed, encouraging the belief that being sexual is only a socially sanctioned activity in late youth and the fertile middle years.

Ambivalent attitudes to young people's sexuality are enshrined in formal legislation, that is, the 'age of consent' and, in a contrasting ruling, the Fraser Guidelines on sex education (details of which can be found in the joint guidance issued by the BMA, GMSC, HEA, Brook Advisory Centres, FPA and RGCP in their booklet *Confidentiality and people under 16*). Probably the most compassionate and humanitarian point of convergence between young people's sexuality and the state is in the guidelines issued by the Law Lords in the wake of the Gillick case. In this 1985 ruling, in response to a parent's request for the right to demand that contraception and sexual health advice should not be given to her under-16-year-old daughter without parental consent, Lord Fraser found that such advice could be given provided that:

- the young person will understand the advice
- they cannot be persuaded to tell their parents, or to allow the doctor to
- they are likely to begin or to continue to have unprotected sex with or without contraception
- their physical or mental health is likely to suffer unless they receive such treatment
- it is in the young person's best interest to receive contraceptive advice.

Age of consent and the law

The age of consent laws also reflect a differential in attitudes towards heterosexual and gay male sexual activity. Lesbians are a strangely invisible phenomenon in this area. The apocryphal explanation for this is that Queen Victoria, when presented with the legislation concerning the age of consent, expressed disbelief and denial that such desire could exist, and the whole issue was therefore omitted. Anecdotally, an alternative parliamentary view from the time claims that the House of Lords debated the issue and was loath to men-tion lesbianism in the legislation lest it should inflame otherwise dormant desires in women!

Therefore a marked contrast has arisen between what young people are *allowed* to do sexually within the law and what they are *supported* to do by health services. Indeed, workers at a local level testify that many doctors and health-care workers remain unaware that they can offer confidential sexual advice and services to young people under 16. It could be assumed that such action would be tantamount to aiding and abetting underage, and therefore illegal, sex. This impression was backed up by a World In Action/FPA survey in 1994 which indicated that 30% of GPs were unaware that it was not illegal to prescribe contraception to women under 16 (a helpful guide to the actual situation can be found in the joint guidance mentioned above).

The arguments for and against an age of consent have been rehearsed in a number of settings,

---

Learning activity 2.3

You are a nurse on a young people's ward in a children's hospital. A young woman of 15 has come in for a routine operation and tells you in absolute confidence that she is on the pill, but is desperate that her parents should not find out. Because of the medical implications of having a general anaesthetic it is your professional duty to inform the medical staff, but you make the circumstances and need for confidentiality very clear when you do so. Immediately the doctor you inform calls down the ward to the young woman, whose parents are sitting on the bed, 'How long have you been on the pill?'

◆ As a nurse, what would you do if this happened to you?

◆ What would you do to set up an environment which ensured that such things would not happen?

◆ What are the political and ethical questions raised by this for (a) the clients, (b) the nursing and medical staff, (c) Trusts?

---

and probably never more vigorously than during the stages leading up to the vote on the Parliamentary Private Member's Bill on the age of consent for young gay men. The arguments commonly put for an age of consent are based on principles of child protection at their most benevolent, and on the immorality of young people who choose to be sexually active at their most fierce.

Freedom and the age of consent

Somewhere in the middle lies the position of liberals, who are torn between their belief in young people's rights and freedoms and their concerns about the potentially deleterious effects of early sexual activity. They see this as an activity which is not equalled by an emotional maturity or the capacity to make healthy choices and decisions.

The questions that need to be considered include: Does the age of consent criminalize young people because of a consensual and natural activity? Is underage sex a victimless crime? Does it protect young people against peer pressure and coercion into sex that they genuinely do not choose for themselves?

There are no simple answers, and whenever two or more workers in the field of sex education or sexual health are gathered together the subject is likely to be revisited. When this happens one area of almost certain agreement is that everyone has encountered emotionally competent and mature 15-year-olds quite capable of a loving and adult sexual relationship free from exploitation or harm. They are equally likely to have met 22-year-olds who wreak emotional and sexual havoc by virtue of their emotional immaturity. The questions therefore remain as to what degree of power the state should exert over people's private sexual choices, and at what stage in their lives people are able to make such choices.

The complexity of this can be highlighted when considering what could justify an unequal age of consent for young gay men. The common response offered is that it is to protect them from a 'phase' of believing they are gay. This supposition is in direct contradiction of much of the evidence, for example in recent research for Avert's publication, *Young gay men and HIV infection*

(Frankham 1996). This demonstrates that young gay men are very clear about their sexuality from early in their adolescence, although they may go through a reverse 'phase' of trying to pass for heterosexual, both to themselves and others, in order to gain social approbation.

At this time, when young men constitute a disproportionate number of new HIV diagnoses, many of them probably infected in their mid-teens, denying them support and education is to condemn many of them to ignorance, danger and fear. These are the very conditions that are most likely to result in unsafe sex. Branding relationships illegal and threatening partners with imprisonment if convicted of having sex with an underage man makes them social pariahs. The consequences of this are all too well known to those working in the field of sexual health. They include isolation, depression, attempted or successful suicide, selfharm, drug and/or alcohol misuse, and generally taking much less than the best possible care of themselves. For people working in the field of HIV prevention this is a cause for great concern, particularly as, understandably, many schools, teachers and other workers with young people may be fearful of attracting negative publicity if they are known to offer information or support to young men who know they are gay or who are questioning their sexuality (Ray and Went 1995).

Looking for a solution

The controversy surrounding legislation related to the age of consent, unpoliceable law or a protective framework will probably never go away. However, it may be worth exploring a wider way of thinking about this, using more imaginative models which do not simply present a cut-off point that makes an act illegal one week and legal the next. One suggestion has been that the age of consent should be lower than 16 – 13 or 14 perhaps – but that sexual relationships would be legal only between two young people less than 5 years apart in age. Such an arrangement, although as difficult to police as the current laws, might at least allow for the lived reality of young people's lives, and not make unnecessary criminals of them while at the same time guarding against exploitation or abuse by adults.

Reflection point 2.4

◆ Thinking about the section that you have just read, try to identify the benchmarks you would use if you were a lawmaker. You might want initially to brainstorm these ideas and then return to each one, giving more thought to where that idea came from and the implications it might have on the sexual wellbeing of the young person.

◆ Design an appropriate law around the age of consent which you feel deals satisfactorily with and answers all the different dilemmas raised by this issue.

Sex and the older person

Another area where the link between age and sex is problematic is that of older people. Unlike sex and younger people, this is more a case of social inhibition. The 1950s song 'Stay young and beautiful if you want to be loved' neatly sums up social attitudes towards older people being sexual. Traditional images have depicted people over a certain age as being asexual and undesirable, but this phenomenon remains unequal between the sexes. For women, youth and beauty are prerequisites to sexual success. Although the boundaries circumscribing the age at which it is allowable to be sexual may be stretching, the sexually active older adult draws responses varying from pity to embarrassment and, at the most extreme, disgust. One place where sexuality and sexual relationships for older adults is examined in more detail is in a booklet produced in conjunction with Age Concern in Sheffield (Adams et al. 1997). Sexual health services for women within the NHS tend to be concerned in the main with obstetrics and gynaecology. The covert message here could be that sexual activity revolves around fertility, resulting in sexual health services for women virtually finishing once they have completed the menopause. This further compounds the view that postmenopausal women have no sexual rights or needs.

Equally, for older men issues of impotence or reduced performance may be dismissed as the inevitable consequence of ageing, with little regard for their impact on emotional and psychological wellbeing. In residential care settings, for example, problems are experienced by both staff and residents when sexual relationships continue or develop. Equally, families may find it difficult to accept an older relative – a father, mother, grandparent – being open and honest about continuing to have a sexual relationship.

It can therefore be said that sexuality in relation to youth and older adulthood is socially controlled. The corollary of course is that if you are between the ages of 20 and 40 then the social expectation is that it is imperative for you to be ultrasexual all of the time. Sex and age seem best described as 'feast or famine', neither of them very balanced or nurturing.

Learning activity 2.4

◆ A nurse working in a nursing home for the elderly arrived for his shift one morning to find that recorded in the log for the previous night was the fact that one of the female residents had been 'caught' masturbating.

◆ Identify the many ways in which this incident signifies poor practice and lack of understanding. Once you have completed this task, try to develop a plan that would ensure an environment that demonstrates respect for person, offers appropriate levels of privacy, and affirms people's lifelong sexuality.

EQUAL OPPORTUNITIES AND SEXUAL HEALTH

Racism and sexual health

In the preceding sections sexual activity and sexual health are shown to be surrounded by legislation, custom, social approval and social taboo, all of which make genuine choices impossible to make without hindrance. Culture, race and ethnicity also play an important part in the construction of sex and sexual health. From proscriptions on interracial relationships to myths about black men being 'studs' and the tabloid demonizing of young black single mothers, this area is fraught with problems.

Most of these are the direct result of institutionalized racism, combined with a tendency to exoticize, sexualize and stigmatize the 'other', the 'incomer' or the 'foreigner'. This sexual xenophobia was graphically demonstrated by the portrayal of American GIs during the second world war as being 'over-sexed, overpaid and over here', and by attempts to insist that HIV came from Africa as a consequence of scarcely veiled insinuations about unspeakable sexual practices with monkeys. Fear of the unknown can so easily lead to prejudice and discrimination. This linking of the 'otherness' of foreigners with sexual disease or depravity is not new, and sexually transmitted diseases have a history of being blamed on incomers, who are seen as importing a sinful and dangerous exoticism (Sontag 1987).

Disability and sexual health

Taboos also surround the area of sexuality and people with disabilities, whether these be physical or learning difficulties. As regards people with learning difficulties the arguments are similar to those on the age of consent; however, in this context they are about the *meaning* of consent for someone with a learning difficulty, and the need for adequate and sensitive protection from potential exploitation and abuse, while at the same time acknowledging the person's human right to sexuality.

People with physical disability may also experience a denial of their sexuality. As well as contending with the challenges faced by able-bodied people, they also face particular challenges, such as finding appropriate sex education, the lack of access to condom machines at wheelchair height, and the difficulty in claiming their right to be sexual at all (Kanga 1995).

This section facilitates the exploration of some of the political identities and factors that may prevent people being able to claim a sense of themselves as sexually equal in an unequal society. Those working in health care and other caring professions need an acute awareness of these in their transactions with service users if they are to be part of the solution, rather than compounding the problems of powerlessness and inequality.

Learning activity 2.5

If working alone, choose one of the following case studies. If working in a group, divide into four subgroups and select one of the following case study outlines each. Then each subgroup discusses the specific issues and implications from one of the following perspectives:

◆ The public

◆ The media

◆ The individuals involved

◆ Nursing and medical staff involved.

Share the main points raised in your discussions with other groups.

Case study 2.1

In 1996 a woman of 59 who had received fertility treatment abroad successfully gave birth, causing great controversy. The issues debated included the correct age for childbearing, the inappropriateness of parenting in years which are more synonymous with grandparenting, and the economics of the situation (the mother was affluent and easily had the means to support the baby).

Case study 2.2

Diane Blood initially lost her court case claiming her right to insemination with her dead husband's sperm, which had been taken from him without his consent (1996). Again this raised a multiplicity of issues, including the right of a widow to bear a child to a dead husband, the ethics of sperm taking without consent, and the financial implications of bringing up the child.

Case study 2.3

The gay couple who had a baby by a surrogate mother and then proceeded to parent her themselves (1996). The controversy in this case revolved around the fitness of gay men to be parents.

Case study 2.4

Mandy Allwood, the woman who in 1996 lost eight fetuses after receiving fertility treatment and refusing selective termination. The key issues, which received much press coverage in this case, were: should a woman who already had a child and whose partner had other children receive fertility treatment? How could such treatment be administered without the father's agreement? What role does chequebook journalism play? In this particular case it was alleged that a national newspaper was willing to pay for a story on a sliding scale according to the number of babies born, which added a potential disincentive to the mother accepting a selective termination to increase the life chances of some of the babies.

It can be seen from these four case studies that the debate and controversy still rages over who is fit to be a parent, and that advances in reproductive and fertility treatment available in the 1990s have created ethical dilemmas previously not encountered.

Sexual practice in private – what is allowed?

The case of 'Operation Spanner' raises issues about what is the role of the state and the judiciary in policing private and consensual behaviour, and which behaviour is selected for such scrutiny. The case, which went to trial in 1990 and resulted in 16 men being imprisoned for up to 4 years, revolved around a group of men who met to take part in sadomasochistic practices. None was a minor, all were consenting, and none was seriously injured during their involvement. More crucially, the men's activities all took place in private and were only exposed when police seized videos and raided homes.

There had been no complaints against the men in relation to the protection of public decency, and they were eventually charged under a 19th-century law forbidding the aiding and abetting of 'assault on oneself'. The result of the convictions had devastating effects on the men's lives, including loss of jobs, loss of partnerships and mental health problems. The ethical question debated in this case, by both the British Courts and the European Court of Human Rights, is whether the state has a legitimate role in judging that what people choose to do in private, with no coercion or infringement of liberty involved, is worthy of punishment. Nicci Gerrard (*Observer*, 20 October 1996) asserts that the key issues are 'about consenting adults' rights to individual privacy and to difference'. Perhaps it is this notion of difference, and intolerance of it, that runs throughout the politics of sexual health.

Reflection point 2.5

Issues raised by 'Operation Spanner' include:

◆ Who has the right to intrude on the choices of consenting adults to private acts?

◆ Does an act's being repugnant to some justify its outlawing to all?

◆ Is the unimaginable also the same as the unacceptable?

◆ Most of the men involved in sexual activities investigated under 'Operation Spanner' were gay. Would the outrage and police activity have been less if they had been heterosexual?

When considering the last point it might be pertinent to think about the antics of senior civil servants and judges seeking humiliation from Julie Walters' portrayal of Cynthia Payne in the film 'Personal Services', and how this was accepted as laughable and amusing. Was their assumed heterosexuality relevant to this response?

Stereotyping nursing: gender

Barbara Windsor's black-stockinged busty nurse in the 'Carry On' films is one portrayal of a famil-

iar caricature of the promiscuous, attractive and available nurse, there for the patients' pleasure. Perhaps this image is rooted in historical perceptions that women nurses could access contraception and termination more freely than others in society, and might therefore feel freer to express their sexuality. Or perhaps it derives from the fact that male patients may feel powerless in their status, and that the only power they can therefore assert is over the women whose role is to care for them, to make them feel better in every sense. Whichever, the chemistry of women nurses, male patients and gender conditioning has tended to make for problematic responses, at their worst expressed as extreme sexual harassment, violence or rape perpetuated against nurses.

Another aspect of this is that assumptions may be made about male nurses in terms of their sexuality. Unless they positively and proactively state that they are heterosexual, they must be assumed to be gay. This does a double disservice to men, as it assumes that a man cannot be both heterosexual and caring, and also that the appropriate role of gay men is to care for others.

Reflection point 2.6

◆ Reflect on your experience of any ways in which you have experienced (or been guilty of) gender stereotyping in nursing.

◆ Then, with your peer group, think of ways in which nurse training could take on and challenge these issues most effectively.

CONCLUSION

It can be seen that all groups treated unequally, whether because of their gender, their sexual preference, their race or their age, are treated less equally than young, white, able-bodied heterosexuals. This is not to say that everyone from this narrow band feels privileged and powerful: clearly that is not the case. However, it is true to say that people who diverge from the norm, either in terms of the group they come from or the practices they participate in, are likely to receive less than full endorsement and approval from the wider society.

REFERENCES

Adams A, Angell D, Bailey J, Brown R 1997 Ageing, loving and sex: a resource for older adults. Sheffield Centre for HIV/Sexual Health and Age Concern, Sheffield

Daly M 1978 Gynaecology: the meta-ethics of radical feminism. Women's Press, London

Davenport-Hines R 1990 Sex, death and punishment: attitudes to sex and sexuality since the Renaissance. Fontana Press, London

Doyal L 1994 AIDS: setting the feminist agenda. Taylor & Francis, London

Frankham J 1996 Young gay men and HIV infection. AVERT, Horsham

Hillin A, Bremner J 1993 Sexuality, young people and care: creating a positive context for training, policy and development. Central Council for the Education and Training of Social Workers, London

Kanga F 1995 Trying to grow. Picador, London
Metcalf A, Humphries M 1985 The sexuality of men. Pluto Press, London

O'Faolain J, Martines L 1973 Not in God's image: women in history. Virago, London

Painter C 1996 Sexual health, assertiveness and HIV. Folens, Dunstable

Palac C 1995 How to have cybersex. Observer, 15 October

Ray C, Went D 1995 Good practice in sex education: a sourcebook for schools. Sexual Education Forum/National Children's Bureau, London

Roberts A, Taylor I 1994 A sensitive question. Nursing Times 90(51): 30–32

Segal L 1995 Straight sex: the politics of pleasure. Virago, London

Sontag S 1987 AIDS as metaphor. Penguin, London

Spender D 1982 Women of ideas. Routledge Kegan Paul, London

Trenchard L, Warren H 1984 Something to tell you. Lesbian and Gay Youth Group, London

Watney S 1987 Policing desire: pornography, AIDS and the media. Methuen, London

Weideger P 1978 Female cycles. Women's Press, London

3

Sexual health abused

Damon Lab

> 'He was all powerful. I was a little boy. I did not recognise that my physical, emotional and other boundaries were being invaded without my consent.' (Richie 1996)

KEY ISSUES/CONCEPTS

◆ Defining sexual abuse

◆ Male victims of sexual abuse

◆ Sexual abuse and mental health

◆ Nurses' attitudes to sexual abuse

◆ Meeting the nurses' needs

◆ Improving service for clients

OVERVIEW

Chapter 3, *Sexual health abused*, focuses on the impact of sexual abuse on a person's sexual health. In the first instance there will be an attempt to define sexual abuse and put it into the context of society today. There will be a specific focus on male sexual abuse and the practitioner's ability to deal with it. The latter part of the chapter will discuss the findings of recent research relating to mental health practitioners offering appropriate intervention to male clients who have suffered sexual abuse.

INTRODUCTION

The preface to this book highlights a number of global issues that present a challenge for health professionals working in the arena of sexual health care. Sexual abuse is a multinational issue and one which creates immense difficulties for many health-care professionals. In 1997 the Criminal Statistics for England and Wales reported 33 200 sexual offence cases, a rise of 6% over the previous year. In spite of this the clear-up rate was the highest for 20 years (clear-up rate is the number of offences that were detected). During the past two decades sexual abuse has been at the forefront of media attention. It can take many forms, both physical and emotional. Apart from rape, it may also include stalking, obscene phone calls, exposure, sexual assault, sexual harassment and female circumcision. Sexual abuse occurs in both childhood (including child prostitution) and adulthood, for both males and females.

Public criticism of the police handling of rape victims, and more recently the numerous inquiries into child abuse in children's homes, have all contributed to a change in social attitude in the way sexual abuse is dealt with in Britain. There are visible moves to tackle some of the problems of sexual abuse, including the setting up of Childline, the Domestic Violence Units and Child Protection Units, with police officers specially trained to work with victims and their families. More recently there has been government acknowledgement of child sexual abuse and the need to strengthen and develop interagency collaboration (DoH 1998). This includes identifying the adverse effects of child sexual abuse, recognizing the methods by which sex offenders gain access to children, and the extent and seriousness of abuse suffered by numerous children living in residential care during the 1980s and 1990s. Despite the increase in opportunities to report sexual abuse, for some victims the fear of reprisal from the abuser outweighs any relief that might be experienced through disclosure, and therefore the abuse and/or the emotional pain and damage continue. There is really no way of knowing how many people have been the victims of abuse during their lives. Contact with health-care professionals may provide an opportunity for those who have been abused to disclose their experience. It is the responsibility of the professional to ensure that they are able to respond in an appropriate and effective way.

DEFINITIONS OF SEXUAL ABUSE

Child sexual abuse

Perhaps the most shocking form of sexual abuse is that of children. On the surface it would appear that society is intolerant of child sexual abuse, yet epidemiological research suggests that it is widespread throughout the world. In the UK there are clearly defined laws on child sexual abuse (see Chapter 7). However, in contrast to legal definitions, the National Association for Prevention of Sexual Abuse Against Children believes it to be:

'Any sexual contact with a child or the exploitation of a child for the sexual gratification of an adult. This may include exhibitionism, fondling of genitals, or request of a child to do so, oral sex or attempts to penetrate the vagina or anus.'

Renvoize (1993) defines it as:

'any type of sexual exploitation of a child or adolescent by an older person or an adult for the stimulation and/or gratification of that person, which is not necessarily confined to physical contact and which may range from exhibitionism or involvement with

pornography to full intercourse or child prostitution; where the developmentally immature victim lacks the authority or power to prevent her/himself being coerced into activities to which she/he is unable to give informed consent, which she/he does not properly comprehend but which – either at the time or later – the victim considers sexually abusive.'

Finklehor, probably the leading researcher in the field of childhood sexual abuse, reviewed a large number of studies investigating the prevalence of sexual abuse (Finklehor 1986). He reported that, depending on the type of study, estimates of prevalence range from 6% to 66% for women and 3% to 31% for men. Studies also show fairly consistently that patients who use psychiatric services are even more likely to have a history of sexual abuse (Wurr and Partridge 1997).

Department of Health figures from the Child Protection Register for the whole of England up to 31 March 1998 show a total of 31 600 children on the Register. At the end of the year there were more boys than girls on the register, a reversal of the position a decade ago.

 Learning activity 3.1

◆ Using the Internet, locate the DoH website http://www.doh.gov.uk/pulic/cprsum98.htm

◆ What percentage of children on the Child Protection Register are aged between 1 and 4 years?

◆ How many of the children on the Register are looked after by local authorities?

◆ What percentage of children on the Register were considered to be neglected?

◆ What percentage of children were sexually abused?

◆ Why do you think the number of child protection cases which are the subject of case conferences is falling?

Female circumcision

Female genital mutilation (also referred to as female circumcision) is the medically unnecessary modification of female genitalia. Estimates suggest that over 120 million girls and women throughout the world have undergone some form of genital mutilation, and that 2 million girls a year are at risk (Dorkenoo 1996). Although there are still many supporters of female circumcision, and the cultural issues involved are not straightforward, the World Health Organization and the World Medical Association oppose the practice, which has numerous unacceptable effects, such as infection, haemorrhage and birth complications (Bayoudh et al. 1995), as well as pain during intercourse and infertility. The psychological impact should also not be overlooked. For health reasons alone female circumcision was outlawed in the United Kingdom in 1985. For many in the western world it is considered a form of child sexual abuse, with many seeing it to be an act of violence against women. The fact that it is outlawed in the UK must not deter us from acknowledging its continued existence in this multicultural society in which we live.

Rape

Rape has little to do with sex and more to do with dominance and power. There are four main classifications of rape:

◆ Stranger rape is when the rapist is not known to the victim.

◆ Acquaintance rape is where the rapist is known well enough by the victim to have their trust.

◆ Date rape is sexual intercourse against the will of one party, where both parties have made some commitment to spending time together.

◆ Marital rape is intercourse forced by one partner on the other in the context of a marital relationship.

A recent research study conducted by the Home Office (Harris and Grace 1999) reveals that the number of recorded rapes has risen threefold since 1985. This most likely indicates an increase in the willingness of victims to report rape rather than an increase

in the actual number of rapes committed. In general, however, the number of incidents of rape committed each year will be much higher than the number reported. A study completed by the Rape Crisis Centre (Rape Crisis Federation 1996/7) identified that only 7% of the women seeking help from Rape Crisis had reported their experiences to the police.

As well as the emotional difficulties in disclosing sexual abuse briefly mentioned earlier, one issue that may be contributing to the apparent lack of reporting rape is the conviction rate for this crime. Of the 7% of the aforementioned women who reported their rape to the police, only 6% of the cases were convicted. Despite a range of initiatives to improve the criminal justice system's response in rape cases, there has been a 15% decline in the conviction rate for rape between the mid 1980s and 1990s (Harris & Grace, 1999).

The above reports relate to female rape only. It is only since the mid 1990s that male rape has been categorized as a separate offence (prior to this it was recorded as buggery). Owing to the even greater stigma associated with being a male rape victim, the level of underreporting of this act is probably even higher than with females. A recent Home Office report indicated that during the period of the financial year 1998/99, there had been 504 reported male rapes in England and Wales (Home Office 1999). Again, this figure is likely to be an underestimation of the true number of rapes committed.

Sexual harassment

Sexual harassment has been defined as 'any deliberate or repeated sexual behaviour that is unwelcome to its recipient, as well as other sex-related behaviours that are hostile, offensive, or degrading' (Fitzgerald 1993). Examples include sexually suggestive jokes, deliberate touching or brushing against a person's body, or pressure to have sex. The US Merit Systems Protection Board (MSPB) 1981 survey, the largest prevalence study in the field, found that 42% of female and 15% of male employees in their sample had been sexually harassed. Most perpetrators (90%) were men and usually in a position of relative power to the victim, such as their supervisor. The psychological impact of sexual harassment on an individual can be significant. Research by Gutek and Koss (1993) revealed that victims often report anger, fear, depression, anxiety, irritability, loss of self-esteem, feelings of humiliation and alienation and a sense of vulnerability. Post-traumatic stress disorder has also been linked to harassment at work (Kilpatrick 1992). There are also practical consequences, such as damage to interpersonal relationships at work, legal battles and possibly loss of employment, all of which are all likely to have a negative impact on psychological wellbeing. In 1975 the Sex Discrimination Act came into force, making it illegal for anyone to be treated differently just because of their sex. Sexual harassment counts as 'discrimination' for the purpose of the Sex Discrimination Act if an employee is treated less favourably than others on the grounds of gender. Sexual harassment of an employee by another employee is an act of misconduct which may justify dismissal of the offending employee, subject to 'normal rules'. In 1991 the European Commission recommended a code of practice on 'Measures to combat sexual harassment', but this does not have the force of the law. However, it should not be forgotten that sexual harassment can be a criminal offence under the Protection from Harassment Act 1997, and remains a widespread problem in the workplace.

Reflection point 3.1

◆ Consider the behaviours and attitudes within your own workplace that can be described as 'normal rules'.

◆ To what extent do they support, condone or prevent sexual harassment?

Possibly the most pertinent issue in the area of sexual abuse is its impact on mental health. Numerous studies have shown that there is a strong correlation between sexual abuse and psychiatric problems. Typically those include depression, anxiety, self-harming behaviour, addictions, relationship problems and sexual dysfunction (Browne and Finklehor 1986). The need to access appropriate services will be recognized for some victims of sexual abuse. Often this requires that

the victim disclose the abuse to their GP. However, sexual abuse is often associated with shame, embarrassment and difficulty trusting others, and many victims will therefore find it very difficult to disclose such personal and sensitive information. It is often up to professionals to ask their clients in a non-judgemental and sensitive manner whether they have been sexually abused.

MEN WHO ARE VICTIMS OF SEXUAL ABUSE

Prevalence

The notion that men can be victims of sexual abuse is relatively new. Studies are now beginning to emerge, however, suggesting that a significant minority of men have been sexually abused. Estimates of the prevalence of sexual abuse in the general population vary greatly from study to study. Because of varying definitions, sampling differences and methodologies, figures have been estimated from as low as 3% to as high as 31% (Peters et al. 1986). As with women, prevalence rates seem to be higher in clinical samples. Swett, Surrey and Cohen (1990) reported that 13% of 124 men at an outpatient psychiatric clinic had histories of sexual abuse. A recent survey of psychiatric inpatients by Wurr and Partridge (1996) found that as many as 39% of the men in their sample reported having been sexually abused. Evidence therefore suggests that a significant proportion of men who use psychiatric services have a history of sexual abuse.

The impact of sexual abuse on mental health

The link between childhood sexual abuse and mental health is now fairly well recognized by professionals. The experience is viewed as a vulnerability factor for developing psychiatric problems (Jehu 1991). Research has started to emerge revealing the consequences of sexual abuse on men.

Emotional and psychological problems, such as anxiety, depression, suicidal feelings, sleep disorders (Briere et al. 1988), obsessive compulsiveness,

Reflection point 3.2

Think about the society in which we live and in particular the expectations of men in that society. Brainstorm what might lead to the promotion of men disclosing sexual abuse, and what might act as a hindrance to that process.

From data on the association between psychiatric morbidity and sexual abuse one would expect that sexually abused men would be frequently identified and managed by mental health professionals. Unfortunately this seems to be far from the case.

Learning activity 3.2

◆ Identify situations from your experience where sexual abuse was suspected.

◆ Identify whether the clients who come to mind were male or female.

◆ What made you suspect that each of these clients had been sexually abused?

◆ What did you do about your suspicions?

paranoid ideation and psychoticism (Fromuth and Burkhart 1989), extreme anger (Olsen 1990) and low self-esteem (Finklehor 1981) have been commonly found in samples of abused men. Links with psychiatric diagnoses, such as post-traumatic stress disorder (Rowan and Foy 1993) have also been made. Another robust finding has been the association often observed between childhood sexual abuse and substance abuse (Dimock 1988, Olsen 1990). Interpersonal difficulties are also a widely reported phenomenon within samples of male victims, as is confusion concerning sexual identity and sexual problems (Dimock 1988).

Avoidance by professionals

Holmes, Offen and Waller (1997) claim that figures from national prevalence studies of sexual abuse in men and women show that approximately 30% of all abuse victims are male. If it is assumed that this proportion is similar in the psychiatric population, one would expect that abused males would represent 30% of the clinical population reporting sexual abuse. However, citing research such as Mendel's (1995) review of the field of sexual abuse in males, Holmes and colleagues concluded that the level of reported abuse by men is actually much lower than this. This leads them to ask the crucial question, 'why is it that health-care professionals identify relatively fewer men with histories of sexual abuse?'

Holmes et al. (1997) propose and comment on a number of reasons that might be offered in answer to this. First, there is the mythical belief among some professionals that sexual abuse has little impact on men. This, Holmes and colleagues largely refute, on the basis of numerous studies already highlighted in this chapter. Secondly, they suggest that owing to the nature of the problems that many sexually abused men manifest, e.g. aggressive and criminal behaviours, many are more likely to come into contact with other services, such as the prison service. Although they find evidence for this, they conclude that it is unlikely to be the whole story. Thirdly, men tend not to disclose their abuse experiences. Holmes et al. suggest that this is almost certainly true and cite a number of possible reasons, including denial that the experience was really abusive, shame, and the feared negative consequences of telling someone. Finally, they suggest that clinicians fail to suspect or enquire about sexual histories of abuse in men.

Holmes et al. (1997) identified four processes that might explain why clinicians are missing male clients who have histories of sexual abuse:

1. Professionals are less likely to hypothesize that a male client's psychiatric problems could be related to sexual abuse. They cite evidence for this from studies such as Holmes and Offen's (1996) experiment, where British clinical psychologists were given identical male and female case vignettes which included phenomena associated with sexual abuse. They found that when asked for hypotheses of aetiological factors for these cases the psychologists were significantly more

Reflection point 3.3

Think back to the previous activity: have you ever asked a male client about past sexual abuse? If yes, think about the way in which you did this and the level of difficulty you found in doing it. If no, think of the reasons why you have not asked.

likely to raise the possibility of abuse if they had been told that the client was female.

2. Professionals do sometimes not believe men's disclosure of sexual abuse.

3. Professionals respond to disclosure in such a way as to contribute, along with the client, to the denial of the experience being abusive.

4. Professionals are failing to ask their male clients about abuse in the first place. The support for this comes from a study by Mills (1993), who found that the majority of men attending a British outpatient clinic reported that they had not been asked about past sexual abuse.

These types of issues are important to investigate as they have implications for the way in which male clients with histories of sexual abuse are handled by health-care professionals. This is particularly pertinent in mental health services. Unfortunately, apart from the research previously cited, no other investigations have ever been carried out which shed light on mental health professionals' views and practice towards the assessment of sexual abuse in men. It was our intention to undertake a research project which would fill this gap.

THE RESEARCH PROJECT

The title of the research is 'Mental health professionals' attitudes and practices towards male childhood sexual abuse' (Lab et al. 2000). The main aim of the study was to test the hypothesis of Holmes, Offen and Waller (1997) that mental health professionals are not asking male clients about histories of sexual abuse. It also aimed to throw light on other important aspects of mental health professionals' attitudes to and practice of the assessment of sexual abuse in male clients. For example, do health-care professionals think men

should be asked about abuse histories? What do they believe are the reasons to ask or not to ask? When they do ask, how do they go about it? What do they do when they learn that a client has been abused? How well informed are they on the prevalence rates? The study also aimed to try and identify the extent to which there is a training need in this area. To investigate this final point, staff were also asked how much training they had received in the area of sexual abuse and whether or not they felt that they had had sufficient training to ask about sexual abuse in male clients.

Brief resumé of methodology

A total of 179 anonymous questionnaires were sent out with a covering letter to 40 psychiatrists, 55 psychologists and 84 nurses of all professional levels working in a large south London teaching

Learning activity 3.3

Before reading the results of the research, try and answer for yourself the questions that were put to the professionals participating in the study.

1. Do you enquire about abuse?

2. What are your attitudes to whether men should be asked about abuse histories?

3. What are your views on the reasons why one should or should not ask?

4. How do you enquire about sexual abuse histories in men?

5. What would you do if a client disclosed a history of sexual abuse to you?

6. Do you believe that disclosure of abuse changes your approach to care?

7. Have you received specific training in the area of sexual abuse?

8. Do you believe that you may have had sufficient training in how to enquire about sexual abuse histories in men?

9. What is the prevalence of male sexual abuse in the psychiatric population?

hospital. The questionnaire asked about their attitudes to and practices regarding male sexual abuse. Of the 179 questionnaires sent out, 111 were completed and returned, yielding an overall response rate of 62%.

Results

Are clinicians enquiring about abuse?

Figure 3.1 provides a breakdown of how often staff enquire about histories of sexual abuse in male clients. One-third (33%) reported that they

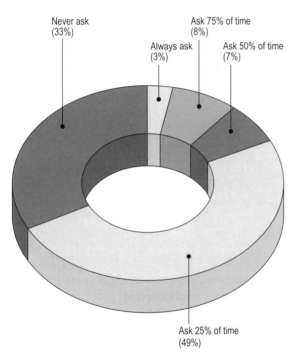

Never ask
(33%)

Always ask
(3%)

Ask 75% of time
(8%)

Ask 50% of time
(7%)

Ask 25% of time
(49%)

Fig. 3.1 How often staff enquire about histories of sexual abuse in male clients.

never ask. About half (49%) reported that they ask only a quarter of the time. Only 18% of staff reported that they ask half the time or more.

What are staff's attitudes to whether men should be asked about abuse histories?

Table 3.1. shows to what extent professionals believe male clients should be asked about abuse histories. It shows that, for staff in general, relatively few thought that men should *always* be asked (15.3%) compared with a much higher proportion (73%) that held the view that men should only be *sometimes* asked. No one responded that one should *never* ask.

What are staff's views on the reasons why one should or should not ask?

Seventeen per cent did not give a reason why they thought men should be asked about prior abuse histories. Of those who did answer this question, all responded that male clients should be asked because sexual abuse has an impact on psychological wellbeing.

Twenty per cent of subjects did not answer why they thought men should not be asked about abuse histories. Of those who did, the two most common reasons by far were that asking can be too intrusive for clients and prevent engagement, and that it is inappropriate to ask clients whose presenting problems are 'irrelevant to sexual abuse', e.g. simple phobias or psychosis. Other less frequent responses included: if the client is too distressed or psychotic; the client could become angry or violent; it is uncomfortable asking; it could worsen the client's condition; one could implant false memories; there

Table 3.1 The extent to which professionals believe male clients should be asked about abuse histories

How often should ask	All staff (%)	Nurses (%)	Psychiatrists (%)	Psychologists (%)
Always	15.3	28.9	4	7.3
Sometimes	73	57.8	96	75.6
Never	0	0	0	0
Not sure	11.7	13.3	0	17.1

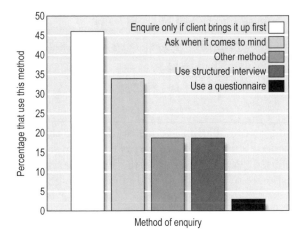

Fig. 3.2 The most frequently used method of obtaining abuse histories.

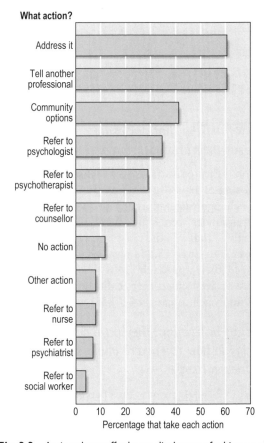

Fig. 3.3 Action that staff take on disclosure of a history of sexual abuse.

may be more pertinent issues to assess in the time given; and there may not be the resources to deal with the consequences of disclosure.

How do staff enquire about sexual abuse histories in men?

Figure 3.2 illustrates the most frequently used method of obtaining abuse histories. It shows that nearly one-half of all staff (46.4%) *enquire when the client brings it up first*. The next most used method was *asking when it came to mind* (34%). The least-used method was a questionnaire (3.1%). Thirty-five per cent of respondents used no other method than *asking when it came to mind*.

What do staff do if they learn that a client has a history of sexual abuse?

Figure 3.3 shows the most common actions taken by staff when they learn that a client has a history of sexual abuse. The most popular action was to address the issue with the client and tell another professional (59%). Other common responses were: to give community options (42.1%), and/or to refer on to a psychologist (34%), a psychotherapist (28%) and/or a counsellor (22.6%). Almost a quarter of psychiatrists (24%) reported that they take no action when they learn that a client has a history of abuse, compared to only 10% of psychologists and 5% of nurses.

Do staff receive specific training in the area of sexual abuse?

Table 3.2 shows the proportion of staff who reported having had specific training in the assessment and/or treatment of sexual abuse: over two-thirds said that they had received *no* training in the assessment of sexual abuse. The 30% who had received training generally reported that it consisted of 1 or 2 day workshops, or was part of their usual professional training. It also shows that there are marked differences in the responses by different professionals, with almost half of psychologists claiming to have had training compared to only 15% of nurses, and psychiatrists falling somewhere in between.

Table 3.2 The proportion of staff who reported having had training in the area of sexual abuse

	All staff	Nurses	Psychiatrists	Psychologists
Percentage who had received training	30	13.3	33.3	46.3
Percentage who felt that they had received sufficient training	30.8	18.6	60	25.6

Do staff believe that disclosure of abuse changes their approach to care?

The majority of staff (65.3%) answered that the disclosure of a history of sexual abuse would *somewhat* change their approach to their client's care. The remainder were split roughly equally between reporting that it did not really change their approach to care (17.8%), and that it significantly changed their approach (16.8%). Of the 18 subjects who responded that it did not really change their approach to care, 14 (78%) were nurses.

Do staff believe that they have had sufficient training in how to enquire about sexual abuse histories in men?

Table 3.2 also shows the percentage of staff reporting that they had received sufficient training to be able to ask about a history of sexual abuse in male clients. It highlights that for staff in general only a minority (30.8%) felt they had had sufficient training. Very few nurses reported having had sufficient training, and only just over a quarter of psychologists felt they had. These figures are in contrast to psychiatrists, where the majority responded that they had sufficient training.

What are professionals' beliefs about the prevalence of male sexual abuse in the psychiatric population?

Table 3.3 shows staff estimates of the prevalence of sexual abuse in the male psychiatric population,

and reveals that on average staff believe that just under a quarter of male clients have been sexually abused. Psychiatrists gave the most conservative estimate of abuse rates, and nurses the highest.

Discussion of the findings

The results from this study show that the vast majority of mental health professionals surveyed either never or only occasionally ask their male clients if they have been sexually abused. This provides strong evidence for Holmes et al.'s hypothesis that one of the reasons why male victims of sexual abuse are not coming to the attention of psychiatric professionals is that clinicians are failing to enquire about their sexual abuse histories. The implications of such unawareness are important with regard to treatment. A fundamental aim of health-care professionals is to understand their clients' difficulties fully, in order to provide the most appropriate care. In practice, the comprehensive formulation of a client's difficulties is an essential component in devising a plan of care and interventions.

The question still remains then, 'why are so few professionals regularly asking men about past histories of sexual abuse?' As previously suggested by Holmes and colleagues, it could be that practitioners fail to acknowledge that their clients could have been abused. Results from this study illustrate that a small number of professionals do not believe that the prevalence rate of abuse in the male psychiatric population is particularly significant. However, most staff actually estimate that a relatively large

Table 3.3 Estimates given by staff of the prevalence of sexual abuse in the male psychiatric population(%)

	All staff	Nurses	Psychiatrists	Psychologists
Mean prediction of prevalence	24	27.5	17.1	24.45
Standard deviation	19.6	23.6	8.9	20.2

minority number of male clients (25% on average) have histories of abuse, indicating that professionals are aware that many male psychiatric clients may have been abused. Whether they use this information in practice is another matter. Nevertheless, this suggests that at least for most staff the reason they do not ask about sexual abuse is not because they do not think that it may have occurred.

Another possible reason is that they do not believe that it is always necessary to ask, and will offer a variety of reasons why. This was supported

Learning activity 3.4

Think of two to four male clients that you have offered care to within your clinical experience. If each of those men had a history of sexual abuse which they had never had the opportunity to disclose, what might be the implications:

(a) for them as an incapacitated person?

(b) on their presenting health problem?

(c) on your relationship with them as care provider?

in the research by the staff's response to question 2, which shows that most practitioners did not respond that male clients should *always* be asked. This interpretation is further supported by the qualitative data, which show that many practitioners report logical reasons why they think clients should not be asked, for example it is too intrusive, and/or that it may be irrelevant to the presenting problem.

A further possibility for why professionals are not asking about abusive histories is that although they believe that they *should* always ask, for vari-

Reflection point 3.4

Think about the things that you might say or believe should happen but that you don't do yourself in practice (for example, engage in clinical supervision). Why don't you practise what you preach? What prevents you from doing so?

ous reasons (e.g. embarrassment) they do not always do so in practice. This explanation is supported by the minority of professionals, mainly nurses, who responded that they thought that one should *always* ask about past history of sexual abuse but reported that in practice they do not. In such cases the reasons appear more related to the actual difficulty of asking.

How do professionals ask about sexual abuse?

The results from this study highlight the ineffective methods used to enquire about abuse histories on the few occasions when practitioners do ask. First, it appears that the most popular method of enquiry relies on the client to bring up the fact that they have been sexually abused first, before the subject is then explored. This is an important finding in the light of research suggesting that clients are more likely to disclose sexual abuse if asked directly (Briere and Zaidi 1989). Furthermore, the

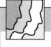

Learning activity 3.5

◆ List any ways that you are aware of that would assist you to enquire into a sexual abuse history in a man. Try to assess how effective each might be.

◆ Thinking about those clients that you identified in Learning activity 3.4, write down ways in which you might begin asking each one whether or not they had experienced sexual abuse.

◆ If possible, test your approach on a colleague. Try to reflect on how difficult or easy it was to initiate, to phrase the question(s), and how comfortable you were in doing this.

second most popular method of enquiry is asking when it comes to mind (one-third of practitioners used this method exclusively), which is a very non-pragmatic method. Taking these two most popular methods together, it seems that the majority of practitioners are using ineffective and non-systematic approaches to enquiring into sexual abuse histories in men.

What do psychiatric services offer men who are victims of sexual abuse?

To date, the focus has been on asking about sexual abuse. Attention now needs to be drawn to what professionals do once they have learnt that a male client has been abused. In general, most health-care professionals seem to be taking appropriate actions, two of the main options being to refer on to other professionals, and/or to offer community options. An exception to this is the one-quarter of psychiatrists who said that *taking no action* was an option they exercised.

One rather striking finding is that over half of all the clinicians (and almost all of the psycholo-

Reflection point 3.5

Consider the last two issues. Brainstorm what you feel the consequences might be for a client who has a history of sexual abuse if:

(a) she or he has disclosed sexual abuse and then it is ignored/no action is taken by the practitioner who received the disclosure

(b) the client is encouraged to continue disclosing and thus reliving the abuse to a practitioner who does not have the level of skill and knowledge to help.

gists) reported that they would address sexual abuse issues directly with the client in therapy, suggesting that they felt competent to do such work. This seems particularly so for psychologists, who are also less likely to refer the client elsewhere, suggesting that they see themselves as competent to treat. Whether professionals are competent or not given the level of training that they have received, however, is an important issue.

Professionals' perception of the prevalence of male sexual abuse

The estimates of prevalence rates of sexual abuse in the male psychiatric population given by pro-

fessionals are interesting. One finding that stands out quite clearly is that these estimates were extremely variable. One interpretation of this could be that, as a group in general, mental health professionals are simply not aware of the prevalence figures. Bearing in mind the little training they have received in the area of sexual abuse, and the lack of good research into the prevalence of male sexual abuse (Mendel 1995), this seems highly likely. It was further supported in the study by a number of professionals leaving this section blank, or often putting a question mark.

Another interesting finding is that on average professionals appear to believe that a fairly high proportion of male psychiatric clients have been sexually abused. This is intriguing in view of how many professionals are actually asking their clients if they have been abused: although they believe that a quarter of their clients have been abused, they rarely actually ask.

Clinical implications and training issues

Approximately two-thirds of professionals reported having had no training in the assessment or treatment of sexual abuse. As these are self-reports, one possibility is that they had actually received training but could not remember it or had missed it. Much more plausible is that there is a lack of teaching on this subject. Perhaps of even more significance is that the majority of professionals feel they have not had enough training to enquire about abuse histories in male clients. Therefore, both objectively in terms of the amount of training they say that they have actually received, and subjectively in terms of whether they perceive themselves as sufficiently trained, the majority of professionals appear under trained in the assessment of sexual abuse of male clients.

There is also a difference in training between the three professional groups: a particularly low percentage of nurses reported having received training, or that they were sufficiently trained; the majority of psychiatrists perceived themselves to be sufficiently trained; and psychologists fell somewhere between the two.

As well as professionals' own view of their training, a number of other findings in this study suggest a lack of training in the area of male sexual abuse. First, there was the lack of knowledge about prevalence rates of sexual abuse in the male psychiatric population. Secondly, professionals did not appear to be using the most effective methods of enquiry about sexual abuse histories. Thirdly, some of the answers suggest that profes-

Learning activity 3.6

Using the prevalence rate of male sexual abuse that you found in Learning activity 3.3, now try and add to your database by finding five research articles which have investigated the effects of sexual abuse on the victim. Once you have completed this task, use the research findings positively to formulate an action plan to enable you to develop a protocol that could be used in your everyday practice. Remember that a protocol may well involve other people doing the same thing. Try to consider how you would introduce the protocol to your colleagues, and what your and their training needs might be.

sionals may not be fully aware of the correlation between sexual abuse and mental health. A good example of this is the fact that many said they would not ask clients about sexual abuse if it was not indicated by their diagnosis, e.g. psychosis. This logic is not consistent with the research by, for example, Wurr and Partridge (1997), who found that many of the men in their sample who had been sexually abused had a psychotic disorder.

A valid concern regarding mental health professionals' inadequate training in the assessment of sexual abuse is the potential for reduced effectiveness in the care that they will be ultimately providing to their clients. Even using conservative estimates of how many male clients have been sexually abused, during the course of their work most professionals will come into contact with a number of such men. One need not elaborate on the benefits of understanding the specific issues surrounding abuse, such as shame or a tendency for

revictimization, in terms of the way these men are treated. It is questionable whether professionals who are untrained in the area of male sexual abuse will be fully aware of these issues. Furthermore, it may be detrimental to the clients' mental health if they are being helped by professionals who are not specifically trained. Despite this, the majority of professionals, and in particular psychologists, said that they themselves would address the issue of sexual abuse in therapy with a client who had disclosed such a history. This is of great concern when less than a third of clinicians reported actually having received specific training in this area, and that fewer regarded themselves sufficiently trained to even enquire about sexual abuse in male clients, let alone address it in therapy. There are clearly generic skills that all health-care professionals learn and can apply to a variety of problems, including those related to sexual abuse, but there is a distinct possibility that someone who is untrained in the specific issues could inflict psychological damage on their clients.

The major implication of this identified lack of training and its probable detrimental effect on the care of sexually abused men is that there is a need for the teaching of this issue to health-care professionals, and in particular mental health professionals. This study has illuminated some of the potential topics that could be addressed in such training, including how best to enquire about sexual abuse. Some professionals would benefit from looking at their own difficulties in the actual task of asking, e.g. dealing with embarrassment or feeling unable to ask in a sensitive manner. For other professionals it might be simply a case of raising awareness of the phenomenon. Teaching the prevalence rates for varying populations might also be useful. In general, learning about the potential consequences of sexual abuse on men would also be useful. There are numerous other issues that could be addressed. What is also important is that this survey suggests that such training would be appreciated by most professionals, and nurses in particular. In the 'comments' section of the questionnaire many respondents identified the need for specific training in this area, demonstrating a willingness to broaden their knowledge and understanding of male sexual abuse.

Learning activity 3.7

Consider what has been highlighted as training needs for professionals who come across male sexual abuse in their client group. Plan a 2-day workshop for your colleagues which would address some of the deficits in their knowledge, skills and understanding of male clients who have been sexually abused.

Summary of research

The topic of male sexual abuse has been described as being at a similar stage as was that of female abuse some 20 years ago (Mendel 1995). The lack of awareness of the issue is exemplified by the response from one psychologist, of lecturer status, who believed that the prevalence rate for sexual abuse in the male psychiatric population was zero. Similarly, a consultant psychiatrist in charge of an acute-stay adult ward and an adult community team commented that in the whole of their career they had never come across a single male client who had been sexually abused. Not surprisingly, this psychiatrist reported that they *never* enquired about sexual abuse histories in male clients. These individuals illustrate, if somewhat extremely, the need for education and training in the clinical aspects of male sexual abuse.

CONCLUSION

This chapter has discussed sexual abuse and how it affects a person's sexual health. Prevalence studies reveal that a significant number of men and women have been sexually abused, but because of underreporting, these figures probably underestimate the extent of the problem. Sexual abuse therefore needs to claim its rightful place on the health agenda. Unfortunately, as shown by the research detailed in this chapter by Lab et al. (2000), professionals who regularly come into contact with men who have been sexually abused may not enquire about abuse and often have little, if any, specific training in the area. This is a problem that probably also applies to female victims of sexual abuse.

In order to work with victims of sexual abuse, professionals need education and training that address the numerous issues in this difficult area. Such training should equip them to offer appropriate care for this client group and, ultimately, provide services that will take into account the range of specific needs of victims of sexual abuse.

Acknowledgement

Research was undertaken with Padmal De Silva, Department of Clinical Psychology, Institute of Psychiatry, London, and Janet D. Feigenbaum, Department of Psychology, University College London, London.

ANNOTATED FURTHER READING

Herman J L (1992) Trauma and recovery. Basic Books, New York

This is an excellent book on the effects of trauma, in particular sexual abuse, on the individual. It also provides an historical account of how the concept of psychological trauma has become incorporated into psychiatry over the years.

Mendel M P 1995 The male survivor: the impact of sexual abuse. Sage, Thousand Oaks

This is perhaps one of the best texts on the phenomenon and impact of childhood sexual abuse on males. It provides up-to-date information on the prevalence and effects of sexual abuse on men. It also gives an excellent account of the importance of seeing male childhood sexual abuse in the context of male socialization. The book's readability is further enhanced by the personal accounts of male survivors that Mendel presents between each chapter.

Finklehor D 1986 A sourcebook on child sexual abuse. Sage, Newbury Park, CA

David Finklehor is a pioneer in bringing the issue of sexual abuse to the attention of the psychiatric

community. This book provides a comprehensive overview of many of the issues relevant to sexual abuse. Finklehor also presents his psychological model, which is useful in explaining how sexual abuse affects mental health.

REFERENCES

Bayoudh F, Barrak S, Ben Fredj N, Allani R, Hamdi M 1995 A study of a custom in Somalia: the circumcision of girls. Medicine Tropicale 55(3): 238–242

Briere J, Evan D, Runz M, Wall T 1988 Symptomatology of men who were molested as children. A comparison study. American Journal of Orthopsychiatry 58(3): 457–461

Briere J, Zaidi LY 1989 Sexual abuse histories and sequelal in female psychiatric emergency room patients. American Journal of Psychiatry 146: 1602–1606

Browne A, Finklehor D 1986 Impact of child abuse: a review of the research. Psychological Bulletin 99: 66–77

Department of Health 1998 Children and young persons on the Child Protection Register, year ending 31 March 1998 (England). Department of Health, London

Dimock P T 1998 Adult males sexually abused as children. Characteristics and implications for treatment. Journal of Interpersonal Violence 3(2): 203–221

Dorkenoo E 1996 Combating female genital mutilation: an agenda for the next decade. World Health Statistics Quarterly 49(2): 142–147

Finklehor D 1981 The sexual abuse of boys. Victimology: An International Journal 6: 76–84

Finklehor D 1986 A source book on child sexual abuse. Sage, Newbury Park, CA

Fitzgerald L F 1993 Violence against women in the workplace. American Psychologist 48: 1070–1077

Fromuth M E, Burkhart B R 1989 Long-term psychological correlates of childhood sexual abuse in two samples of college men. Child Abuse and Neglect 13: 533–542

Gutek B, Koss M P 1993 Changed women and changed organizations: consequences of and coping with sexual harassment. Journal of Vocational Behaviour 42: 28–48

Harris J, Grace S 1999 A question of evidence? Investigating and prosecuting rape in the 1990s. Home Office Research Study 196. Home Office, London

Holmes G R, Offen L 1996 Clinicians' hypotheses regarding clients' problems: are they less likely to hypothesise sexual abuse in male compared to female clients? Child Abuse and Neglect 20: 493–501

Holmes R, Offen L, Waller G 1997 See no evil, hear no evil, speak no evil: why do relatively few male victims of childhood sexual abuse receive help for abuse-related issues in adulthood? Clinical Psychology Review 17: 69–88

Home Office 1999 Home Office Statistical Bulletin: Recorded Crime Statistics for England and Wales 1998/99. Home Office, London

Jehu D 1991 Clinical work with adults who were sexually abused in childhood. In: Hollin C R, Howelles K (eds) Clinical approaches to sex offenders and their victims. Wiley, Chichester, pp 229–260

Kilpatrick D G 1992 Treatment and counseling needs of women veterans who were raped, otherwise sexually assaulted, or sexually harassed during military service. Testimony before the Senate Committee on Veterans' Affairs

Lab D D, Feigenbaum J, De Silva P 2000 Mental health professionals' attitudes and practice towards male childhood sexual abuse. Journal of Child Abuse and Neglect 24: 3

Mendel M P 1995 The male survivor: the impact of sexual abuse. Sage, Thousand Oaks

Mills A 1993 Helping male victims of sexual abuse. Nursing Standard 7: 36–39

Olsen P E 1990 The sexual abuse of boys: a study of the long-term psychological effects. In: Hunter M (ed) The sexually abused male. Vol. 1, Prevalence, impact and treatment. Lexington Books & D. Heath & Company, Lexington, MA, pp 137–152

Peters S, Wyatt G, Finklehor D 1986 Prevalence. In: Finklehor D (ed) A sourcebook on child sexual abuse. Sage, Newbury Park, CA, pp 15–59

Rape Crisis Federation 1996/7 Rape Crisis 5 Statistical Survey Annual Report 1996/7. Rape Crisis Federaton, Nottingham

Renvoize J 1993 Innocence destroyed. A study of child sexual abuse. Routledge, London

Richie B 1996. In: Read J, Reynolds J Speaking our minds. An anthology. Open University Press, Milton Keynes, p. 10

Rowan A B, Foy D W 1993 Post-traumatic stress disorder in child sexual abuse survivors: a literature review. Journal of Traumatic Stress 6(1): 3–20

Swett C, Surrey J, Cohen C 1990 Sexual abuse and physical abuse histories and psychiatric symptoms among male psychiatric outpatients. American Journal of Psychiatry 147(5): 632–636

US Merit Systems Protection Board (MSPB) 1981 Sexual harassment in the federal workplace: is it a problem? US Government Printing Office, Washington DC. In: Salisbury J, Ginorio A B, Remick H, Stringer D M 1986 Counseling victims of sexual harassment. Psychotherapy 23: 316–324

Wurr C J, Partridge I M 1997 The prevalence of a history of childhood sexual abuse in an acute adult inpatient population. Child Abuse and Neglect 20(9): 867–872

2

Part Two
What influences professional practice in sexual health?

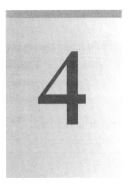

4

Sexual health and professional practice

Kevin Corbett

> 'The responsibility of the writer as a moral agent is to bring the truth about **matters of human significance** to **an audience that can do something about them.** This is part of what it means to be a **moral agent . . .'** (Chomsky, 1996, p. 56. Emphases in original)

KEY ISSUES/CONCEPTS

◆ Multidisciplinary and multiagency approaches

◆ Shared care and community care planning

◆ Clarifying roles and responsibilities

◆ Networking and liaison

◆ Collaboration in care and prevention

OVERVIEW

Chapter 4, *Sexual health and professional practice*, introduces multidisciplinary and multiagency approaches to professional practice in the field of sexual health, using the professional experiences of the author to aid further understanding. The focus is on shared care, care planning, interprofessional and interagency collaboration. It is proposed that the assessment of sexual wellbeing should be part of mainstream practice, rather than the preserve of specialists. The key issues for practitioners are the range of practice settings for sexual health promotion, professional development and lifelong learning, the clarification of roles and responsibilities, and network and liaison activity. Examples are drawn from different practice settings, including the clinic, community health and local authority settings.

INTRODUCTION

'Profession means that one professes to be able to help another. A professional not only makes **choices** affecting the good of the other, but in making those *choices*, also affects his own being and thus contributes his own *identity* . . .

. . . replacing practice with technique not only threatens the identity of nursing but makes it impossible to **establish her/his identity by making choices** within her/his chosen profession.' (Bishop and Scudder 1990)

Orthodox medicine may be considered an 'applied' science where physicians are the technologists. In such a design, the danger for nursing is that of being reduced to 'technicians . . . appliers of techniques' developed by medical technologists (Bishop and Scudder 1990, p. 68). Medical predominance over health care may attempt to categorize nursing in a similar vein, preventing nurses from establishing a unique professional identity and eroding clinical decision making. In order to develop an understanding of nursing's potential for promoting clients' sexual wellbeing, the meaning of concepts such as sexual health and professional practice need to be explored.

PROFESSIONAL PRACTICE AND SEXUAL HEALTH

Sexual health has been defined in terms of a social and a personal ethic:

'. . . *the integration of the somatic, emotional, intellectual and social aspects of sexual beings in ways that are positively enriching and enhance personality, communication and love.*' (World Health Organization 1975)

Few (1997) discusses the lack of reference in such definitions to issues of power. Ingram-Fogel (1990) reflexively defines sexual health in terms of individual capacities and freedoms. Often such definitions discuss neither experience, enjoyment or pleasure, nor the plurality of sexual orientation and its expression. Ekeid (1992) defines sexual health in terms of a rights discourse. This appears similar to the debate on 'new nursing' (Salvage 1990), government guidance on health promotion (Department of Health 1993), and that of the health-care 'market' (Seedhouse 1993).

Modern health rhetoric positions the patient as a service user, a consumer or a 'client'. In the ethics of the health and social care market, the client or service user has rights and responsibilities over their entitlement to the delivery and the quality of care. Aggleton and Tyrer (1994, p. 72) formulate a socially conscious definition of sexual health, which is '. . . more than the absence of STDs and unwanted pregnancy . . . it implies more positively the pleasures of sexual relationships and emotional closeness and . . . of taking responsibility for oneself and others'.

Reflection point 4.1

◆ In Reflection point 1.2 you were asked to create your own definition of sexual health.

◆ Looking back at your definition, try to identify the values you think you implied when you created that definition.

Defining nursing practice

Generic nursing practice has been defined in phenomenological terms as embodying the opposite of theoretical knowledge. In Box 4.1 it is defined as a 'practical' knowledge or 'know-how' devel-

Box 4.1 Phenomenological definitions of nursing as practice

Nursing is:

'. . . know-how or knowing how. It is the opposite of theoretical knowledge' (Benner and Wrubel 1989, p. 411)

Nursing is:

'. . . knowledge development in an applied discipline . . . practical knowledge (know-how) through theory-based scientific investigations and . . . know-how developed through clinical experience in the practice of the discipline' (Benner 1984, p. 3)

Nursing is:

'. . . a practice which is founded on the moral imperative to foster the physical and psychological well-being of persons, especially when ill, by caring for them in personal relationships' (Bishop and Scudder 1990, p. 171)

oped through experience. The regulation of nursing practice in the UK is through the Central Council (UKCC). It is also regulated by the power relationships that exist between the health-care consumer and the physician. It is assumed that nursing practice in the field of sexual health can be developed through experience and education. This requires practitioners to undertake educational development in order to sustain appropriate standards of practice (ENB 1994a,b, 1995).

Today there is a greater understanding about the creative interaction between the work environment and the practitioner (Schon 1983, Palmer et al. 1994). The rationale for continually seeking to improve the standard of practice is well established, and has led to thinking about professional development as a process of lifelong learning (ENB 1994b, 1995). English National Board (ENB) guidelines for developing practice-oriented preregistration nursing focus on the practitioner. Nurses are seen as having greater responsibility for progressing professional achievements and delivering high standards of care by responding quickly and flexibly to client need (ENB 1994a). Health-care professionals further their professional knowledge and skills by flexibly reconstituting their roles to meet the changing needs of clients. Likewise, a client's wellbeing may be enhanced if professionals can reflect upon and improve their practice. Such a dialectical relationship with the client (often called 'empowerment') is, '. . . a process of helping individuals develop a critical awareness of the root causes of their problems and a readiness to act on this awareness' (Gibson 1991, p. 356).

Nursing practice in the field of sexual health occurs in the context of professional understanding about the 'positive pleasures of sexual relationships and emotional closeness' which enables or empowers individuals to take responsibility for 'oneself and others' (Aggleton and Tyrer 1994, p. 72). Following on from this understanding, such practice is not the preserve of the specialists but should occur in generic health and social care settings. In many settings power relationships can directly or indirectly influence practice. For example, Englehardt conceptualizes nursing as having an 'in-between' position. In practice, the nurse is under the gaze or scrutiny of the client and the physician (Englehardt 1985). In health care today, the scrutiny of the client is increasingly one of a consumer of services and the scrutiny of the physician is that of diagnostician and prescriber of treatment. However, nurses are developing practitioner roles in first-line diagnostics and treatment management (Mullen 1995, Harris et al. 1996).

Nursing practice and sexual health

There are a range of settings for sexual health practice. People can access health professionals in a diverse range of formal and informal contexts, for example when receiving instruction about medication, or for the diagnosis and treatment of sexually transmitted infections. Irwin (1997) states that sexual health practice means promoting sexual wellbeing or the psychosocial aspects of sexual health. Weeks (1995) believes that sexuality, intimacy and sexual behaviour are also important identity constructs of postmodern culture.

Therefore, it is essential that the range of practice settings should extend beyond the medical taxonomies of genitourinary medicine (GUM) to include generic settings.

The UKCC (1992b) Scope of Professional Practice regulates nurses' professional behaviour to ensure that working practices accord with the health needs of individuals. It acts as a realistic framework for promoting more independent professional judgement. In such a framework, 'principles for practice' have replaced 'certificates for tasks' (Walby et al. 1994). Today nurses are better able to undertake clinical decision making and to develop autonomous judgement. This represents a form of professional **agency** and supersedes the previous system of '. . . minute certification' (Walby et al. 1994, p. 82). In this way the professional growth of nursing is constructing a true 'professional identity' (Bishop and Scudder 1990, p. 69).

Reflection point 4.2

Thinking about your practice, consider how you make clinical decisions. How are these affected by:

(a) other professional groups, e.g. physicians and allied professions?

(b) the policies and practices of employers, e.g. management procedures?

(c) statutory or government bodies, e.g. UKCC, Department of Health?

COLLABORATION IN PRACTICE

Two aspects of interprofessional collaboration are task and process. Braye and Preston-Shoot (1995) define collaboration as 'both a task to be achieved and a process to be understood'. They go on to suggest that 'obstacles lie in the path of developing a shared sense of purpose . . . and looking anew at services which will realise the full potential of empowerment and partnership with users'.

Gray (1989) defines collaboration as 'a process through which parties who see different aspects of a problem can constructively explore their differences and search for solutions that go beyond their limited vision of what is possible'. Clause 5 of the Code of Professional Conduct (UKCC 1992a) requires nurses to collaborate and cooperate with other professionals. Research into the work of sexual health clinics shows that professional boundaries and responsibilities are not clear. In a national survey of genitourinary medicine (GUM) clinics by Allen and Hogg (1993), nursing roles were found to overlap with those of other staff. Many nurses wished to take over elements of medical practice, such as microscopy, cryotherapy and venepuncture, or administering intravenous therapy and undertaking physical examinations.

Developing a shared sense of purpose

Walby et al. (1994) examined working relationships between nurses and physicians and described them as a balance between elements of hierarchy and symbiosis which involved a combination of 'complex relations' between the professions. Such collaboration did not fit neatly into a particular model. They described nursing as shedding its 'handmaiden' role without having achieved a professional status equal to that of medicine. This shifting relationship is perceived as one where both professions may assume different positions at different times (Walby et al. 1994).

Looking anew at services

Nursing practice has to be seen within the framework of policy guidance. For example, in one official framework for health promotion it is unclear how nursing practice relates to working in 'healthy alliances', which are '. . . imaginative and flexible approaches to local inter-agency cooperation, working across boundaries with the objective of improving the health of the population, as well as **increasing collaboration** between differing agencies and within the NHS . . .' (Department of Health 1993, p. 13. Emphasis added).

Policy guidance that encourages working across boundaries may be problematic. In reality, professionals may be challenged to negotiate and coordinate between themselves. For example, policy guidance in the framework of the *Health of the Nation* and the NHS and Community Care Act emphasizes a 'search for solutions' which are important for effective collaboration. Such guidance concentrates on service developments rather than professional and sectoral interests or funding streams, and focuses on how to best meet client needs. Following on from Gray's definition of collaboration, such guidance seeks solutions to problems which go beyond any one sector's vision of the possible. It would appear from reading such official guidance that the meeting of client needs is a combination, or synergy, of sectoral inputs surpassing that which any one sector can deliver. Finally, the ideological and philosophical consequences of applying cost-effectiveness and measurable indicators to health are ignored by policy guidance (Haydock 1992, McDonnell 1994).

Empowerment and partnership in bureaucracies

In health and local authorities the organizational cultures and management structures can negatively affect collaboration with the voluntary sector. Between professional groups power differentials can affect working practices and collaboration.

In order to better understand the ethical context of nursing work, Englehardt (1985) describes the in-between position of the nurse. This is considered to be a practical or collaborative context where the nurse prescribes and delivers care, advice or information. In respect of advancing practice it represents a situation where nurses can potentially exercise professional agency. It is through the individual actions of the professional, or professional agency, that many 'different aspects of a problem' (Gray 1989) can be examined. Giddens (1991, p. 175) discusses the environment of actions in the postmodern world:

'one cannot argue . . . that while the micro-settings of action are malleable, larger social systems form an uncontrolled background environment.'

For health practitioners this 'uncontrolled background' may be the bureaucracy of the service. A common perception is that such bureaucracy limits nurses' ability to care. The potential for transforming such systems may lie in what Engelhardt (1985) conceives of as nursing's in-between position. From this position, one may view all sides of an issue and seek practical solutions which achieve collaboration between differing professional ideologies. This position is further strengthened by nurses adopting 'principles for practice' (UKCC 1992 a,b Walby et al. 1994,), which acknowledge the complexity of the working environment and the need to make clinical decisions for optimal care. This reorientation of nursing towards the consumer through flexible working predates the NHS reforms and represents a genuine strengthening of clients' wellbeing (Walby et al. 1994).

Reflection point 4.3

◆ How do you experience collaboration with physicians? How would you describe your working relationship? Do you take on 'different positions at different times'?

◆ What do you think about the 'in-between' position of the nurse? How far does this concept describe some of your experiences with physicians? Can you describe other positions that exist for nursing in relation to other professionals?

NURSING IN THE SEXUAL HEALTH CLINIC

*'In the hospital, the patient is the **subject** of his disease, that is, he is a **case**; in the clinic, where one is dealing only with **examples**, the patient is the accident of his disease, the transitory object that it happens to have seized upon.'* (Foucault 1963, p. 59. Emphases added)

Overcoming medical predominance

Bennet (1992, p. 37) describes the difference that key professionals made in the 1980s growth of sex-

ual health services. Creative and innovative developments came from the 'product champion(s)', who were necessary for the 'innovation process'. Product champions were characterized as having autonomy, which helped them assume lead roles in service development (Bennet 1992). Innovative services were developed by such professionals, who set up visionary initiatives. Bennet characterizes such practice as going '. . . beyond the narrow confines of . . . specialities' (Bennet 1992, p. 37).

In order to understand how sexual health nursing can develop in the context of the health-care market it is useful to consider how innovative product champions could arise in the GUM clinic setting. Such nursing practitioners could develop practice which goes beyond that of medically dominated GUM clinics. Such medical predominance has far-reaching effects. Even though many innovative and autonomous nursing roles have been established – for example clinical nurse specialists and nurse-led clinics – the literature cites few examples in GUM of such practice (Pearson 1988).

Developing nursing practice in the clinic

Vaughan (1990) discusses the potential for nursing knowledge to develop practice by addressing the 'theory–practice' gap. This is considered necessary in order for nursing to develop its practice base and effect a shift in attitudes towards practice.

Vaughan discusses three important issues that need to be addressed before any shift can occur. These include the knowledge required for practice; the new ways of learning or gaining knowledge and insight about the professional 'self'; and the way nursing work is organized. Specific issues related to the politics of collaboration with physicians in the GUM context must be addressed if clinic-based nursing is to further its practice base and product champions are to emerge.

First, there is the issue of the knowledge required for practice. Informal means of learning are needed to professionally develop experienced practitioners.

In their survey Allen and Hogg (1993) found that over half the senior nurses and three-quarters of the staff nurses sampled had not undertaken any educational development appropriate to inform their practice. Consequently, nursing practice in those settings was not considered as being developed. Many frameworks and philosophies exist which are appropriate and may be applied to clinical practice. Berridge's (1995, p. 60) analysis of AIDS policy in the 1980s cites the 'holistic' framework that British nurses developed in response to HIV/AIDS and its focus on the 'whole person' as opposed to 'carrying out technical procedures under medical direction'. Such holistic care may be in opposition to medicalized or task-oriented approaches, which tend to elide the individual as a whole by focusing upon their diseased 'parts'. It is seen as non-participative and 'disempowering' (Salvage 1990).

The second area for consideration is knowledge of the self or the 'professional self'. In order to function at an optimum level any professional must perceive themselves as equal to other professionals, and as possessing autonomy, accountability and effectiveness. In the GUM clinic this is especially important, given the close proximity to physicians, whom Allen and Hogg describe as having 'traditional autonomy' over determining the clinic organization and structure (Allen and Hogg 1993, p. 44). In much of the literature about nursing in the sexual health clinic there is an absence of nurse-led or holistic approaches, except for HIV/AIDS care (Faugier and Hicken 1995) and in the discourse of educational resources (ENB 1994a).

Allen and Hogg (1993) showed how professionals' working roles and responsibilities varied across differing sexual health clinics. The variation was greater for nursing than for any other group, which was the result of medical custom and practice dictating clinic organization and practice. Nursing roles were found to be constrained by the multiplicity of other roles, such as that of the health adviser.

Thirdly, the manner in which nursing work is organized in the clinic requires consideration. Allen and Hogg found that more than half of the nurses sampled (n = 98) wanted to take on extra working roles. Such wished-for responsibilities also varied, and included microscopy, cryotherapy, venepuncture and the examination of female clients. Sixty-two per cent of medical staff supported the idea of nurse-run clinics. Support among nurses was variable for nurse-led wart therapy clinics (55%) and cytology clinics (8%), although 86% of senior nurses favoured such developments (Allen and Hogg 1993, p. 63).

The structure and organization of the clinic

The research illustrates how the clinic setting and its professional proximity to physicians affects nursing practice (Allen and Hogg 1993). Physicians appear to heavily influence, if not actually define, the nature of nursing practice. Box 4.2

Box 4.2 Structure and organization of the clinic vist		
Personnel	**Client assessment**	**Outcomes**

◆ Receptionist
◆ Nurse
◆ Physician
◆ Health adviser
	◆ Assessment and examination of urethra, vagina and anus:
	  – externally
	  – internally
	◆ Cytology:
	  – specimens
	  – speculum
	  – proctoscopy
	  – colposcopy
	◆ Microscopy and culture of discharge for in situ diagnostics
	◆ Blood and drug monitoring
		◆ Diagnosis and treatments
		◆ Referral
		◆ Return visit(s)
		◆ Information giving

shows the structure and organization of a typical clinic visit (Corbett 1994). The traditional autonomy of GUM physicians to determine the organization and structure of GUM clinics is due to their geographical and professional isolation (Allen and Hogg 1993). Nurses must negotiate the boundaries of their practice with this well established power base.

Allen and Hogg's survey also shows that many developments in nursing have not affected practice in the sexual health clinic. For example, there was no 'nursing process' or any documentation of nursing care in care plans, yet many nurses considered continuity of client care a deciding factor for choosing to work in GUM clinics (Allen and Hogg 1993, p. 49). There was little evidence that continuity of care was addressed, either from a service-user or a professional perspective, or even embodied as a value in practice.

From this research the clinic emerges as a mechanical or production-line experience for any client. The structure of the visit positions the 'client' as the patient, who forms the input at one end and is physically processed by swabbing, diagnostics and prescription drugs, and discharged at the other end. In between, clients experience several professional roles which may appear unrelated to each other. The professionals focus on the diseased part of the client, who becomes 'the accident of his disease . . . the object that it happens to have seized upon' (Foucault 1963, p. 59). For the professionals, the psychosocial aspects of the client's visit can appear almost secondary to the defining biomedical aspects that give structure to it. This understanding may inform Allen and Hogg's overall perspective when they recommend a review of the aims and objectives of GUM clinics and their position '. . . within the wider health service' (Allen and Hogg 1993, p. 219).

The quandary of clinic practice

The underdevelopment of nursing practice in the sexual health clinic setting remains a quandary, especially given recent developments. In other settings nurses are working in collaboration with physicians, with a greater semblance of continuity of care and clarity in role and responsibility. For example, there are nurse-led clinics for patients with rheumatological conditions (Hill 1997) and diabetes, and many Nursing Development Units (NDUs) (Pearson 1988). However, the King's Fund database of NDUs cites few references to sexual health, GUM or HIV/AIDS.

When considering such issues there are several factors that constrain the development of nursing practice for this setting. Palmer et al. (1994, p. 1) describe the alienation experienced due to the contemporary 'high-speed' manner in which nurses have to care for clients. This 'high-speed' work in GUM settings is a result of client numbers and the production-line structure of the service. The medical structure in this physician-oriented environment is that of task allocation. A transformation is required in the politics of collaboration with physicians in order to move away from task allocation. This would involve nurses assuming both the assessment and the diagnostic roles, which would also address the issue of continuity. In this new structure the nurse would become the Consultant and the physician a technician.

Implications for practice

The health-care market has opportunities to develop roles that maximize nursing skills using business management and cost-effectiveness. There are new ways for organizing work, for example primary nursing (Pearson 1988) and 'new nursing' (Salvage 1990), which represent a greater professional autonomy. These developments arose alongside the perception of the client as an active consumer, as opposed to a passive recipient of care. The philosophical and ideological effects on nursing practice have resulted in an increased emphasis on health. In 'new nursing' the professional–client relationship changes from one of paternalism to one of participation: the client becomes the client of the provider. For health nursing it is not so much '. . . what the nurse does, but how she (he) does it which counts' (Macleod Clark 1993, p. 258), clearly embodying the 'whole person' approach witnessed in HIV/AIDS nursing (Berridge 1995, p. 60).

If clinic-based nursing, implemented by clinical nurse specialisms and nurse-led clinics, is to

Reflection point 4.4

◆ How can nurses become 'product champions'
for GUM/sexual health settings? What do you
consider to be the factors that prevent
nurses assuming lead roles in such settings?

inform approaches to care and prevention, then
the dissonance between the level of care nurses are
allowed to deliver, as opposed to that which they
are educated to provide, must be addressed. A
shift in attitudes is required in the sexual health
clinic setting in order to further the development
of personalized or therapeutic care. Several
methodologies may be useful in such developments, including evidence-based practice, quality
assurance and cost-effectiveness.

HOME CARE PLANNING FOR A CLIENT WITH AIDS

*'The boundaries between home and hospital
care are constantly shifting. Care in the
community for people with long term
dependencies, an increasingly sophisticated
primary care service and the expansion of
outreach and day surgery have all contributed
to a reassessment of the central role of the
hospital.'* (Marks 1991, p. 4)

Responsibility for care

The balance between home and hospital was
expected to change in the 1990s (Marks 1991).
The expectation was for the provision of intensive
care at home for the chronically ill, called 'hospital care at home' (HCH). HCH is defined as a
hospital level of care in the home setting (Marks
1991, p. 4). This is different from the social and
rehabilitative care that is commonly known as
community care.

When HCH was compared with hospital care
for several medical conditions it was found to be

both clinically safe and organizationally and
financially viable (Marks 1991). When AIDS was
first diagnosed there was already an awareness of
the role for home care. The British Minister for
Health said that such clients '... did not need or
want continual hospital care', as care was '... better in the home' (Williams 1987, p. 4). The major
barrier to the expansion of HCH was not the lack
of technology, nor the provision of care, but the
problem of 'transferring responsibility for acute levels of care to the home setting' (Marks 1991, p. 9).
For AIDS care this transfer was the responsibility of
community nurses, who had to coordinate the
input of 'health services, local authorities and voluntary organisations' (Williams 1987, p. 26). Case
study 4.1 details the professional communication
and care planning required from different sectors.
In this example, the nurse-led planning successfully transferred acute levels of care to the home
setting. Through the professional agency of the
nurses, the client is supported by the primary and
secondary health sectors in a coordinated fashion
(Corbett 1997).

Enabling consumer choice

The importance of providing consumer choice is
seen as informing the growth in home care (Marks
1991). Many AIDS clients are young and have certain expectations:

> '... we have a very vocal group of people who
> expect ... to have a very big **voice** in what
> happens to them during their care ... they
> aren't passive people, they come in and tell
> you what they want ... the clients wanted to
> direct *their care ...'* (Scott 1994, p. 40.
> Original emphasis)

The planning of care in a true spirit of partnership with clients must take note of those clients'
'voice'. This has implications for any philosophy
of care. A facilitative or enabling approach can
match client expectations about wanting to direct
their care. In Case study 4.1 the client preferred
non-institutional care (Corbett 1997) and the philosophy of care facilitated and enabled his choice.

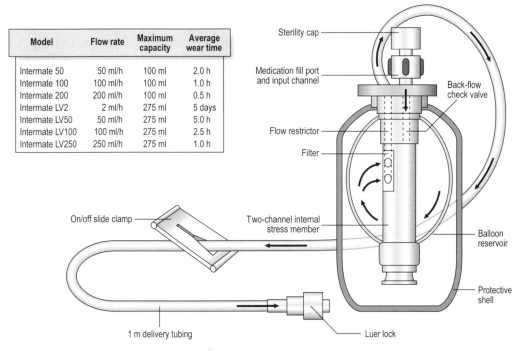

Model	Flow rate	Maximum capacity	Average wear time
Intermate 50	50 ml/h	100 ml	2.0 h
Intermate 100	100 ml/h	100 ml	1.0 h
Intermate 200	200 ml/h	100 ml	0.5 h
Intermate LV2	2 ml/h	275 ml	5 days
Intermate LV50	50 ml/h	275 ml	5.0 h
Intermate LV100	100 ml/h	275 ml	2.5 h
Intermate LV250	250 ml/h	275 ml	1.0 h

Fig. 4.1 Intermate ambulatory infusion system. (Reproduced with kind permission of Caremark Ltd.)

Sharing the care between sectors

In Case study 4.1 the benefits of an infusion technology that fosters self-care were discussed by nurses with the client and the GP. The nursing service was instrumental in developing and sustain-

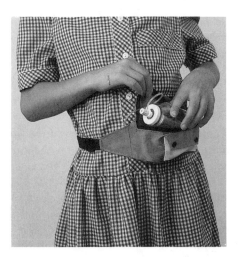

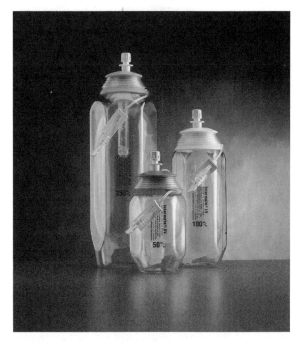

Fig. 4.2 Baxter elastomeric infusion technology. (Reproduced with kind permission of Baxter Healthcare.)

ing a shared care package between sectors. Bennett et al. (1994) describes several models of shared care, all needing close collaboration between sectors so that appropriate client management and decision making can occur. They found that such relationships develop when neither sector feels dominated by the other.

Case study 4.1

*John requires intravenous (i.v.) therapy (amphotericin) for the treatment of his chronic candidiasis. He requests home-based care (Corbett et al. 1993, Livingston et al. 1993, Corbett 1997). Each preprepared dose is self-administered using an elastomeric **Intermate** ambulatory infusion system (Fig. 4.1).*

Elastomeric infusion technology facilitates empowerment by promoting mobility and self-care. Electrical devices and drip stands are not required (Fig. 4.2) (Wonke and Fielding 1992, Duncan-Skingle and Bramwell 1993, Steel et al. 1995). Venous access was achieved using a central venous access device, a Port-a-Cath (Fig. 4.3).

Kidney function is a key indicator of drug side-effects and John's serum creatinine was measured regularly. John was prescribed an alternating regimen of twice- and thrice-weekly doses of intravenous amphotericin 50 mg reconstituted in 5% glucose (Chavenet et al. 1992) for a period of 17 months.

Nurse instruction in both the Intermate and Port-a-Cath devices was given to John in hospital (Corbett et al. 1993) and at home by the practice and home nurses (Corbett 1997). Nurse instruction and coaching for clients is cited as an important community role, along with assessment and care planning (Department of Health 1994). John's clinical response to therapy was maintained at home without side-effects such as chills, fever and significant nausea (DataPharm 1991).

The infusion protocol involved John having regular venepuncture from the practice nurse to assess serum creatinine levels. Communication between the community nurses and the hospital ensured that appropriate and speedy decisions were made for John to self-administer safely. Through the professional agency of the community nurses John was advised about the drug dosage and side-effects.

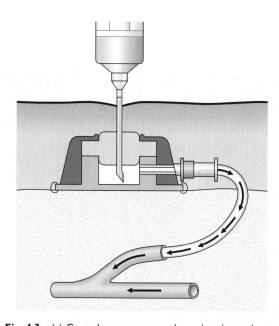

Fig. 4.3 (a) Central venous access: chest-placed portal location. (Reproduced with kind permission of SIMS Deltec Inc., St Paul, Minnesota). (b) Central venous access: an implantable central venous access device called the Port-a-Cath. Fluids can be injected through the Port-a-Cath system and into the bloodstream. (Reproduced with kind permission of SIMS Deltec Inc., St Paul, Minnesota).

AIDS-related candidiasis

The acquired immune deficiency syndrome (AIDS) may predispose a person to fungal infections as a result of failure of cell-mediated immunity, thought to occur after the development of antibodies to the human immunodeficiency virus. Clients so diagnosed are considered at greater risk for developing fungal infections commonly caused by *Candida albicans*, which may affect the skin, nails, mouth, oesophagus, lower gastrointestinal tract, genitalia and rectum (Gallis et al. 1990).

Candida oesophagitis is diagnostic of AIDS and involves erythematous lesions, pseudomembraneous areas and/or ulcerations of the oesophagus. It can cause severe problems such as difficulty and/or painful swallowing, retrosternal pain, and nausea and vomiting. Initial treatment is with systemic oral or topical medications. Intravenous therapy may be useful if infection becomes clinically unresponsive. Lifelong administration may be required.

Reports suggest therapy failure, incomplete response and decreasing susceptibility to azole medications such as ketoconazole, fluconazole and itraconazole (Diamond 1991). Liposomal amphotericin remains the standard i.v. treatment for systemic or resistant mycoses (Gallis et al. 1990). Inpatient experience of this drug's known toxicity may act as a limiting factor against initiating home-based therapy.

The politics of health resources

Case study 4.1 describes the benefits of portable elastomeric technology for a client using the Intermate system. Figure 4.1 illustrates the potential of this system for self-care. Its consumer friendliness is well documented (Wonke and Fielding 1992, Duncan-Skingle and Bramwell 1993, Steel et al. 1995). Elastomeric infusion technology does not rely on gravity feed or electronically programmed delivery systems. The drug is aseptically prepared and presented in a ready-to-use form (compounded) within an elastomeric balloon reservoir. The Intermate works through positive pressure being exerted as the balloon deflates.

This pushes the drug-in-solution through a flow restrictor and combines with the pressure of the balloon to dictate the infusion flow rate. The Intermate is primed like any other i.v. giving set, and the infusion pack is then connected to the client's venous access device.

Unlike gravity-feed or electronically programmed delivery systems, which limit both activities and environments, such technology allows a client to undertake a fuller range of activities while receiving their medication: they are not confined to one environment, and retain more control over the drug administration procedure. The Intermate is lightweight and does not require programming. Research shows its suitability for home use (Wonke and Fielding 1992). It eliminates the anxiety of pump alarms and maximizes a client's independence. Figure 4.2 shows the variety of Intermates and the range of flow rates available.

There are difficulties with prescribing this technology for NHS clients. Steel et al. (1995) describe a community-based i.v. service using elastomeric infusions for clients with AIDS: they focus on cost as an important consideration in service provision, and so caution the use of this technology, talking about 'responsible' and 'appropriate' use because this technology is 'very expensive' (Steel et al. 1995, p. 328). This professional discourse conveys important attitudes towards self-care and client-administered therapy. Often professional paternalism can influence perceptions about 'expensive' or 'appropriate' treatment modalities. This results in professional attitudes determining the parameters for client choice and hence which actual treatments are offered. Official guidance on high-tech home therapies speaks about choice (Department of Health 1995a). The consumer may experience difficulty in gaining access to information and in exercising choice over the options that are available. In the UK issues over funding and professional attitudes to self-care may negatively affect access to such consumer-friendly technology.

More discussion is needed about the regional variations in access to innovative health technology. Hutton (1995) describes the NHS as always being free at the point of use for those in need. The development of the NHS Trusts has been guided by the ethos of market economics.

There thus has been a danger that differences may emerge in the treatment of clients across regions. The character of health-care provision has had the potential of becoming a lottery, dependent upon differing purchasing policies in different districts (Hutton 1997). This would negatively affect people's ability to access so-called high-tech resources. However, modernization of the NHS has moved the emphasis away from the internal market. As the new Primary Care Trusts develop, one can only speculate about the effects on community health service provision in this area. In the short term some innovative treatment modalities, such as elastomeric technology, may appear expensive. Hutton discusses how 'privatization of the public domain' produces perverse attitudes and quick-fix solutions (Hutton 1995, p. 218). By taking a longer perspective and factoring in significant measurable parameters (self-care efficacy, reduced number of hospital admissions, lack of nosocomial infections), 'expensive' options may emerge as being the most cost-effective.

Reflection point 4.5

◆ In your experience is a limit ever applied on grounds of cost to the therapies needed by clients?

◆ How do you think the cost of treatment influences clinical decisions?

Learning activity 4.1

A client you are visiting is refused high-cost treatment by her GP. She approaches you for help and advice to seek an alternative to her current GP (i.e. reregistration). What would your response be? What sources of information and advice are available in the community to enable a person to reregister?

HEALTH AND THE LOCAL AUTHORITY

'. . . if the major determinants of ill health are rooted in wider social and economic relationships **practice has to be explicitly geared to changing those relationships . . .'**
(Moran 1986, p. 124. Emphasis added)

Before 1974, health education units were under local authority management but after this time became the responsibility of the health sector (Moran 1986), which holds technocratic and professional values in greater esteem than 'political' values. Initiatives from the health sector tend to individualize risk-taking and personal behaviours. In contrast, local authority health initiatives are couched in grass-roots or corporate terms (Department of Health 1993). Moran (1986) discusses the methods whereby local authorities may 'reinvent' public health (often featured in policy guidance on HIV/AIDS). These include consolidating links with local communities, reviewing the health implications of council activities, funding local groups working on health-related issues, and making specialist skills accessible (Moran 1986).

Radical initiatives that alter power relationships in health care or challenge health-damaging relationships do not usually come from within the mainstream, as shown by the example of the women's health movement (Grace 1991). Factors influencing the origin of such innovation are the predominance of medicine, which silences criticism of its practice, and the health sector's professional embargo against political activity.

The needs of young gay, bisexual and lesbian people

Research has linked negative societal attitudes about sexuality and ill health (Samaritans 1996, Gray 1997). Homophobia is defined as an intense fear or hatred of gay sexuality, and includes 'levels of prejudice, discrimination or aggression' (Besner and Spungin 1995). The different kinds of homophobia are: personal (believing in the 'wrongness'

Table 4.1 Range of harassments faced by young lesbians and gay men (*n* = 140) (Rivers 1996)

Name calling	80%
Peer and teacher ridicule	69%
Rumour mongering	55%
Physical attack	59%
Regular teasing	49%
Frightening behaviour	45%
Property theft	45%
Verbal isolation	23%
Sexual assault	8%

of gays or lesbians), interpersonal (fear or hatred of those perceived as gay or lesbian) and institutional (ways in which institutions discriminate against gays or lesbians). Greene and Herek (1994) also discuss internalized homophobia, thought to be common among many gay men and lesbians, causing self-inflicted psychological distress as well as parasuicide and suicide.

Rivers (1996) researched the problem of homophobic abuse at school and its long-term effects upon the mental health and the social development of lesbians and gay men. The research findings in Table 4.1 show that young gay men and lesbians become targets for bullying at school: in over 140 cases lesbians and gay men reported severe forms of regular daily harassment. As many as 40% of the sample reported one or more suicide attempts while coping with the daily and the long-term effects of bullying (Rivers 1996).

The experience of bullying has been so damaging for many young gay men and lesbians that they seek counselling and psychiatric support (Stonewall 1994, Rivers 1996, Golding 1997). This research underlines their need for support and protection, and further identifies a need for practical interventions that support young people 'as they come to terms with their sexuality' (Rivers 1996, p. 19) and illustrates how negative societal attitudes act as determinants of ill health that should be addressed by health promoters.

The 'Staying Out' Project (SOP)

The Staying Out Project seeks to positively affect the sexual health and wellbeing of young gay men

Table 4.2 Staying Out Project. Services for young people

Weekday	Provision
MONDAY	SUPPORT, INFORMATION, ADVICE & COUNSELLING
Information/counselling Support 'Forbidden fruit'. Gay and bisexual group	By appointment or drop-in to explore issues/problems: safer sex, relationships, health, homelessness, family and social services, education, employment and prostitution
TUESDAY	SEXUAL HEALTH, HEALTH & WELLBEING
Information/counselling Support Sexual health Helpline* Drop-in (wellbeing) Homework drop-in 'Staying Out'. Lesbian, bisexual, gay group	In response to needs of young people to address deficits in school sex education. Space to talk through safer sex information and explore related issues and pressures: poverty, homelessness and self-esteem
WEDNESDAY	HOMEWORK SUPPORT & DROP-IN
Information/counselling Support Homework drop-in Creative arts workshops: drama photography painting	Space for members to come in from school to do work in relaxed, supportive environment with staff, free of bullying and homophobia
THURSDAY Information/counselling Support Homework drop-in 'Diaspora' people of colour	GROUPS Group-led specific activities: quizzes, debates, discussions, photography, video-making, music and trips
FRIDAY Information/counselling Support Homework drop-in 'Divas'. Women's group Brook	CREATIVE ARTS Workshops for sexual health and wellbeing and advertising imagery; expressive learning experience; peer education programme from London

*Joint appointment funded by East London and The City Health Authority and jointly managed by Hackney Council and City and

and lesbians who form its membership. This project is managed by Hackney Council's Youth

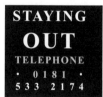

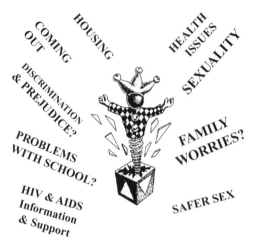

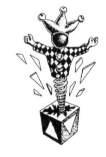

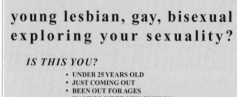

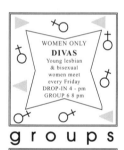

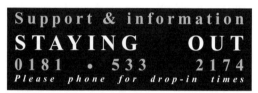

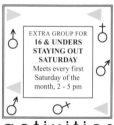

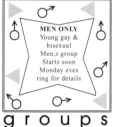

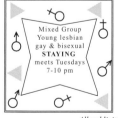

Fig. 4.4 Staying Out Project. Flyer for members. (Reproduced courtesy of London Borough of Hackney.)

Service and forms part of the borough's Directorate of Education, Learning and Leisure Services. Table 4.2 describes the services available for young people.

SOP emphasizes the development of the 'whole' person, as seen by the members' flyer in Figure 4.4. The range and nature of member-led activities are significant: they foster an ethos of self-help and individual responsibility. For example, many studies suggest that the academic underachievement shown by some gay men and lesbians is linked to school-based harassment (Sears 1991, Telljohn and Price 1993, Stonewall 1994, Rivers 1996). A homework support session is therefore provided at the Project.

SOP is staffed by full- and part-time qualified youth workers. The skills needed for such work are those of counselling about homophobic oppression and self-harm, HIV prevention and health promotion. The training and professional supervision of staff address these issues. The Project also acts as a focus for local activity and developments, which include peer education and support undertaken by London Brook through funding from the Council's Environmental Services Department.

The Project has potential for partnership working with the health sector. Research shows a difference between professional working methodologies: for example, Few et al. (1996) investigated school nurses' sex education practice and found problems in the methodology commonly used in schools. There was a mismatch between the teaching of safer sex and the teaching of practical communication and negotiation skills. It is noteworthy that SOP members specifically requested such input from within this Project.

SOP has developed sex education methodologies that address the needs of gay men and lesbians. Although the Project may be less formal an environment than the school classroom, it is no less rigorous or demanding. The methodology comes from a peer-led and facilitative approach to sex education which the members experience as less top-down. In accordance with the Youth Service curriculum the environment is participative and facilitative. Furthermore, this methodology combines expertise from local health professionals such as GUM nurses, health advisers and educators experienced in working with young people. The latter are seen as significant for effecting school-based sex education (BMA Foundation For AIDS 1997).

The Project represents an opportunity for school nurses to develop their sex education methodologies, based upon equal partnership, mutual trust and total confidentiality with members. Research cites the latter as problematic for school nurses and other nursing disciplines and professionals (James et al. 1994, Few et al. 1996).

SOP focuses on the local provision of health promotion and HIV prevention for gay men. It is informed by government policy guidance and the need for effective targeting of resources (King 1993, Department of Health 1995b). There is added value in making such support available within the pro-health values of the Youth Service. Research clearly indicates that younger gay men's sexual risk behaviour appears to conform far more to safer-sex guidelines than that of other risk groups (Coxon 1996). It is unrealistic to expect younger gay men to be affected by sexual health education and community responses from the past, and so this Project provides young gay men with ongoing and targeted advice about safer sex and relationships.

Much debate was generated by Clause 2A in Section 28 of the Local Government Act 1986, which attempted to ban the 'promotion' of homosexuality as 'pretended family relationships'. The Act was in response to government perceptions of poor school management. Norrie (1988) states that the Act is legally meaningless; Weeks et al. (1996) describe its negative effect on educational initiatives. However, its practical effect may be rhetorically prohibitive (Thomson 1996, p. 100). It created a climate of self-censorship that negatively affected school sex education.

Local authorities can legally target resources at areas of perceived need. Over the last 10 years consistent legal advice indicates that this Act cannot prevent service developments that address gay and lesbian needs. The Department of the Environment supports the rationale for providing positive environments for gay, bisexual and lesbian people by focusing on the 'needs of homo-sexuals' (Department of Environment 1988). Mental health services such as MIND have encouraged the development of self-help and peer methodologies, which are better able to provide appropriate and confidential access to health and social care professionals without stigmatizing or pathologizing one's sexuality.

SOP operates on a basis of absolute confidentiality, but makes an exception in any case of abuse, or suspected abuse, of underage members, who are referred to senior management in the Youth and Social Services. Young people are apprised of this policy so as to inform their choice of counselling. Where young people decide to tell their parents about their attendance at the Project, itself a confidence, there exists a productive relationship with parents.

Local authority initiatives, such as the *Staying Out Project*, provide an important focus using positive empowerment and choice that enhance the sexual health and wellbeing of young lesbian, gay and bisexual people. As such, the Project represents an example of local authorities reinventing public health by advancing fundamental or so-called 'radical' health initiatives in practice (Moran 1986).

 Learning activity 4.2

Highlight the professional issues faced by registered nurses working within a project such as 'Staying Out'. Consider how a nurse would practise within this context. Write a job/person specification and advertisement for a school nurse to be employed in the Staying Out Project by the local authority.

 Reflection point 4.6

In what other ways do you think local authorities could play a significant role to positively influence people's health?

CONCLUSION

This chapter has discussed multidisciplinary and multiagency approaches in the field of sexual health. There are implications for the nature of professional collaboration and for awareness of the social determinants of ill health. First, the practice discussed requires significant collaboration between professionals across differing sectors. Collaboration is an essential characteristic of modern-day practitioners.

Secondly, the potential for professional action or agency of the in-between position of the nurse was identified. This professional context may foster client empowerment and increase capacity for decision-making. Such agency is facilitated through professional insight and educational development. Therefore, in order to acquire such essential qualities, practitioners must first enable themselves by investing in approaches such as lifelong learning.

Thirdly, awareness of sexual health has created new practice settings as the promotion of sexual wellbeing moves away from specialist centres and towards the community health and local authority settings. Further opportunities for partnerships arise, for example with the neighbourhood infrastructure of general practice clinics, schools, youth services and the voluntary sector. Practitioners can use this generic infrastructure for sexual health promotion. It is well positioned to influence both behavioural and attitudinal determinants of ill health.

Finally, purchasing for health and social care services may be used to innovate practice. It was described how policy guidance fostered a synergy between sectors. Professionals are now asked to work in flexible, non-hierarchical relationships based on a positive regard for each other's expertise. Nursing has encouraged such flexibility through policy guidance, which frames responsibility to clients within standards of professional practice (UKCC 1992a,b). The result should be a greater sense of responsibility, accountability and professional identity. In the longer term, full responsibility for professional development, or lifelong learning as opposed to in-service training, will devolve to individual practitioners. If practice can be developed in the light of such implications, it may afford a better opportunity to address the social determinants of ill health and to promote the wellbeing of individuals, families and communities.

ANNOTATED FURTHER READING

This list relates directly to the themes and issues discussed under each subheading in the chapter. A short description is given including any specific characteristics.

Professional practice

Davies C 1995 Gender and the professional predicament in nursing. Open University Press, Milton Keynes

Davies examines gendered understanding of nursing practice. Reference is to the health-care market, education reform and professionalism. The author draws on her experience as policy officer for 1980s British nurse education. Includes a literature review of gender and nursing.

Professional collaboration

Beattie J et al. 1996 The politics of collaboration as viewed through the lens of a collaborative nursing research project. Journal of Advanced Nursing 24: 682–687

The authors analyse the meaning and politics of collaboration. A theoretical framework is used which can be useful for analysing collaboration in other settings.

Home and community care

Baldwin S 1993 The myth of community care. An alternative neighbourhood model of care. Chapman & Hall, London

Baldwin deconstructs the model of community care, preferring the less-valued model of neighbourhood care. The history of British community care is described before and up to 1980s restructuring of the British welfare state.

Holmes S 1995 Ideology underpinning the issue of community care. British Journal of Therapy and Rehabilitation 2(5): 246–250

Holmes reviews the change in British community care and its political ideology. Influences reviewed are managerialism, deprofessionalization, consumerism and privatization. Points relevant to practice are summarized.

The health needs of gay, bisexual and lesbian people

Thinking it through. A new approach to sex, relationships and HIV for gay men, 2nd edn: Camden and Islington Health Promotion Unit, London. Available from Camden and Islington, 4 St Pancras Way, London NW1 0PE. Tel: 020 7530 3912, or Resource Sales: 020 7530 3922

A booklet for use as an adjunct to advising gay men about HIV antibody tests, safer sex and relationships. Includes a short list of HIV services in the British Isles and abroad.

MIND file Policy 1. MIND's policy on lesbians, gay men, bisexual women and mental health. MIND, London. Available from Mind Publications, 15–19 Broadway, London E15 4BQ. Tel: 020 8519 2122

A short policy document for mental health professionals working with lesbian, gay and bisexual people that focuses on mental ill health caused by discrimination. Sections include legislation and working in healthy alliances.

REFERENCES

Allen I 1991 Family planning and pregnancy counselling projects for young people. Policy Studies Institute, London

Allen I, Hogg D 1993 Work roles and responsibilities in genitourinary medicine clinics. Policy Studies Institute, London

Aggleton P, Tyrer P 1994 Sexual health. In: Aggleton P, Rivers, K, Warwick I, Whitty G Learning about AIDS. Scientific and social issues, 2nd edn. Churchill Livingstone, London

Benner J, Wrubel J 1989 The primacy of caring. Stress and coping in health and illness. Addison-Wesley, Menlo Park, CA

Benner P 1984 From novice to expert: excellence and power in clinical nursing practice. Addison-Wesley, Menlo Park, CA

Bennet C 1992 HIV/AIDS: some organizational and managerial issues. Journal of Management in Medicine 6(4): 36–40

Bennett L, May C, Wolfson D J 1994 Sharing care between hospital and community: a critical review of developments in the UK. Health and Social Care 2: 105–112

Berridge V 1995 AIDS in the UK. The making of policy, 1981–1994. Oxford University Press, Oxford

Besner H J, Spungin C J 1995 Gay and lesbian students. Understanding their needs. Taylor & Francis, London

Bishop A, Scudder J 1990 The practical, moral and personal sense of nursing. A phenomenological philosophy of practice. State University of New York Press, Albany, New York

Braye S, Preston-Shoot M 1995 Empowering practice in social care. Open University Press, Milton Keynes

British Medical Association Foundation For AIDS 1997 Using effectiveness to guide the development of school sex education. British Medical Association Foundation For AIDS, London

Chavenet P, Garry I, Charlier N et al. 1992 Trial of glucose versus fat emulsion in preparation for amphotericin for use in HIV infected patients with candidiasis. British Medical Journal 305: 921–925

Chomsky N 1996 Powers and prospects. Reflections on human nature and the social order. Pluto Press, London

Corbett K, Meehan L, Sackey V 1993 A strategy to enhance skills: developing intravenous therapy skills for community nursing. Professional Nurse 9(1): 60–63

Corbett K 1994 Developing reflective practice through focus group methodology within the outpatient sexual health clinic. Unpublished paper given to 'Lecturer practitioners – the vital link'. Foundation of Nursing Studies and The Nightingale Institute, King's College, London, 21 May, 1994

Corbett K 1997 Community HIV/AIDS services and 'Health of the Nation': an analysis of the infrastructure promoting healthy alliances across health and social care sectors. In: Bright J (ed.) Health of the Nation: health promotion in clinical practice. Baillière Tindall, London, Chapter 4

Coxon A 1996 Between the sheets. Sexual diaries and gay men's sex in the era of AIDS. Cassell, London

DataPharm 1991 APBI Data Sheet Compendium 1991–1992. Associated British Pharmaceutical Industry, London

Department of the Environment 1988 Local Government Act 1988. Circular 12/88. Cardiff: Department of the Environment, Welsh Office. In: Colvin M, Hawksley J 1989 Section 28. A practical guide to the law and its implications. National Council for Civil Liberties (Liberty), London

Department of Health 1993 Health of the Nation. Key area handbook. HIV/AIDS and sexual health. Department of Health, London

Department of Health 1994 Implementing Caring for people. Community care for people with HIV and AIDS. Heywood, Lancashire, Department of Health

Department of Health 1995a Purchasing high-technology health care for patients at home. Department of Health NHS Management Executive EL(5)5. Department of Health, London

Department of Health 1995b HIV and AIDS health promotion. An evolving strategy. UK Departments of Health, London

Diamond R 1991 The growing problem of mycoses in patients infected with the human immunodeficiency virus. Review of Infectious Diseases 13: 480–486

Duncan-Skingle F, Bramwell E 1993 Home help. Nursing Times 88(51): 34–35

Ekeid R 1992 Opening statements. In: Curtis H (ed) Promoting sexual health. Health Education Authority, London

Engelhardt H 1985 Physicians, patients and health care institutions – and the people in between: nurses. In: Bishop A, Scudder J (eds) Caring, curing, coping: nurse, physician and patient relationships. University of Alabama Press, Alabama

English National Board 1994a Caring for people with sexually transmitted diseases, including HIV disease. English National Board For Nursing Midwifery and Health Visiting, London

English National Board 1994b Creating lifelong learners. Partnerships for care. English National Board For Nursing Midwifery and Health Visiting, London

English National Board 1995 Creating lifelong learners. Partnerships for care. Guidelines for programmes leading to qualification of specialist practitioner. English National Board For Nursing Midwifery and Health Visiting, London

Faugier J, Hicken I (eds) 1995 HIV/AIDS: the nursing response. Chapman & Hall, London

Few C 1997 The politics of sex research and constructions of female sexuality: what relevance to sexual health work with young women? Journal of Advanced Nursing 25: 615–625

Few C, Hicken I, Butterworth T 1996 Partnerships in sexual health and sex education. School of Nursing, Midwifery and Health Visiting, University of Manchester, Manchester

Foucault M 1963 The birth of the clinic. Routledge, London

Gallis H, Drew R, Pickard W 1990 Amphotericin B: 30 years of clinical experience. Review of Infectious Diseases 12: 308–328

Gibson C 1991 A concept analysis of empowerment. Journal of Advanced Nursing 16: 354–361

Giddens A 1991 Modernity and self-identity. Polity Press, Cambridge

Golding J 1997 Without prejudice. MIND lesbian, gay and bisexual mental health awareness research. MIND, London

Grace V M 1991 The marketing of empowerment and the construction of the health consumer: a critique of health promotion. International Journal of Health Services 21(2): 329–343

Gray B 1989 Collaboration. Jossey Bass, London

Gray P 1997 Young male and suicidal. Healthlines December 1996/January 1997

Greene B, Herek GM (eds) 1994 Lesbian and gay psychology. Theory, research and clinical applications. Psychological perspectives on lesbian and gay issues. Vol. 1. Sage, London

Harris R, Ferguson H, Brooks V 1996 Imaginative solutions: a nursing-led unit's story. Nursing Development News 16 September, 6–7

Haydock A 1992 QALYs – a threat to our quality of life? Journal of Applied Philosophy 9 (2): 183–188

Hill J 1997 Patient satisfaction in a nurse-led rheumatology clinic. Journal of Advanced Nursing 25: 347–354

Hutton W 1995 The state we're in. Vintage Books, London

Hutton W 1997 The state to come. Vintage Books, London

Ingram-Fogel C I 1990 Sexual health promotion. WB Saunders, Philadelphia

Irwin R 1997 Sexual health promotion in nursing. Journal of Advanced Nursing 25: 170–177

James T, Harding I, Corbett K 1994 Biased care? Nursing Times 90(51): 28–30

Jessop L 1988 Lessons for the teenage parent. Health Service Journal 98(5104): 646–647

King E 1993 Safety in numbers. Safer sex and gay men. Cassell, London

Livingston J, Parker N, Corbett K 1993 Homecare for intravenous treatment of HIV-related candidiasis. At Home. The Newsletter for Homecare Therapy Initiatives 5: 6–7

Macleod Clark J 1993 From sick nursing to health nursing: evolution or revolution? In: Wilson-Barnett J, Macleod Clark J (eds) Research in health promotion and nursing. Macmillan, London: pp 256–270

Marks L 1991 Home and hospital care: redrawing the boundaries. King's Fund, London

McDonnell S 1994 In defence of QALYs. Journal of Applied Philosophy 11(1): 89–97

Moran G 1986 Radical health promotion: the role of local authorities. In: Rodmell S, Watt A (eds) The politics of health education. Routledge, London, pp 121–138

Mullen C 1995 Delivering health care in a nurse led practice development unit. NHS Executive Value For Money Update 14: 3

Norrie K 1988 Symbolic and meaningless legislation. Journal of the Law Society of Scotland, September, 310–331

Palmer A, Burns S, Bulman C 1994 The reflective practitioner. The growth of the professional practitioner. Blackwell Science, Oxford

Pearson A (ed) (1988) Primary nursing. Nursing in the Burford and Oxford Nursing Development Units. Chapman & Hall, London

Rivers I 1996 Young, gay and bullied. Young People Now, January, 18–19

Salvage J 1990 The theory and practice of new nursing. Nursing Times 86(4): 42–45

Samaritans 1996 Key facts report on young people and suicide. The Samaritans, London

Schon D 1983 The reflective practitioner. HarperCollins, San Francisco

Scott C 1994 The care and treatment of people with HIV disease and AIDS: a nursing perspective. Daphne Heald Research Unit, Royal College of Nursing, London

Sears J 1991 Educators, homosexuality and homosexual students: are personal feelings related to professional beliefs? Journal of Homosexuality 22: 29–79

Seedhouse D 1993 Fortress NHS: John Wiley, London

Steel S, Sinclair L, Timbrell H 1995 A home infusion service from community pharmacies. Pharmaceutical Journal 254: 327–328

Stonewall Lobby Group 1994 Arrested development?: Stonewall survey on the age of consent and sex education. Stonewall Lobby Group, London

Telljohn S K, Price J H 1993 A qualitative examination of adolescent homosexuals' life experiences: ramifications for secondary school personnel. Journal of Homosexuality 26: 41–56

Thomson R 1996 Sex education and the law: working towards good practice. In: Harris N (ed) Children, sex education and the law. National Children's Bureau, London, pp 99–112

United Kingdom Central Council 1992a Code of professional conduct. United Kingdom Central Council for Nursing, Health Visiting and Midwifery, London

United Kingdom Central Council 1992b Scope of professional practice. United Kingdom Central Council for Nursing, Health Visiting and Midwifery, London

Vaughan B 1990 Knowing that and knowing how: the role of the lecturer practitioner. In: Kershaw B, Salvage J (eds) Models for nursing 2. Scutari Press, London, pp 103–113

Walby S, Greenwell J, Mackay L, Soothill K 1994 Medicine and nursing. Professions in a changing health service. Sage, London

Weeks J 1995 Invented moralities. Sexual values in an age of uncertainty. Polity Press, Cambridge.

Weeks J, Donovan C, Heaphy B 1996 Families of choice: patterns of non-heterosexual relationships. A literature review. No 2. Social Science Research Papers. South Bank University, London

Williams S (ed) 1987 Caring for people with AIDS in the community. A report of a conference held at the Institute of Education University of London on 25 March 1987. King Edward's Hospital Fund for London: Department of Health and Social Security

Wonke B, Fielding D 1992 Novel delivery system for continuous desferrioxamine infusion in iron overloaded patients. Lancet 882(340): 790–791

World Health Organization 1975 Education and treatment in human sexuality: the training of health professionals. Technical Report Series No. 572. WHO, Geneva

Sexual health for sale

5

John Hooker   Barbara Wallace

'You can't put a price tag on love, but you can on all its accessories.'   (Melanie Clark)

KEY ISSUES/CONCEPTS

- ◆ The context of sexual health purchasing
- ◆ Strategy development, needs assessment and priority setting
- ◆ Strategic vision
- ◆ Funding arrangements
- ◆ Clinical effectiveness
- ◆ Effective purchasing
- ◆ The nurse's role and 'managing up'

OVERVIEW

Chapter 5, *Sexual health for sale*, covers the epidemiological context within which the purchasing of sexual health services is carried out. It provides broad definitions of purchasing and examines the way in which purchasers develop strategies, set priorities and carry out needs assessment. It looks at the processes for the development of funding and how clinical effectiveness informs the whole process. It also gives models of effective purchasing, and explores the role of the nurse in developing services, along with the concept of 'managing up'.

INTRODUCTION

The purchasing of health services is a concept which has only been in use since the health service reforms of the 1990s. Along with the developments in purchasing and commissioning comes a new range of terminology and processes. With the future direction marked out since the change of government in 1997, some definitions are needed. These are the main definitions which will be used in this chapter:

- ◆ **Purchasing** – the activity involving a health agency, e.g. health authority contracting with a service provider for an agreed service defined in terms of quantity, quality or cost. Purchasing is a systematic process identified in Box 5.1.

Box 5.1 Health purchasing as a systematic process (analogous with the nursing process)	
Subjective and objective	Givens
	Prioritization
	Needs assessment
	Clinical effectiveness
Assessment	Consultation
Planning	Strategy
Implementation	Service specification
	Contract/service-level agreement
Evaluation and re-evaluation	Contract monitoring
	Service reviews
	User feedback
	Research/formal evaluation
	Financial review

Box 5.2 Comparison between the 'old' and the 'new' NHS		
	The reformed NHS 1991–98	The new NHS 1999+
Process	Purchasing	Commissioning
Vehicle	Contracts	Service-level agreements
Duration	1 year	3 years+
Purchaser(s)	HAs/GPFHs	PCGs/HAs
Purchaser/ provider relationship	Separation	Cooperation

◆ **Commissioning** – compared to purchasing, a more active development of a service, whether existing or new, seeking out the best provider for it and involving more agencies, including providers, in the process

◆ **Contract** – the agreement that specifies the service to be provided in terms as above (see purchasing), and which may also include a service specification

◆ **Service agreement** – since the government decided that contracts were not legal agreements, they should perhaps more accurately be described as service agreements. In future, **service-level agreements** will replace contracts and will be of longer duration (several years instead of the yearly contract) and include explicit quality standards and indicators

◆ **Service specification** – a detailed breakdown of the service into measurable elements which may well include quality indicators

◆ **Purchasing strategy** – a statement of intent on the part of the purchasing authority which should include the values underpinning the strategy, key goals and expected outcomes

◆ **Mission statement** – a statement of purpose which communicates who the organization is, what its boundaries are, what its business is, and how that business will be carried out. It may also contain some of the values of the organization, e.g. the public service ethos

◆ **Contract monitoring** – any activity, mainly on the part of the purchaser, to oversee how the service

is matching up to the contract. The provider may also cooperate in this process, and this is likely to be a key element in the more collaborative health service of the future

◆ **Consortium contracts** – low-volume contracts, such as for HIV treatment and care in low-prevalence areas, and GUM services in large cities that draw clients from a large hinterland, are often purchased by a group of health authorities with one of them acting as **lead purchaser**

◆ **Health improvement programmes** – local strategy for improving health and health care. Have become a statutory responsibility of health authorities, with a duty of partnership of all NHS bodies. Local authorities are responsible for promoting the economic, social and environmental wellbeing of the area.

Box 5.2 highlights the comparison between the 'old' and the 'new' NHS.

GP fundholding is no longer an issue, having been abolished in 1999 (DoH 1997). Nevertheless, GPs continue to have a major influence on commissioning through Primary Care Groups (PCGs) as well as being providers of some sexual health services, e.g. family planning.

There is no such thing as purchasing in its purest sense in the NHS. The market is managed to favour NHS providers and ensure their survival, and there are many other processes at work and influences on the purchasing decision.

With hindsight, the reforms of the 1990s can be seen as an attempt to bring rigour and discipline to the business of managing developing (and in some areas diminishing) health service activity. There is no doubt that such rigour will continue.

'Purchasing is about change. It is ludicrous to think that the NHS should be doing today exactly what it was doing in 1948, or that it should be doing in another 45 years exactly what it is doing today. As people's needs change, so must their health service.'
(NHSME 1993a)

SEXUAL HEALTH IN CONTEXT

Sexual health is a major concern of international organizations such as the World Health

Organization (WHO). The Family and Reproductive Health Division of WHO brings together programmes that promote the overall health and development of families, children, adolescents and women. The aim of this more integrated approach is to link health and human development with people's needs for reproductive health at key stages in their lives.

WHO defines reproductive health as follows: **Reproductive health** is a state of complete physical, mental and social wellbeing and not merely the absence of disease or infirmity, in all matters relating to the reproductive system and to its functions and processes. **Reproductive health** therefore implies that people are able to have a satisfying and safe sex life and that they have the capability to reproduce and the freedom to decide if, when and how often to do so. Implicit in this last condition is the right of men and women to be informed and to have access to safe, effective, affordable and acceptable methods of family planning of their choice, as well as other methods of their choice for regulation of fertility which are not against the law, and the right of access to appropriate healthcare services that will enable women to go safely through pregnancy and childbirth and provide couples with the best chance of having a healthy infant. In line with the above definition of reproductive health, reproductive health care is defined as the constellation of methods, techniques and services that contribute to reproductive health and wellbeing by preventing and solving reproductive health problems. It also includes sexual health, the purpose of which is the enhancement of life and personal relationships, and not merely counselling and care related to reproduction and sexually transmitted diseases. (WHO Family and Reproductive Health 96.1).

Reproductive health has been given priority by the WHO because it:

◆ addresses major reproductive health problems
◆ responds to people's needs
◆ has a significant impact on health status
◆ addresses prevention as well as cure
◆ is cost-effective
◆ aims to improve equity, particularly gender equity.

Box 5.3 Reproductive ill health in the world	
Couples with unmet family planning needs	120 million
Infertile couples	60–80 million
Maternal deaths per year	585 000
Cases of severe maternal morbidity per year	20 million
Perinatal maternal deaths per year	7.2 million
Unsafe abortions per year	20 million
Adults living with HIV/AIDS	20.1 million
New cases of HIV infection per year	2.75 million
Cases of curable sexually transmitted diseases per year	333 million
Women living with invasive cervical cancer	2 million
New cases of cervical cancer per year	450 000
Women with female genital mutilation	85–110 million

Although the global AIDS pandemic has received the most attention from the international press in recent years, HIV is only one of the problems affecting reproductive health. Some of the major problems are listed in Box 5.3.

Reflection point 5.1

How do the problems listed in Box 5.3 relate to problems in your clinical area? Consider the ways in which the local picture relates to the global picture. What does this tell you about local priorities?

The agenda for sexual health in Britain has been shaped by the Health of the Nation (the health strategy for England) (DoH 1992). The Health of the Nation targets for sexual health were:

◆ to reduce the incidence of gonorrhoea among men and women aged 15–64 by at least

Learning activity 5.1

The following organizations all provide differing types of public information related to sexual health:

◆ Health authority

◆ General practitioners

◆ NHS Trusts

◆ NHSE regional offices

◆ Voluntary organizations

◆ Education authorities.

Knowing how to access this information is vital for planning, implementing or evaluating local services.

Find out the addresses of the above organizations: look in telephone directories, libraries, health centres, citizens' advice bureaux, local press for details. Once you have found them, try to determine what sources of information they have and how this might help service planning or delivery.

How is this information presented to the public? Do they provide summaries of reports and documents? Do they have newsletters? Do they use patient panels to gather information?

How easy is it to access the material, and how 'user friendly' is it?

Feedback on Learning activity 5.1

Did you find any of the following information?

The local health authority purchaser will have documents and reports relevant to sexual health. These may include:

◆ the most recent health strategy

◆ annual reports

◆ report of the Director of Public Health

◆ Health of the Nation updates

◆ needs assessment or survey work

◆ service specifications and contracting documentation.

The local Trusts will have documents and reports relevant to sexual health. These may include:

◆ annual reports

◆ annual business plans

◆ service descriptions and contracting documentation

◆ statistics provided to the Department of Health

◆ surveys of consumer satisfaction

◆ service monitoring data.

Larger local GPs or PCGs will have documents and reports relevant to sexual health. These may include:

◆ practice profiles

◆ practice charters or patient information leaflets

◆ specific information (e.g. letters inviting adolescents for a health check).

See if you can find out about any major voluntary organizations with a sexual health remit and ask them for a leaflet on their services.

Finally, ask your local education authority for any policy documents or other information laying out their position on sex education.

This information should help you to build a comprehensive picture of sources of sexual health information in your area, and will be useful for Learning activity 5.2.

20% by 1995 (from 61 new cases per 100 000 population in 1990 to no more than 49 new cases per 100 000)

◆ to reduce the rate of conceptions among the under-16s by at least 50% by the year 2000 (from 9.5 per 1000 girls aged 13–15 in 1989 to no more than 4.8 nationally).

The Health of the Nation target for cervical cancer was to reduce the incidence of invasive cervical cancer by at least 20% by the year 2000. There were also targets for reducing the sharing of equipment used by injecting drug abusers, to reduce HIV transmission through needle sharing. The Health of the Nation strategy gave a tremendous impetus to improving sexual health programmes, particularly those aimed at teenagers. Although it contained no specific targets for sexual health, the Green Paper 'Our Healthier Nation' (DoH 1998a) placed greater emphasis on addressing the well known links between poverty, unemployment, lack of educational attainment and early childbearing. The sexual health agenda for purchasers has also been shaped by the report by the Social Exclusion Unit (1999) which heralds a major drive to reduce the socially disadvantaging effects of teenage pregnancy through the goals of:

◆ halving the rate of conceptions in under-18s by 2010

◆ getting more teenage parents into education, training or employment.

Teenage pregnancy was similarly emphasized in the White Paper 'Saving Lives: Our Healthier Nation' (DoH 1999) as a major area for action. The increase in sexually transmitted infections among teenagers in the 1990s was also highlighted and chlamydia, with a 45% increase among 16–19-year-olds, targeted for a response.

The impact of other policies and legal landmark decisions has been more mixed. For example, the Gillick judgement raised major concerns among health professionals and adolescents themselves about the legal aspects of prescribing contraception to young people under 16 without their parents' knowledge or consent. The British Medical Association has subsequently made the position much clearer and reassured health professionals in their document *Confidentiality and people under 16* (BMA 1993). This document stated that health professionals owe as great a duty of confidentiality to a person under 16 as to any other person. It also said that any competent young person can seek medical advice and give consent to medical treatments independently, regardless of age. A doctor would be justified in prescribing contraceptives to a girl under 16 without parental consent, provided:

◆ the doctor cannot persuade her to inform her parents or allow him to do so

◆ she is likely to begin or continue having sexual intercourse

◆ if she does not use contraceptives, her physical and/or mental health is likely to suffer

◆ she understands the advice

◆ her best interests indicate that she should receive advice and treatment without parental consent.

Case study 5.1: Tackling fears about confidentiality

Dr McAndrew, a GP in a busy inner-city practice, noticed that very few of her consultations were with younger teenagers. The few adolescents who did visit the surgery asked her about skin problems, weight, minor illnesses and other concerns, but almost never raised the question of contraceptives. This began to worry Dr McAndrew when she got into a conversation with the nurse who worked at a nearby comprehensive school and was told that the school had had nine pregnancies to girls under 16 in the past year. The GP and her practice nurse reviewed recent research about adolescent sexual behaviour and found that almost 75% of 16-year-olds feared that their GP would not preserve confidentiality if asked for contraception.

Dr McAndrew discussed the problem with her partners and the nursing team, and they agreed to reserve an evening each week for young clients. The whole team underwent a training day with a local youth service so that they could make the surgery more adolescent friendly. They then wrote out to all young people aged 16 to invite them for a general discussion with their GP, and assuring them of confidentiality.

The school nurse and the practice nurse carried out focus groups with young people in the comprehensive school and found out why they were reluctant to attend their local surgery, what would reassure them, and what types of services they would like. This formed the basis for a practice guide for adolescents, which was agreed by the practice team and posted prominently in the surgery. It covered emergencies, confidentiality, contraception and emergency contraception, counselling and general services.

Nearly 50% of the adolescents invited attended, giving Dr McAndrew and her team a chance to address their young clients' concerns and proactively offer advice on sexual health and contraception to those who needed it. A stronger link was also forged with the comprehensive school, so that health promotion programmes and health services could reinforce each other.

Reflection point 5.2

Think back to your pre-16 experience: if you had been sexually active, how would you have felt about consulting your family doctor or the nurses at that practice about contraception? What might have inhibited you or encouraged you to go to them for advice? How could you use that experience in your current area of practice?

YOUNG PEOPLE AND SEX

In other chapters reference has been made to organizations such as the WHO, which indicates that the sexual activity of the majority of young people follows a particular pattern, for example:

◆ Sexual relations begin in adolescence, within or outside marriage.

◆ Unprotected sexual relations increase the risks of unwanted pregnancy and too-early childbirth, unsafe abortion and sexually transmitted diseases (STDs), including HIV, resulting in AIDS.

◆ Lack of knowledge, skills and access to contraception, and vulnerability to sexual abuse puts adolescents at the highest risk of unwanted pregnancy.

◆ Worldwide, about 10% of all births are to adolescent women.

◆ Adolescent abortions are estimated at between 1 and 4.4 million per year.

◆ Each year more than 1 in 20 adolescents contracts a curable STD, not including viral infections.

◆ Of the estimated 330 million STDs that occur in the world every year, about 165 million occur in young people under the age of 25, and 110 million in those below the age of 20.

◆ Worldwide, more than half of all new HIV infections occur among people aged 15–24.

Learning activity 5.2

What are the sexual health problems of young people in your area?

Using the sources of information from Learning activity 5.1, find the source of statistics for abortions, pregnancies and sexually transmitted diseases in your local area and then identify sources for national statistics using the Internet.

Feedback on Learning activity 5.2

Did you find the national information you required?

Sources of statistics could include:

◆ health and personal social services

◆ health survey for England

◆ mortality statistics

◆ social trends

◆ population trends.

Your library will contain guides to official statistics and you will be able to get help accessing sources of information you require.

Professionals often think they understand the needs of their client group. They may also believe that their client group is not aware of or does not understand its needs, and so has no role to play in deciding what services are appropriate and how they should be delivered. Adolescents in particular are rarely asked for their opinions about their needs and the services they receive, as many professionals sincerely feel they would have little to say.

WHY BOTHER WITH SEX?

Sexual health has become a big issue in the planning processes of the purchasers of health services in the last few years. Central to this development

Learning activity 5.3

Using your information sources and focusing on the needs of young people, try to establish to what extent local education programmes and sexual health services have understood and addressed the needs and problems of teenagers in your local community.

You could check by asking the following questions:

◆ Have consumer surveys or focus groups been undertaken with young people to identify their attitudes, sexual behaviour and need for education and services?

◆ Were the findings turned into meaningful action?

◆ How are young people involved in planning and evaluating services?

◆ Are there local sexual health clinics or services aimed specifically at young people?

◆ Are these run by one agency, or by a number of agencies working in partnership?

◆ Has there been any attempt to train or involve GPs and primary health-care teams in improving their sexual health services to young people in their practice?

◆ How are the most vulnerable young people in your community reached with sexual health services and education?

◆ What services are made available to young people in care, for example young people excluded from school, or pregnant teenagers and schoolgirl mothers?

Reflection point 5.3

If you find that very little work is going on in any of the above areas, you could consider how you can contribute to the development of the agenda and influence others.

was the publication of the White Paper *Health of the Nation* (DoH 1992), with HIV/AIDS and sexual health as a key target area. The consultative Green Paper that preceded it (DoH 1991) described HIV and AIDS as 'the greatest new threat to public health this century'. But during the consultation period it became clear that HIV and AIDS could not be viewed alone, and the White Paper therefore included targets for the reduction of HIV incidence, the incidence of sexually transmitted diseases and teenage pregnancies.

Health authorities are the bodies responsible for planning and shaping health services in their localities, increasingly in conjunction with general practitioners, who will be closely involved in primary care groups along with primary care nurses. Developing strategies for individual services such as sexual health is central to this process. Strategies must also be incorporated into the health improvement programme (DoH 1998a).

As well as global targets such as those in the *Health of the Nation*, health authorities also receive annual priorities and planning guidance from central government. These are turned into specific targets in the health authority's annual accountability agreement with the NHS Executive. To achieve these targets, action is often required of Trusts, and so specific requirements may be included in Trust business plans and service-level agreements. In this way, a broad strategic purpose is turned into real action and meaningful health improvements.

'Effective organisations know where they are going. "The secret of success", said Benjamin Disraeli, "is constancy to purpose". Organisations that drift – like much of British industry in the past – are prone to disappear. Organisations that have strategies can concentrate on what they do best and devote resources (which are always limited) accordingly. . . . Setting a strategy also forces people to look to the future, making it more likely that they will see emerging opportunities early and be able to exploit them and notice the spot on the horizon that is an express train coming to destroy them – giving them a chance to get out of the way.'   Richard Smith (1991)

Box 5.4 Considerations in developing a sexual health strategy

◆ Performance data: comparison of local data against national targets

◆ Problem recognition: identification of particularly vulnerable groups

◆ Choice of effective interventions

◆ Value for money

◆ Determination of scope and priority for services

◆ Prevention: early intervention which may lead to improved physical and mental health later, e.g. prevention of HIV, psychological morbidity

◆ Coordination and consistency of services and education

◆ Provision of equivalent services in different geographical areas and consistency of health messages

◆ Ability to audit and monitor agreed priorities and quality standards

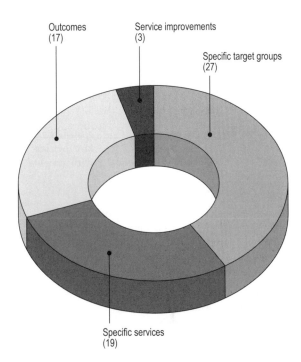

Fig. 5.1 Health authorities' priorities by type.

A strategy has to be selective and must inevitably set priorities (Box 5.4).

In order to find out what are the current priorities for health authorities in their sexual health purchasing strategies, a simple questionnaire was sent to all 124 health authorities and health boards in the UK via the Public Health Link (Epinet); 31 completed questionnaires were returned, a return rate of 25%. The responses are analysed overleaf and in Figures 5.1 – 5.6.

From this survey, you can see that most authorities who responded had already developed a sexual health purchasing strategy. There were recurring themes – of targeting vulnerable groups, of developing better-integrated, user-sensitive services, and of attempting to set and reach local targets in line with the national agenda.

Strategies had been developed through needs assessment, listening to user views, expert advice, and often through multiagency collaboration.

Needs assessment plays an important part in sexual health strategy development. Local needs

assessment may be complicated because of the difficulty for purchasers in accessing the views of potential service users. In many cases, user views on their sexual health needs are fed into the planning process through an intermediary, usually a voluntary or non-statutory agency. Large-scale anonymous surveys may yield much useful information. There is also much value in consulting regional or national health needs surveys, such as *Health purchasing, HIV prevention and gay men* (HEA 1994) and *The sexual health needs of HIV positive gay and bisexual men* (Court et al. 1996).

For many authorities, sexual health strategies have grown organically from the HIV/AIDS strategies developed in the mid-1980s. They are a natural development paralleling movements within the health and personal social services to mainstream HIV, and more open attitudes to discussing sex and sexuality in society and, in particular, in schools. The publication of the *Health of the Nation* (DoH 1992), which officially bracketed HIV with sexual health, gave impetus to this process.

1. What are your authority's key local priorities for sexual health?

Three authorities were either developing/reviewing strategy or failed to list key priorities. Of the remainder, priorities fell into several categories (Fig. 5.1).

Specific target groups (Fig. 5.2)	**Number of authorities with targets**
Young people	21 (75%)
Reduction in teenage pregnancy rate	11
Sex education/prevention work in schools	3
Family planning for young people	2
Improve awareness of current services	2
Extend/develop existing services	1
Non-specified target	2
Men who have sex with men	8 (28.6%)
Specific men's sexual health project	1
Increase safe sex practices	1
Non-specified target	6
Multiethnic communities	3 (10.7%)
Provision of sex education	2
HIV prevention in African communities	1
The general public	3 (10.7%)
Rights of all to sexual health	1
Non-specified target	2
Women at high risk	1 (3.6%)
Non-specified target	1
Sex workers	1 (3.6%)
Increase safe sex practices	1
Drug users	1 (3.6%)
HIV prevention by needle exchange	1
Vulnerable groups in general	1 (3.6%)
Gay and bisexual men/learning difficulties	1

Specific services (Fig. 5.3)

AIDS/HIV prevention	7 (25%)
Integrated family planning/GUM	4 (14.3%)
Family planning	2 (7.1%)
Emergency contraception availability	2 (7.1%)
Work with primary care	2 (7.1%)
Provision of drop-in facilities	1 (3.6%)
Prompt treatment for STDs	1 (3.6%)

Outcomes (Fig. 5.4)

Decrease in STDs (including HIV)	9 (32.1%)
Decrease in unwanted pregnancies	3 (10.7%)
Health of the Nation targets	2 (7.1%)
Decrease in TOPs past 12 weeks	1 (3.6%)
Increase in positive sexual health	1 (3.6%)
Decrease in NSU/chlamydia incidence	1 (3.6%)

Service improvements (Fig. 5.5)

Improve targeting of family planning	1 (3.6%)
Coordinate STD services in primary/ secondary care	1 (3.6%)
Improve information/education/outreach	1 (3.6%)

2. How were they determined? (Fig. 5.6)

30 authorities responded to this question.

Local needs assessment	13
Multidisciplinary interagency consultation	13
National imperatives, e.g. Health of the Nation	10
Public consultation (user groups etc.)	7
Local epidemiology/demographics	4
Specific sexual health steering group	3
Local specialist advice	2
Good practice elsewhere (benchmarking)	2
Service reviews	2
Authority commitment to providing locally relevant service	1
Commitment to providing a quality service	1
Local resource constraints	1

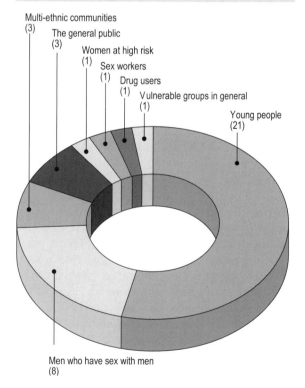

Multi-ethnic communities (3)
The general public (3)
Women at high risk (1)
Sex workers (1)
Drug users (1)
Vulnerable groups in general (1)
Young people (21)
Men who have sex with men (8)

Fig. 5.2 Specific target groups.

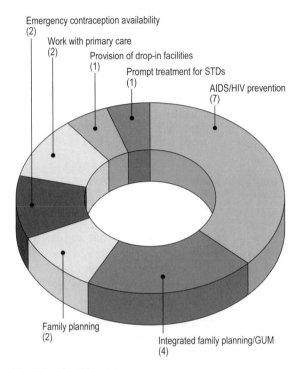

Fig. 5.3 Specific services.

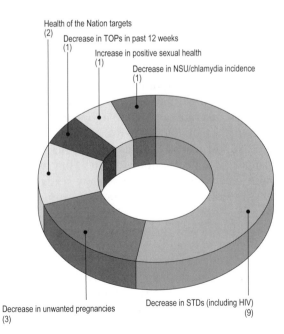

Fig. 5.4 Outcomes.

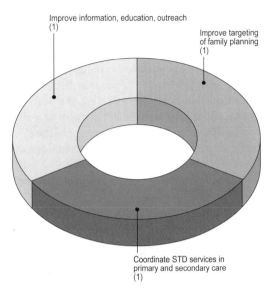

Fig. 5.5 Service improvements.

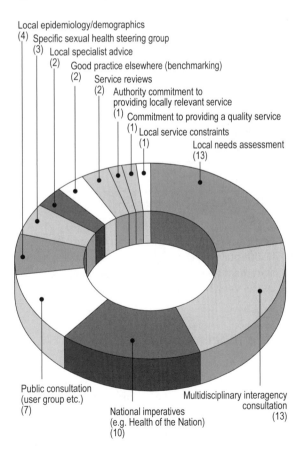

Fig. 5.6 How priorities were determined.

Learning activity 5.4

Try to find out about how the sexual health strategy was developed in your area. Your first port of call would be to contact a health-care commissioner for sexual health services at your local health authority. Alternatively, published strategies may be available through contacts in Trusts, e.g. the District HIV Prevention Coordinator, or Manager of the Family Planning Service.

Some questions to ask:

◆ Who was involved in strategy development, and which agencies were represented?

◆ How were user views sought?

◆ Was there a consultation exercise, and if so, how easy was it for groups and individuals to respond?

◆ Does the strategy contain expected outcomes which are measurable, time-limited and auditable?

◆ How could you make sure that the strategy happens?

◆ How, in your view, could the strategy be improved?

Reflection point 5.4

Look at your local health authority's sexual health purchasing strategy: does it contain a value statement and, if so, how does this measure up to the WHO definition of sexual health?

Value judgements

A sexual health strategy which does not have values underpinning it would run the risk of lacking focus and charges of bias could be levelled against it by user groups. Many health authorities have developed mission statements that reflect the overall standards that apply to the conduct of their business. However, sexual health is such a special-ized part of the health service, and demands such a level of interagency working, that a statement of the principles and values of the organizations involved in both purchasing and provision of sexual health services is essential.

The starting point may be to agree a definition of what sexual health is. One of the commonly used definitions is that of the WHO (1972), described elsewhere in this book.

The benefits of strategic vision in planning any health services are that:

◆ the key values of the purchasing authority are made explicit

◆ a global framework for planning is created

◆ a focus for policies and objectives is provided

◆ motivation factors are incorporated into planning goals (Edwards et al. 1994).

However, a value statement or mission statement will be unusable if it incorporates 'unmeasurable qualities or unrealistic expectations', or is created without involving or being communicated to all of the team members, thereby being divisive (Edwards et al. 1994).

FUNDING ARRANGEMENTS

Paying for sex

The arrangements in the reformed health service demand that money changes hands to pay providers for an agreed set of services. So, for example, a Trust may be paid a defined price per client for carrying out hip replacement operations. Similarly, small-volume items of health care, or those for which no contract exists, may well be costed and paid for individually. However, it is immediately obvious that not many sexual health services fall into either of these categories, other than in- and outpatient HIV services. So, the majority of sexual health services will be funded in a different way and the service specifications in the service-level agreement will reflect this. The emphasis is much more likely to be on an agreed set of activities, objectives or outcomes.

The question of where money comes from is also important. Although virtually all health authority funding is derived from taxation and allocated by the Department of Health or the equivalent in Wales, Scotland and Northern Ireland, in practice it is placed into various 'pots', some of which are earmarked for certain services. Local authorities are funded from council taxes, as well as grants from central government.

The main 'pots' which are used to fund sexual health services, and the ways they can be used, are shown in Figure 5.7.

Funding for HIV work has traditionally been separate from the main health authority allocation. There was an obvious need for this in the early years of the epidemic, to ensure that services were developed at a time when predictions of the size of the problem in the UK were pessimistic. This thinking has persisted even though treatment and care monies are no longer ring-fenced. Nevertheless, prevention monies are still ring-fenced and should not be used for anything other than HIV prevention work. A proportion may be put into genitourinary medicine (GUM) services, as it is assumed that up to 30% of GUM activity is HIV related. Authorities are obliged to account for how both funding streams have been used under the AIDS (Control) Act 1987 (HMSO 1987).

HOW WAS IT FOR YOU?

Change is always difficult, and the changes resulting from the NHS reforms have had mixed reviews from providers of sexual health services. The head of an HIV/AIDS prevention team sums up her experiences:

'Initially I and my service were severely disadvantaged by the purchaser/provider split. I had been a member of a unitary health authority and met regularly with the Director of Public Health. I had direct influence over the way the AIDS allocation was spent. After the reforms I was designated a "provider" and this influence was lost. It took over two years to reach my current position as a provider with an explicit role in advising the purchaser. These two years were the most frustrating of my whole professional life.

'The merging of two health authorities, the separation of health promotion and HIV prevention services, and the cross-district working of these two agencies from differently managed Trusts, have all added to the complications of the change.

'The initial purchaser/provider divide sent repercussions throughout the NHS locally. I saw a weariness in all staff. Job insecurity and role uncertainty diminished energy at all levels and in all jobs. New roles and tasks were expected of staff who had no clarity, preparation or training. Many processes were "muddled through", leaving staff unsure of channels of communication or responsibility.

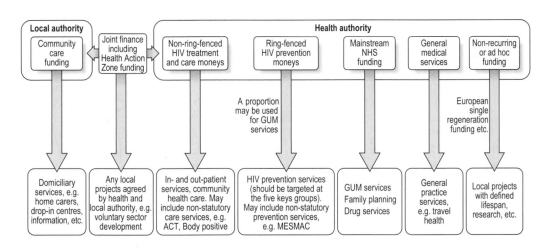

Fig. 5.7 Sources of funding for sexual health services.

'At the same time there have been major changes in local authorities (especially in education and social services) and in the voluntary sector (especially in the amount of funding available and the rules for accessing it). Possessiveness and competition have sometimes been more apparent than the alliances and collaboration which are needed. Essentially, too many changes have been imposed on too many people, too quickly, leading to confusion, anxiety and exhaustion . . .

'What has not changed is a professional's reliance on the good will, commitment and personalities of those in positions of power – whether in Trusts or in the health authority. These key relationships have been strengthened by the issuing of the Health of the Nation White Paper. The single most positive influence on my service has been the Health of the Nation – particularly, of course, the targets for sexual health.

'Following the stress and demotivation caused through the process of change, my service is now developed and well supported by both purchaser and provider. The continued ring-fenced allocations are key to our service, as is my explicit advisory role to the health authority.' Patricia Tyson, HIV Prevention and Sexual Health Coordinator, Gateshead and South Tyneside.

A family planning doctor also related her experience of the dramatic changes in the purchasing and provision of sexual health over recent years:

'Isaac Asimov wrote 20 years ago: "It is change, inevitable change, that is the dominant factor in society today." The Family Planning Association Clinics of yesterday have gone from a Cinderella specialty, staffed by the twin-set and pearls brigade, to a modern contraception and sexual health service run by a well trained team of clerks, nurses and doctors. The transformation from a service for married couples (or those intending to be) to one serving any sexually active person has been dramatic. The advent of AIDS, a younger starting age for sexual intercourse, multiple sexual partners, increase in teenage pregnancies and sexually transmitted diseases are some of the factors which have initiated change. The post-Thatcherite business ethos with the language of contracts, currency (client contacts), projections and management have placed extra demands for adaptation through the purchaser/provider structure. This jargon is now the everyday slang of the health service. Patients no longer fork out their pounds, shillings and pence for contraceptives. The state now recognises the value of unhindered and free access to contraception. Targets set by the Government in the Health of the Nation statement emphasise the importance of this policy. The service is now increasingly, however, subject to financial constraints. Few services are as accessible with "open access" to regular clinics scattered in the community. Demand has increased by 60% within the last two years in South Tyneside. This is the down side of being too popular! Whilst setting targets and figures projecting the future service and demand, we are beset by external factors, the weather, which team is playing football on TV, and potentially a change in government!

'Asimov concluded: "No sensible decision can be made any longer without taking into account not only the world as it is, but the world as it will be . . ." and so do I!' (Dr Janet E. Gallagher, SCMO, Contraception and Sexual Health Service Manager, South Tyneside Health Care Trust.)

WHERE'S THE ACTION?

Why do purchasers and providers bother developing strategies for sexual health, and what difference does it make?

The filing cabinets of health authorities are lined with health strategies of various vintages. At the time when each strategy was produced it was clearly felt to be important; however, the only obvious health benefit from many of these strategies was the tremendous stress reduction experi-

Reflection point 5.5

Review the documents from the health authority, Trusts, GPs and other agencies that you were able to collect from previous learning activities in this chapter, answering the following questions if you can:

◆ How easy was it to gain an overview of the strategy for sexual health in your area? Are there any obvious gaps or inconsistencies in the information available? How important is sexual health to the health authority, compared with other priorities?

◆ How important was sexual health to the provider?

◆ What are the main settings where sexual health practice is taking place?

◆ What are some key roles being undertaken by nurses in developing sexual health policy and practice in your area?

enced by those concerned when the process was over and a document was produced.

> ' "Sir," said Sir Percivale, "I am of King Arthur's Court, and a knight of the Table Round in the quest of the Holy Grail, and here I am in great duress, and never like to escape out of this wilderness."'

Strategy production can be like the quest for the Holy Grail: inspiring commitment and exhaustive effort, but with the goal only dimly perceived and never reached. Statements in some strategies reflect the ideals of a quest: 'To promote attitudes that challenge sexual exploitation' or 'To continue to work together, to coordinate services, reduce inequalities, promote understanding, prevent ill health and promote wellbeing'.

With the slimming down of health authorities and the constant changes experienced by all services it is important to have a similarly slimmed-down, practical and dynamic approach to strategy production which leads to improved performance across agencies. The end-point of a strategy should be real change as perceived by service users, rather than simply the production of another glossy document.

There can be a number of reasons for producing a strategy on sexual health. A case study from one health authority in the North of England illustrates the reasons that were important to them: Gateshead and South Tyneside Health Authority's rationale for a sexual health strategy is set out in Case study 5.2.

Case study 5.2

◆ *Performance data: National targets have been set (Health of the Nation) and local data (e.g. on adolescent fertility) are significantly worse than national data.*

◆ *Problem recognition: A number of problems have been recognized by several agencies, and in some cases also by the public. For example, there is shared concern about adolescent mothers and about vulnerable groups such as young people in care. Young people say they could have much more effective sex education programmes than at present. Gay men report that some health services are not always user friendly for them.*

◆ *Value for money: There is a substantial amount of money ring-fenced for HIV/AIDS and sexual health. Decisions for spending this money need to be made, including a review of whether the money already spent on genitourinary medical services is purchasing the style of service required.*

◆ *Comparative data: Information from other places indicates scope for doing better. For example, data from other parts of the UK and other countries indicate that a further increase in the use of condoms could prevent STDs.*

◆ *Prevention: Early intervention in sexual health may lead to improved health in later life. For example, the majority of people with AIDS worldwide were infected in their teens or early 20s. A review may highlight areas where 'investment in the future' could be made.*

Learning activity 5.5

This learning activity can be undertaken on an individual or a group basis. If you are in a group you may wish to share the questions.

Strategy for sexual health

Try to obtain a copy of your health authority's strategy for sexual health. If your area does not have a strategy, obtain one from a neighbouring authority.

Review the strategy against the following questions:

◆ What are the aims of the strategy (what does it hope to achieve?)

◆ What are the problems it seeks to address?

◆ What are the values underpinning the strategy?

◆ What agencies and groups took part in producing the strategy?

◆ Was there a clear lead agency or individual?

◆ What is the scope of the strategy (what population of groups and services are included?)

◆ What background information on the current situation was gathered? For example, are data and information included on health problems of different groups, patterns of existing services, health-care provider views and consumer views?

◆ What information on effectiveness of interventions was gathered to guide decisions about the right combination of interventions to be supported?

◆ Is the strategy explicit about priorities and availability of funding?

◆ Is there an action plan for implementing the strategy? An action plan should include specific targets, and each target should have a clear lead individual or agency, a timescale, identified resources and a means of measuring whether it has been achieved.

◆ How will the implementation of the strategy be coordinated?

◆ How will the longer term benefits to health and quality of life (outcomes) resulting from the strategy be measured?

◆ Has the strategy been agreed by the heads of the agencies involved, and are they signed up to implementing the action plan?

◆ Does the strategy reflect the needs and views of the people it is supposed to benefit?

If you have done this as a group exercise, once you have answered the above questions you can go on to discuss the following points:

◆ How does the strategy measure up? What are its main strengths and weaknesses?

◆ If you were in charge of strategy production, is there anything you would have done differently?

◆ What is the role of nurses in each stage of the strategy process?

IF IT FEELS GOOD ...

Over the past few years there has been an increased emphasis on evidence-based health care (NHSME 1993b, NHSE 1994). The objective is to ensure that all involved in health care, both purchasers and providers, work together and in partnership with clients to 'increase the proportion of clinical services which have been shown by evidence to be effective' (Welsh Office 1995). This initiative continues to be given the highest priority and is now underpinned by the National Institute for Clinical Excellence (DoH 1998b).

Evidence-based health care is the explicit use of current relevant research evidence to make decisions about health interventions. Good evidence of effectiveness will be required by most purchasers before they will consider funding new health interventions, and they will increasingly ask for the evidence to justify current practice.

Box 5.5 Agenda setting: Clinical effectiveness

'Clinical effectiveness has been defined as "the extent to which specific clinical interventions when deployed in the field for a particular patient or population do what they are intended to do, i.e. maintain and improve health and secure the greatest possible health gain from the available resources.' (NHSE 1996)

What is the evidence on sexual health? Recently, reviews by the BMA Foundation for AIDS and by the York Centre for Health Economics have highlighted the following evidence for effective sex education and sexual health programmes for young people:

◆ The most effective approach to HIV risk reduction in young people lies in the provision of practical information and support in a non-didactic way, based on an accurate, qualitative assessment of young people's needs (Oakley and Fullerton 1994).

◆ School-based sex education can be effective in reducing teenage pregnancy rates, especially when linked to access to family planning services. There is no evidence that it increases either sexual activity or pregnancy rates (NHS Centre for Reviews and Dissemination 1997).

◆ The availability of contraceptive clinic services for young people is linked with reduced pregnancy rates. Services should be based on local needs assessment and should provide accessibility and confidentiality (NHS Centre for Reviews and Dissemination 1997).

Sources of information to promote clinical effectiveness

How do you set about finding information on clinical effectiveness without spending days carrying out literature searches and reviewing papers? The NHS Executive (1998) has produced a reference pack to guide you through the maze. This lists all the main sources of information and how to access them. The following is a checklist:

◆ Bulletins/Journals: *Bandolier, Effective Health Care, Effectiveness Matters, Evidence-Based Medicine, MeReC Bulletin, Journal of Clinical Effectiveness, Clinical Effectiveness in Nursing*

◆ Guidelines/Reports, e.g. epidemiologically based needs assessment reviews, Health of the Nation Key Area Handbooks, Clinical Standards Advisory Group reports, Health Technology Assessment reports

◆ Cochrane Library Cochrane Database of Systematic Reviews, Database of Abstracts of Reviews of Effectiveness (Centre for Reviews and Dissemination, University of York), Cochrane Controlled Trials Register

◆ Medline. Use as a last resort. Not easy to find reliable 'gold standard' evidence, much of which will anyway have been published in another format.

To access this sort of information, a starting point would be to consult a librarian at a university with a good health faculty. Approaches to the public health department of your local health authority and the Royal College of Nursing library might also be useful.

Reflection point 5.6

The philosophy of clinical effectiveness is unarguable. However, the evidence can sometimes conflict with people's beliefs or attitudes. For example, many people are uncomfortable with the idea of sex education in school, particularly for younger adolescents and children, because they think this encourages experimentation. The evidence says otherwise.

Faced with a hostile group of school governors or a concerned group of parents, how would you use the evidence from research and from consumer work with young people themselves to make a case for sex education *before* young people become sexually active? How would you use information to make the case for telling young people how to access sexual health services?

SO WHAT NOW?

Starting with the background to health-care purchasing, an examination of the ways in which health purchasers develop strategies for sexual health has illustrated commissioning in action. The sources of funding for both mainstream health service provision and jointly commissioned services have also been identified, followed by a look at the centrality of clinical effectiveness in driving purchasing strategy.

This process cannot and should never be carried out by a purchaser in a complete vacuum. Health improvement programmes are central to this, and epitomize the collaborative nature of service delivery and development, consulting with providers, primary care groups and other primary care professionals, partner organizations, especially local authorities, and the public (DoH 1997, 1998a).

The sorts of activities intrinsic to comprehensive and effective purchasing can be judged by the sets of questions in Boxes 5.6, 5.7 and 5.8.

Target setting

Setting targets or objectives can appear deceptively simple. In practice, however, the opposite can be the case. To begin with, whose targets are they and how have they been arrived at? In the context of a sexual health strategy, targets should be integral to the process. This implies that all of the agencies involved in strategy development should be engaged in setting targets. The first step for many strategy groups is to consider what national imperatives there are. Many of the health authorities who responded to our survey (see above) saw the Health of the Nation (DoH 1992) targets as of paramount importance. Others had obviously picked up on the key groups identified in *HIV & AIDS health promotion an evolving strategy*:

Key groups targeted for HIV health promotion
◆ Gay men
◆ Bisexual men and other men who have sex with men
◆ Men and women who travel to, or have family links with, high-prevalence countries where the predominant mode of transmission

---

Box 5.6 Purchaser's checklist

1. Have you consulted with:
   ◆ The Director of Social Services?
   ◆ The Director of Education?
   ◆ Voluntary organizations that work with target groups, e.g. young people, gay men?
   ◆ User groups?

2. Are you aware of your responsibilities arising from:
   ◆ The Children Act 1989?
   ◆ The Education Act 1993?
   ◆ The AIDS (Control) Act 1987?

3. Do you know what resources are currently deployed in sexual health services?

4. Do you have the information, knowledge and alliances to develop a strategy which:
   ◆ is jointly agreed?
   ◆ is based on needs assessment?
   ◆ has agreed priorities?
   ◆ has a specification?
   ◆ includes a process for achieving necessary change?
   ◆ has evaluation methods built in?
   ◆ can cope with rare, expensive referrals?
   ◆ is reviewable in the light of practice?

5. Does your strategy consider sexual health in a comprehensive manner?

6. Do you have a provider(s) with whom you can work to achieve your strategy?

7. Do you have separate service-level agreements specifically for sexual health?

8. Are your contracts for defined services rather than being based on FCEs (finished consultant episodes)?

9. Do your service-level agreements specify levels of in-service training?

10. Are you confident that the staff of the provider organizations with whom you are in

contract are sufficiently knowledgeable about sexual health issues and provision?

11. Is the sexual health service that is delivered to the populations for which you are responsible an integrated service in which the various components and providers play acknowledged, coordinated roles?

Box 5.7   Provider's checklist

1. Do you have a clear management structure in which sexual health services are integrated?

2. Do you understand your purchaser's sexual health strategy?

3. Does your purchaser's strategy consider sexual health services in a comprehensive manner?

4. Do you understand your purchaser's sexual health priorities?

5. Do you understand the way in which your purchaser perceives the contribution of your service to the delivery of comprehensive sexual health services?

6. Do your purchaser's perceptions of the role of your service within the overall provision of sexual health services match your own?

7. Do you have a contact person in the purchasing authority who holds specific responsibility for sexual health services?

8. Do you have a method of delivering sexual health services at the primary service level?

9. Do you have a multidisciplinary sexual health team or a network of separate service elements?

10. Are the management and clinical roles of your service clear with respect to which are:
   - based on multidisciplinary teams?
   - integrated into service networks?

11. Is the composition of your service appropriate in respect of:
   - the number and type of the professional disciplines?
   - staff levels within all service components?

12. Do you have an operational policy for sexual health services?

13. Do you have a business plan for sexual health services?

14. Do you have an adequate information system geared specifically to sexual health services?

15. Do you have clear floors and ceilings for your contractual commitments?

16. Do you have a recognizable and separate budget for your sexual health services?

17. Have you avoided different professional groups or service components competing with each other?

18. Do members of your sexual health services have good relationships with:
   - the social services department?
   - the education department?
   - the police?
   - voluntary agencies?
   - each other?

19. Does your sexual health service provide an out-of-hours service?

20. Do you audit work done by your sexual health service?

21. Do you have training programmes specifically for staff working in sexual health services?

22. Are secretarial and reception staff working in sexual health services trained for their roles?

---

is sex between men and women, for example in sub-Saharan Africa
- People diagnosed with HIV and AIDS
- Injecting drug users.
  (UK Health Departments 1995).

Targets may be soft or hard. An example of a soft target would be 'To improve sexual negotiating skills in young people'. On the other hand,

---

Box 5.8 Multiagency checklist

1. Is there a multiagency group with enough seniority and 'clout' to plan the approach to sexual health in the district? Are all key partners represented in the group?

2. Does the group identify clear and specific priorities for action on an annual basis?

3. Are the priorities supported by a detailed action plan which can be monitored regularly?

4. Are the views of young people, particularly vulnerable groups, incorporated into the group's planning process?

5. Are the priorities for action picked up in the business plans and individual performance targets of all member agencies?

6. Does the group produce and distribute an annual report and work to secure the support of key decision makers?

---

a hard target might be 'To increase the awareness of safer sex methods in injecting drug users attending Clinic X from 50% to 75% by December 19 . . .'.

In the main, managers tend to use the 'SMART' principle when drawing up targets or objectives (Upton and Brooks 1995). This rule of thumb is a useful one to remember. Targets or objectives should be:

Specific: Precise and concerned with an individual aspect or service, not the totality

Measurable: Anyone can tell whether the target has been achieved or not

Achievable: Ideals are wonderful things, but in the real world there are resources and constraints. There is nothing more demotivating than to have targets that are never met

Relevant: The targets are ones which are important to the organization

Timed: Everyone knows when the effort is expected, and definite review dates can be built in.

The benefits of using the SMART principle are that:

◆ Everyone is clear about what they are expected to achieve.
◆ Measures for evaluating work performance are agreed.
◆ Timescales are clearly understood.

However, all targets should in essence be derived from the mission statement or statement of intent in the strategy, and must reflect the underlying values.

Action planning

Strategic health objectives are the outcomes you are trying to achieve. For example:

◆ Reduce dropout rates in secondary school due to unwanted pregnancy from 3% to 1.5%
◆ Offer in-service training on adolescent sexual health to 50% of family planning staff
◆ Reduce the incidence of new STDs in people attending GUM clinics from 50% to 30%
◆ Increase the family planning clinic attendance of 16-year-old girls from 2% to 10% of the population (one-third of the sexually active population of 16-year-old girls)
◆ Establish a peer education programme for gay men aged 18–25.

Change does not occur overnight. Many programmes suffer from short-term planning, which is insufficient to bring about lasting change. This is often because purchasers want 'instant' results. Your action plan should define all the things that will need to happen over the next 5 years to bring about your strategic health objectives. For example, in order to increase the family planning clinic attendance of 16-year-old girls who are sexually active, you might need to:

◆ identify ways to reach sexually active 16-year-old girls who still attend school/no longer attend school
◆ identify barriers to the use of existing family planning services
◆ work with young girls to develop a plan for a more appealing service

- work with family planning service providers to implement the plan
- train service providers in adolescent sexual health
- develop a publicity and outreach strategy
- establish funding to support the changes you want to introduce.

Strategic activities are what you will actually do to carry out the different components of a 5-year plan. For example, in identifying the barriers faced by 16-year-old girls in using existing family planning services, you might need to:

- interview service managers to identify major problems in reaching this age group, from their perspective
- develop a structured interview plan with the help of young people and service staff to identify the psychosocial 'costs' (e.g. embarrassment, staff attitude, fear) of using the service
- interview a representative sample of 16-year-old girls
- interview staff to find out whether their perceptions about the problems match those of the young people interviewed
- collect objective information about aspects of the service that might affect its use by young clients, such as types and costs of transport, opening times, information provided.

Case study 5.3

A combined hospital–community Trust wanted to set up a family planning service specifically for young people. They convened a group composed of a senior manager, the family planning doctor, a consultant gynaecologist and the family planning nurse to draw up the plans for the service.

At the first meeting of the group, discussion about the model of service was becoming quite heated when the family planning nurse intervened. She pointed out that none of the people in the group was under 30, and none lived anywhere near the council estate where the service would be based. Even she, who frequently visited

schools to talk about family planning, did not know what sort of service young people wanted.

Although one of the doctors claimed that he knew better than young people what sort of services they needed, the majority of the group supported the nurse. They connected up with local voluntary and youth groups who had direct contact with young people, including vulnerable groups such as children in care, drug abusers, schoolgirl mothers and gay or bisexual young people, and using focus groups asked 'What sort of advice and services would young people like about sex?'

The results were used to shape a very different model of service from that which had been envisaged. Instead of family planning alone, the service offers a one-stop shop for counselling, contraception and other problems such as drug abuse. The service has formed the core of a multiagency action group to improve young people's sexual health.

THE NURSE'S ROLE

Nurses need to be sure that their activities are likely to achieve their strategic objectives. For example, if you are trying to change behaviour or develop new skills, you are unlikely to achieve this through the production and distribution of an information leaflet alone. Information is not usually sufficient to change behaviour: your activities will also need to include work with small groups.

If you are trying to create a more user-friendly health clinic, you may not achieve this by redesigning the physical layout of the clinic alone. The attitudes of the reception staff may also be a major barrier to using the service: your activities should include staff retraining or redeployment.

The management of change is becoming increasingly central to health services, and nurses now have to come to grips with change management in a number of ways (McPhail 1997). Nurses working in sexual health may experience a considerable level of change arising from the rapid advances in treatments, epidemiological developments and changed client demands. Changes to service configuration may be imposed by national directives or, more likely, by changes in health-care purchasing. Such imposed change creates uncertainty and anxiety, and one reaction to incessant change, common in nursing, is to retreat into familiar patterns and situations. Change thus has to be managed both individually and collectively. A possible remedy is for nurses working in sexual health to feel part of the shared vision of the service. Purchasers ought to include service providers in the planning process, but on grounds of sheer impracticality this will inevitably fail to include all staff.

Managing up

Managing up is about closing the gap between the nurse at the sharp end and the planners, so that the former can influence the latter. There is no mystique in achieving influence in reverse: the 'junior' person simply uses the tools of management, and the first rule is that information equals power. So, what tools will you need?

A 'managing up' toolbox

Information
- ◆ Who are the people to influence? Find out who the key contacts are in the health authority primary care groups and the provider.
- ◆ Arm yourself with copies of all the relevant reports. Remember that most health authority, Trust and local authority planning documents, strategies and reports are in the public domain. Most will be available on request from the organization concerned. Otherwise, use your key contacts.
- ◆ Review the evidence on clinical effectiveness. A proposal backed up by sound research is far more likely to be accepted than one based on feelings, views or anecdotal evidence.
- ◆ Find out the meetings and groups that discuss changes to services and new service developments. Good ones might be a sexual health strategy group or steering group, a district HIV/AIDS committee or a community care planning group.

Planning
Think carefully about how to get your views heard and how to present them. Who can you use as allies?

Presentation
- ◆ Be prepared as early as possible to produce a written proposal, backed up by the evidence.
- ◆ A written proposal should be as brief as it can be without omitting the essentials: the benefits to the service, to users and, if the case, in financial terms (new service developments need not cost more!).

Persuasion
- ◆ Gain support among your colleagues. Be ruthless about using people who have standing and influence.
- ◆ Seek the support of other agencies – voluntary groups, people with influence in the local authority.
- ◆ Try to get your proposal on the agenda of one of the groups with a planning or service development remit (see above).
- ◆ Seek to meet your key contacts as soon as your presentation is as polished as you can make it.
- ◆ Project the right image – confident without cockiness, assertive without aggression, and polished without glibness.

'Knowledge for its own sake. But also, and perhaps still more, knowledge for power . . . Increased power for increased action. But finally and above all, increased action for increased being.' Pierre Teilhard de Chardin

Case study 5.4
A local community in the West Midlands was concerned about problems among its young people and carried out a survey to find out what people felt most strongly about. This initiative was strongly supported by two school nurses and a health visitor. The survey showed that the three issues the community wanted action taken about were crime, teenage pregnancies and drug taking. The genitourinary nurse counsellor became involved, thought through what was needed and set about convincing the purchasers. As a result, a health project worker was appointed with a remit to particularly address the needs of the disenfranchised. The project worker then took on the mantle of pushing for new services and driving forward several new

initiatives, such as working with the school nurse on contraception.

Of course, it may be easier to convince purchasers if the lead on sexual health services is a nurse. A nurse working in a health authority public health department as their HIV/AIDS and sexual lead said:

'A nursing background certainly helped me in the experience of developing a sexual health strategy. Having a nursing background with a wide-ranging experience helped with strategic thinking. It also helped to understand the NHS culture. There is a challenge to nurses to get involved in sexual health strategy and purchasing. However, they must try to avoid getting into the "provider mode". At their best, nurses bring an understanding of health and the problems that clients and their carers face.'

 Reflection point 5.7

If you were to explain to a member of the public what possible benefits they could derive from sexual health services being planned and managed through a purchasing framework, how would you do it?

How would you see the sexual health purchasing agenda moving on in the next few years, given the change of government and new policy directions? And how can you prepare for the changes ahead?

CONCLUSION

This chapter has set sexual health services within the context of the health service of the late 1990s. It has demonstrated that the separation of purchaser from provider has posed problems, but has also helped to clarify priorities. With the emphasis on increased collaboration, some thoughts on how commissioning will develop have been offered.

The process of purchasing for sexual health has been followed, from strategy development and needs assessment to making purchasing decisions. The importance of selecting clinically proven interventions has been discussed. Although some nurses may be unconvinced of the merits of the purchaser/provider model of health-care management, few could argue professionally against evidence-based care. It is important that all nurses working in the sexual health field get to grips with this aspect.

Although many nurses working at the 'sharp end' may feel alienated from the decisions that affect their working lives and their clients' wellbeing, a potential remedy lies in using knowledge of the management of change to influence decision making. This can be called 'managing up', an apt description of the mechanism. It is up to 'ordinary' nurses to make the lives of sexual health planners and purchasers interesting and ensure that they have a say in the shape of the services of the future.

'What's happened has happened. Poisons poured into the seas cannot be drained out again, but everything changes. We plant trees for those born later.'   Cicely Herbert

RESOURCES AND ANNOTATED FURTHER READING

NHS Confederation website: http://www.nhsconfed.net/

Department of Health website: (to download strategy documents) http://www.doh.gov.uk/

Clinical effectiveness reference pack. NHS Executive, Leeds, 1998. Available from NHS libraries or via the NHS Response Line, tel: 0541 555455
Achieving effective practice: a clinical effectiveness and research information pack for nurses, midwives and health visitors. NHS Executive, 1998. Available via the NHS Response Line, tel: 0541 555455

Family Planning Association publications include FPA's guide to commissioning sexual health services, available from FPA, PO Box 1078, East Oxford DO, Oxfordshire OX4 5JE. (Price £9.99 plus £1.50 p&p per copy.)

BMA Foundation for AIDS, BMA House, Tavistock Square, London WC1H 9JP. Publications include Towards a sexual health strategy for England, 1998. Website: http://www.bmaids.demon.co.uk/

SASH (Society for the Advancement of Sexual Health), PO Box 17, Cheltenham GL54 2YU. Regular newsletter for members

The King's Fund website: http://www.kingsfund. org.uk/default.htm

The Health Services Management Centre (part of the School of Public Policy at the University of Birmingham) website: http://www.bham.ac.uk/ HSMC/

Ham C 1991 The new national health service. NAHAT, Oxford

A brief but eloquent account of the NHS reforms of the 1990s.

Ham C 1994 Management and competition in the new NHS. NAHAT, Oxford

This picks up on Chris Ham's earlier book to show how the reforms are working in practice. Again, pithy and packed with useful information.

Levitt R, Wall A 1992 The reorganised national health service, 4th edn. Chapman & Hall, London

For those wanting to view the present management arrangements in the NHS against the backdrop of its development and policy changes since its inception, this book could prove a valuable source of information.

NHS Management Executive 1993 Contracting for specialised services. A practical guide. NHSME, Leeds

Useful for insight into the smaller-volume services such as HIV treatment and care, which need to be contracted for on a consortium basis.

Paton C 1998 Competition and planning in the NHS, 2nd edn. Stanley Thornes, Cheltenham

Recently updated, this text examines the NHS reforms from a historical perspective. It also critically analyses their consequences for the future NHS.

Plant R 1987 Managing change and making it stick. HarperCollins, London

An excellent starter on change management, this book is packed with handy exercises to help the reader focus on practical ways of effecting or managing change.

Upton T, Brooks B 1995 Managing change in the NHS. Kogan Page, London

More specific to the NHS and contains some helpful insights into the ways in which the enlightened manager should manage change.

REFERENCES

British Medical Association 1993 Confidentiality and people under 16. Guidance issued jointly by the BMA, GMSC, HEA, Brook Advisory Centres, FPA and RCGP. BMA, London

Court P, Holt R, Vedhara K et al. 1996 The sexual health needs of HIV positive gay and bisexual men. Northern and Yorkshire Regional Health Authority, Newcastle upon Tyne

Department of Health 1991 The health of the nation. HMSO, London

Department of Health 1992 The health of the nation. A strategy for health in England. HMSO, London

Department of Health 1997 The new NHS. Modern. Dependable. HMSO, London

Department of Health 1998a Our healthier nation. HMSO, London

Department of Health 1998b A first class service. Quality in the new NHS. HMSO, London

Department of Health 1999 Saving lives: our healthier nation (Cm 4386). HMSO, London

Edwards P, Jones S, Williams S 1994 Business and health planning for general practice. Radcliffe Medical Press, Oxford

Health Education Authority 1994 Health purchasing, HIV prevention and gay men. NAM Publications, London

Her Majesty's Stationery Office 1987 AIDS (Control) Act 1987. HMSO, London

McPhail G 1997 Management of change: an essential skill for nursing in the 1990s. Journal of Nursing Management 5: 199–205

NHS Centre for Reviews and Dissemination 1997 Preventing and reducing the adverse effects of unintended teenage pregnancies. Effective Health Care 3(1): 1–12

NHS Executive 1994 Improving the effectiveness of the NHS [EL(94)74]. NHSE, Leeds

NHS Executive 1996 Promoting clinical effectiveness – a framework for action in and through the NHS. Department of Health, Leeds

NHS Executive 1998 Clinical effectiveness reference pack. NHSE, Leeds

NHS Management Executive 1993a purchasing for health. A framework for action. NHSME, Leeds

NHS Management Executive 1993b Improving clinical effectiveness [EL(93)115]. NHSME, Leeds

Oakley A, Fullerton D 1994 Risk, knowledge and behaviour: HIV/AIDS education programmes and young people. Report for North Thames Regional Health Authority. University of London, London

Smith R 1991 First steps towards a strategy for health. In: Smith R (ed) Health of the nation. The BMJ View. BMJ Publishing, London

Social Exclusion Unit 1999 Teenage pregnancy (Cm 4342). HMSO, London

UK Health Departments 1995 HIV and AIDS health promotion. An evolving strategy. Department of Health, London

Upton T, Brooks B 1995 Managing change in the NHS. Kogan Page, London

Welsh Office 1995 Towards evidence-based practice. A clinical effectiveness initiative for Wales. Welsh Office, Cardiff.

6

Sexual health: sense and sensibility

Robert Tunmore

'*I came to realize that the study of organizations is not to do with predictive certainty . . .*' (Charles Handy 1993)

KEY ISSUES/CONCEPTS

◆ Organizational culture

◆ Handy's types of organizations

◆ A gender typology of organizational culture

◆ The gender culture

◆ What is a successful organization?

◆ Sexual harassment

◆ Bullying

◆ Possible solutions to sexual harassment and bullying

◆ An action plan

OVERVIEW

Chapter 6, *Sexual health: sense and sensibility*, covers sexual health in terms of cultures, relationships and behaviours that are characteristic of work organizations. It aims to increase an understanding of how organizational culture may affect the sexual health of practitioners. It explores the impact of organizational culture and behaviour on the development of sexual health-related policies and practice developments, highlighting the sexual health needs of its clients. It focuses on equal opportunities, sex discrimination, sexual harassment and bullying from the perspectives of both employee and practice.

INTRODUCTION

There are as many types of organizational culture as there are organizations. However, an insight into the different classification systems and frameworks supports and aids understanding. Organizations may be seen in terms of common sex roles and sexual stereotypes. Each type of culture will emphasize different relationships and behaviours. The concept of the gendered culture provides a framework for understanding any type of organization in terms of gender issues and sexual health characteristics.

Organizational culture embraces characteristics of organizations, including structures and hierarchies, systems, policies and procedures. It also includes less tangible aspects of organizational life, for example the values and beliefs, behaviours and practices, customs and traditions of the work environment. Each of these factors has an impact on the sexual health of the organization. For example, behaviours involving sex discrimination, sexual harassment and bullying have a major influence on the sexual health of individuals within that organization. This chapter will address these behaviours in terms of the organizational dynamics involved in the process of exclusion.

Throughout the chapter different activities are suggested. These are intended to assist you to examine your organization and to identify the implications for sexual health policy and practice in the work setting.

ORGANIZATIONAL CULTURE

The culture of the organization is dynamic and interactive, a matrix of relationships between formal and informal organizational processes, individual attributes and the world outside the organization. Different types of organization have different types of culture. This section identifies these different types and different ways of looking at organizations.

A popular means of studying organizations and organizational cultures involves the identification of characteristics common to different types of organizations. Both Handy (1985) and Mintzberg (1989) take this approach. Handy (1985) identifies various factors that may determine or influence the structure of an organization and describes four different types of organizational culture. Likewise, Mintzberg (1989) reports six basic organizational attributes (Table 6.1) and seven different types of organization. There are many similarities between the two approaches. Each type of organization is based on underlying assumptions about how those organizations work. Different types are not necessarily pure, i.e. completely distinct from others. Where Handy describes a 'mix of cultures', Mintzberg outlines how one configuration of the basic attributes or characteristics may overlie others. They are described in this way to aid understanding of the similarities and differences between different organizations. Both

authors suggest there may be a prevailing culture within an organization. Individuals each have their personal way of perceiving the culture, and may have a preference for a particular type or mix of attributes and characteristics. This approach may be extended to gender cultures in organizations. The following section looks at these in more detail.

MINTZBERG'S TYPES OF ORGANIZATION

The entrepreneurial organization

This type of organization is often new or just starting up. It is simple and informal, with a small management hierarchy. There is a highly centralized power system, power and control being set with the leader, who is often visionary and charismatic. Their clear sense of mission and purpose is conveyed to and shared by staff. Strong personal leadership is evident through close direct supervision of staff. Loose division of labour reflects a simple and dynamic environment. The small size and strong, focused but flexible leadership enable the entrepreneurial organization to respond quickly to pressures from the external environment. Some of these characteristics may appear in large established organizations, for example during a time of crisis.

The machine organization

This type has a relatively large bureaucracy. Mintzberg uses the term 'technostructure' to describe the elaborate body of administrative personnel, planners, accountants, quality assurance officers etc. in this type of organization. Control through standardization, rules and regulations plays a central part. Efficiency, reliability and consistency are crucial to the smooth running of the organization. Communication is formalized and set in the strong management hierarchy. Administration is elaborate, with sharp divisions of labour. The technostructure, despite lacking formal authority, is a powerful factor pervading the whole organization. Considerable power and

Table 6.1 Common characteristics of organizations

Handy (1985)	Mintzberg (1989)
History and ownership	The operating core: the operators or workers who produce the goods or
Size	provide the service.
Technology	The strategic apex: here is the top
Goals and objectives	manager, executive etc.
Environment	Middle line: a management hierarchy between the core and the apex.
The people	Technostructure: thisconsists of people involved inadministrative duties, planning and controlling the work of others.
	Support staff: internal services, e.g. canteen, portering, information technology, public relations.
	Ideology: some prefer the term culture (Handy)to refer to the values and traditions,beliefs and practices within the organization

authority are set centrally at the strategic apex (Table 6.1). Management alone knows how the whole organization works.

Organizations of this type include those where the work is simple and repetitive, e.g. mass production companies, small manufacturers, banks and insurance companies; those where external control and accountability are paramount, e.g. government departments, tax offices; those regulatory agencies where routine control and safety are key features, e.g. the prison service, police, the military, aircraft carriers, firefighting services.

The diversified organization

A central administrative headquarters presides over several service- or market-based divisions, directorates or units, each of which is a semi-autonomous business and functions independently from the others. At the management apex headquarters has specific functions through which it exercises power over the units. These include the development of an overall corporate strategy – a portfolio of business within the organization; management of funds between the units; the design and implementation of performance control systems, based on measurable operational goals; hiring and firing of unit managers; and the provision of support services shared across all units, for example occupational health services or corporate public relations departments.

The professional organization

Here a decentralized professional bureaucracy draws on the knowledge and skills of professionals to produce standardized products or services. Training and indoctrination are incorporated in a lengthy process of socialization. Once qualified, many professionals complete a period of preceptorship, internship or on-the-job training. Professional codes of practice hold individual professional practitioners responsible for keeping themselves up to date with recent developments in their field.

The application of this standardized knowledge and skills is complex. Professional responsibility incorporates wide-ranging discretion and judge-

ment. Categorization or diagnosis and intervention are two fundamental tasks of the professional organization, involving the use of standardized knowledge and skills, programme and interventions.

The technostructure and middle-line hierarchy is minimal, although there is increased use of support staff for the professionals, e.g. libraries and archives, information technology, computing and statistics, printing and publishing services. These organizations are normally services such as universities, hospitals, public accounting firms and social work agencies.

The innovative organization

Innovation involves breaking away from the established conventional approach. The innovative organization consists of multidisciplinary project teams, task forces involving a disparate range of experts, each with highly developed knowledge and skill in a particular field. They are temporary organizations with short lifespans, set up for a specific reason and a given time, and are most effective in providing new approaches and different ways of working. Standardization, unity of command, bureaucracy, a sharp division of labour, planning and control systems do not have an important part to play in this type of organization.

Adhocracy is the term used to describe the structure of innovative organizations which are characteristically complex and unpredictable. In this configuration – a matrix structure – experts act in a liaison capacity, working with others from different backgrounds or different expertise. Two forms of adhocracy are identified: the operating adhocracy – contract project work – where innovative solutions are found for clients' problems; and the administrative adhocracy, which undertakes a similar problem-solving approach to serve itself, for example bringing new ideas and activities to the organization.

Power tends to be based on expertise rather than formal authority. Decision making based on this expertise is dispersed across the organization, depending on the nature of the project or issue at hand. Examples include consultancy firms and manufacturing companies that make products to order.

The missionary organization

The missionary organization is distinguished by its strong, clear and focused sense of mission and tradition, often associated with charismatic inspiring leadership. Each individual's identity is shaped by the organization and loyalty is reinforced by traditions and practices. Selection and indoctrination play an important part in the socialization process. Intangible value and belief systems have a unifying power, often taking the place of close supervision, standardization of output and skills. Individuals conform to beliefs and practices – the standardization of norms holds this organization together. The prevailing ideology itself is not challenged, although different interpretations may be the focus of debate. This configuration may coexist with others, particularly the entrepreneurial, innovative, professional or machine organization. Examples include various religious orders, kibbutzes, or Alcoholics Anonymous.

The political organization

Like the missionary organization this configuration usually coexists with the more conventional patterns, but may be strong enough to stand alone. In some organizations politics is the dominant system. Political activity pitches individuals or groups against the organization's systems of influence, different systems against each other. The lack of any preferred form of order, structure or coordination typifies the political organization. Although the nature of the conflict may vary in terms of intensity, pervading influence and endurance, the exercise of technically illegitimate, informal power is central to the conflict. Conflict manifests itself in political games, and is often motivated by self-serving self-interest.

HANDY'S TYPES OF ORGANIZATIONS

The power or club culture
(Handy 1985, 1988)

This type of organization is often small and entrepreneurial, with a central power source exercising influence and control through the selection of key individuals who share the leader's values, views and vision. The organization may be an extension of the head or founder dictatorship. For those who belong to 'the club' it is rich in personality and most exciting. Trust and empathy are important factors in the organization, which invests in individuals rather than committees, rank or position. There are few rules and procedures. Individuals have freedom of manoeuvre, are motivated, power oriented, politically astute risk takers.

These are political organizations in that decision making is based on influence and networking, rather than procedure or logic. These organizations are competitive, able to react quickly in a changing environment. They may appear tough and abrasive, or proud and strong. They are highly dependent on the person or people at the centre, which is the site of power and influence, but this may also be their main source of weakness. Expectations are constantly high. There may be low morale and high turnover among staff.

The role culture

Organizations are represented as a hierarchical arrangement of different roles with a uniform definition of responsibilities. Routinization of work occurs across and within roles. The arrangement of roles may be altered, and individuals may move or be moved from one role to another within the organization. Communication systems are formalized though policies and procedures, rules and regulations.

The task culture

This type of organization focuses directly on a project, problem or task. Work is usually planned based on the sharing of skills within a collaborative team approach to problem solving. Individuals with different skills make specific contributions to various aspects of the work. They are often expensive, may be short-lived, and are demanding in terms of energy, commitment and enthusiasm. Examples include consultancy companies, project development, advertising companies, construction work.

The person culture

This differs from the others in that the organization serves the purpose of the individual. The skill and talent of the individual is central, and management exists to support and enable their work. Approaches to work may involve persuasion, or influence used in conjunction with professional knowledge and skills. Examples include barristers in chambers, doctors in practices, professors in university faculties. Table 6.2 lists the various types according to Handy and Mintzberg.

Table 6.2 Types of organization

Handy (1985)	Mintzberg (1989)
The power culture/	The entrepreneurial organization
The club culture	The machine organization
The role culture	The diversified organization
The task culture	The professional organization
The person culture	The innovative organization
	The missionary organization
	The political organization

 Learning activity 6.1

This provides a simple means for analysing the organization and identifying individual preferences from the practitioner's perspective.

(a) Of all the types of organization identified in the different typologies, which best describes your organization? How many different types of organization are you involved in? Identify similarities and differences. Do you have a preferred type of organization?

(b) Can you identify different ways of representing your organization? Draw a diagrammatic representation of your organization – an organizational chart or map. If you have identified positions or key roles, mark those occupied by men and women with the symbol ♂ or ♀ respectively. Do any patterns emerge? What is the significance of this result?

(c) Can you identify:

the percentage of women and men in senior appointments?

the percentage of women and men in staff grades (e.g. G or H grades)?

the percentage of women and men part-time/full-time?

(d) For each area can you find out the percentage of male and female job applicants? The proportions of successful candidates? Does anyone keep this kind of information? Who monitors issues relating to equal opportunities within your organization?

 Learning activity 6.2

Sex and the four big Ps: Pressure, Position, Possibilities and Proposals

Organizations may be described in terms of an external **Pressure**

their **Position** (in the marketplace, local community etc.)

Possibilities: the way things could develop

Proposals: plans for future courses of action.

Use the four Ps to define and analyse an organizational pressure in sexual health. Identify two or more responses, and take the best one. Devise a short-term course of action incorporating key concepts and theoretical frameworks from the rest of the text.

A GENDER TYPOLOGY OF ORGANIZATIONAL CULTURE

The means of identifying the different types of organization provided by both Handy and Mintzberg provide insights into the culture of the organization. However, the implications for the sexual health of the organization are not directly addressed, even though gender issues are implicit in common characteristics. Each type of organization is gendered: for example, the power culture replicates and maintains a specific ethos by key individuals choosing others who think like them and share the same values. Usually it is men who hold these positions of power, i.e. at the apex: hence the 'old boys' network', where policies, procedures, practices, experience and expectations defined by male value systems are reinforced and perpetuated.

Sexual stereotyping emphasizing heterosexual male stereotypes has been used to describe the attributes of different groups of worker and types of employee. For example, Kanter (1989) identifies 'corporate characters', such as organization man, corprocat, maverick and cowboy. Maccoby (1976) also identifies corporate types in terms of sexual stereotypes (Box 6.1). The exclusion of women from the analysis of the organization is apparent. Kanter (1975) addresses power relations between men and women, emphasizing the strong influence of paired stereotypes, including macho man/seductress; chivalrous knight/helpless maiden; possessive father/pet; tough warrior/nurturing mother.

Like Handy and Mintzberg, Parkin and Maddock (1995) have developed typology to help understand how organizations work. However, this is a gender typology of organizational culture based on the views of women working in public sector organizations. Here each type of culture has a particular mindset or approach which sets expectations and influences the motivation and self-confidence of women:

◆ **The gentlemen's club** This appears a polite, kind and humane, protective and civilized culture. However, it may be experienced as patronizing, overprotective and restrictive. Men act as if they have the best interests of women at heart. This leads to overprotection and the active exclusion of women from certain areas of work, for example physical danger, violence, dirty or physically demanding tasks. Women are valued for playing their part in the organization, but are kept in their place. The traditional sex roles of women as housekeeper and mother and men as breadwinner are reinforced.

◆ **The barrack yard** This is a hierarchical type of organization with a strong and obvious chain of command. It takes after a military model, relationships between employees being defined in terms of their rank or position. Power is invested in higher positions. Abuse of this power leads to compliance among subordinates. Often experienced as a bullying, authoritarian culture where subordinates are treated with little respect by their superiors. Women will seldom reach senior positions. All those in lowly positions, regardless of their sex, are seen as weak and of little value or significance in the overall scheme.

◆ **The locker room** A matrix of heterosexual male relationships, perspectives and assumptions from which women are excluded characterizes this type of organization. Sexual harassment, including groping, leering, offensive overfamiliar remarks and pornography are commonplace and are seen as

---

Box 6.1 Corporate types (Maccoby 1976)

The jungle fighter – The environment is tough. The jungle fighter needs to be powerful, to win battles and skirmishes, destroying or defeating enemies, rejecting losers. He is portrayed as fiercely protective, often domineering and defensive.

The company man – Corporate identity and loyalty to the organization are paramount. Often focusing on the social aspects – people working together towards a shared goal – the company man may become engulfed in organizational politics, engrossed with procedure and policy, regulation and routine.

The gamesman – A skilled strategist and a risk taker. New approaches to problems and challenging issues drive him. A competitive team player who, if given the chance, will shape the approach taken by others. Simple solutions may be overlooked, as he thrives on complexity.

The craftsman – This creative individual has high personal standards and is often better working alone. However, he may be a good teacher if others are prepared and able to follow his instruction.

harmless. Male bonding, involving talk of sport and sexual conquests, and sexual teasing of women, asserts the heterosexuality of male participants.

◆ **The gender blind** Gender issues are completely overlooked and neglected in this type of organization. Everyone is treated the same, regardless of any real differences. It is not only gender issues that are ignored, but also differences associated with, for example, physical disability and race. Everyone is treated as if they are male, white and able bodied. There is a blind spot associated with any difference and diversity among the membership of the organization. Working conditions and work practices are not addressed in terms of the needs of individuals, nor identifiable groups of workers.

◆ **Lip service, feminist pretenders and equality experts** Individuals may be self-serving and assume respectability under the auspices of equal opportunities while discouraging any real change. They may, for example, develop a range of equal opportunity policies promoting women's equal rights, but do little or nothing to raise awareness nor alter the prevailing culture of the organization.

Some organizations become highly politicized: the extensive use of politically correct language and the promotion of minority interests become ends in themselves. These highly moralistic cultures may develop equality experts in a hierarchy of oppression, featuring, for example, women, blacks, gays, the disabled, disfigured and so forth. Often this leads to restrictive practices, as individuals are expected to conform to alternative radical stereotypes regardless of their needs and point of view.

◆ **The smart macho** These are highly competitive organizations where individuals are under constant pressure to achieve targets and goals in the name of efficiency, effectiveness and profit. The culture favours those who are able to work excessively long hours and deliver at a rate and pace that others cannot maintain. Single-minded, ruthless, and aggressive behaviours are personal characteristics often associated with extreme competitiveness.

THE GENDER CULTURE

These approaches are helpful in understanding different aspects of organizational life but do not specifically address issues pertaining to the sexual health of the organization. Itzin (1995) takes an alternative approach, describing 'the gender culture', a culture common to all organizations. Here gender issues and sexual health characteristics provide a framework for understanding the organization. Usually this culture remains unarticulated. It is regarded as natural, the way of things and inevitable: *it is natural so you cannot change it.*

The gender culture includes each of the following characteristics:

◆ Hierarchical and patriarchal
◆ Sex-segregated
◆ Sexual division of labour
◆ Sex-stereotyped
◆ Sex discriminatory
◆ Sexualized environment
◆ Sexual harassment
◆ Sexist
◆ Misogynist
◆ Resistant to change
◆ Gendered power.

These will all be present in some form or another and have different implications for both men and women within the organization (Table 6.3). The extent and form of expression for each characteristic will vary between organizations in relation to other internal and external factors. An understanding of how these characteristics, together with those described by Handy and Mintzberg, shape an organization is a prerequisite to the successful management of organizational change.

 Learning activity 6.3

Look at Table 6.3. Consider the gender culture of your organization. Write down as many different factors as you can relating to the 11 characteristics of the gender culture. Try this exercise with groups of men and women. What would you expect from the different groups? Compare the results. Are they similar to what you expected? If not, how are they different?

ASSUMPTIONS ABOUT ORGANIZATIONS

Typologies are helpful in developing an awareness of how organizations function. They help to explain the relationships between organizational structures and cultures and the values and practices of the people who work in them. However, one of the main problems with any typology or classification system is that it may limit, restrict or define the way in which things are viewed within the classification. Views may be based on assumptions associated with the way it has been classified, rather than on the attributes of the organization itself.

Newman (1996) is critical of models of organizational culture found in traditional management texts and identifies a number of erroneous assumptions that underlie such models. These assumptions need to be addressed and challenged as a prerequisite to understanding organizational change.

Table 6.3 The gender culture

Characteristic	Men	Women
Hierarchical and patriarchal	Top of the hierarchy: positions of power and influence Have access to information Control information Gatekeepers to training and promotion opportunities	Lower down the hierarchy: subordinate social, political and economic positions
Sex-segregated	Higher wages: architecture, engineering, business development and planning	Lower wages: cleaning, catering, caring, teaching, home care
External sexual division of labour	Full-time work Continuity of employment Variety of career opportunities	Part-time work Breaks in employment Restricted career opportunities Domestic responsibilities Child care, elder care
Sex-stereotyped	Breadwinner	Supportive to male partners and family
Sex discriminatory	Favours men	Covert/overt barriers to recruitment, training and career opportunities
Sexualized environment	Represents heterosexual male interests	Sexualized in the workplace Sexual language Portrayal of sex objects 'Pin-ups' and pornography
Sexual harassment	Perpetrators	Victims/recipients
Sexist	More valued and valuable	Less valued and valuable
Misogynist	Men and masculinity are the norm	Women and femininity associated with negative attributes
Resistant to change	Maintain barriers to equal opportunities through subversion and sabotage	High personal cost of change Difficult to influence and effect change
Gendered power	Determined and exercised by men Maintains subordination of women Difficult to be 'one of the boys' and break ranks against male power	Women excluded

Assumption 1: Cultures are 'closed societies'

Often organizations are examined as if they existed in a bubble or vacuum, separate or sealed off from the world outside. This may lead to intro-spection: a disproportionately narrow focus on the internal issues, conflicts and concerns of the organization.

Assumption 2: Cultures are 'integrated wholes'

The idea of a 'corporate culture' suggests that all areas within an organization are unified and integrated under one overarching cultural umbrella. Overemphasis on this homogeneous organizational culture leads to neglect of the influence of subcultures. There may be strong organizational boundaries between different groups. Organizational divisions, departments and sections, various functional and professional groupings, different sites, areas and geographical locations may each develop a 'house style', adopt various interpretations of practices and procedures, promoting their values and beliefs. There may be 'cross-cutting cultures' that evolve because of or in spite of the formal organizational boundaries. Examples include the child care social activities involving parents, special-interest groups, sports clubs or teams. The dynamic interplay of subcultures may allow boundaries to shift and change, and ultimately affect the wider organizational culture.

Assumption 3: Cultures 'are consensual'

The notion of a 'corporate spirit' implies shared values, with consensus and continuity across the organization. However, organizational politics, conflict and revolutionary factors play a key part in many if not all organizations. Tensions at the margins or between groups often becomes the defining characteristics of those groups. Tension and conflict, for example, between new values and traditional values, or resistance against authority, are most apparent during periods of organizational crisis and change.

Assumption 4: Culture 'is objective reality'

The culture of an organization may be seen as something separate and distinct from those who work in that organization. Culture is seen as if it exists and has a life of its own, regardless of any human effort or intervention.

Assumption 5: Culture 'is static'

Culture is treated as if it is an inanimate object, ready to be taken and shaped by those with authority. This is very different from saying culture is resistant to change. Just as there are forces for change, equally there are forces against change. However, these are active dynamic processes. Something may go through a process of change but the core elements or key factors may remain: the form is transmuted and reinvented.

Assumption 6: Culture 'can be changed through new symbols'

Symbols may provide a powerful representation of an organization, for example a leader, a figure-head, publication of the visions, value or mission statement, upgrading of interior decor, standardization and revision of publicity materials, and the introduction of new uniforms. Attempts to change the organization by changing these symbolic representations alone are unlikely to be effective. Organizational symbols, practices and values need to be addressed together in a coordinated attempt to bring about organizational change.

WHAT IS A SUCCESSFUL ORGANIZATION?

Different factors associated with successful organizations include the general environment, management style, human resources and organizational structure (Table 6.4). For example, the structure of the organization may be 'narrow', with a steep hierarchical structure, or 'wide' with a flattened hierarchy. There are advantages and disadvantages associated with each type of structure (Table 6.5).

Reflection point 6.1

Sexual health encompasses a number of rights (RCN 1996):

1. The right to be a sexual being

2. The right to access appropriate information and resources to enable sexual safety, and to access appropriate services

3. The right not to be at the mercy of other individuals' sexual attitudes

4. The right not to be sexually harassed, exploited or assaulted

5. The right to confidentiality and sensitive information gathering.

In your reflective journal, write down how you might challenge each of these assumptions in relation to the rights of sexual health.

Assumption 1: Cultures are 'closed societies'

Assumption 2: Cultures are integrated wholes

Assumption 3: Cultures are consensual

Assumption 4: Culture is objective reality

Assumption 5: Culture is static

Assumption 6: Culture can be changed through new symbols.

The successful organization depends on the dynamic relationship between the common at-tributes and characteristics described above. It is the arrangement of these factors in relation to each other that makes an organization success-ful, rather than the presence or absence of particu-lar factors or the effect of a single factor. A successful organization will adapt and survive in a changing environment. It can change itself and survive by promoting internal consistency and integration between and within these common factors.

Viewed in this way it is clear that, in order to survive, organizations need to change as their environment changes. Successful organizations are those that can manage change and manage to change successfully. Mintzberg (1989) suggests that organizations change through periodic revitalization, quantum leaps and strategic revolu-tion from one configuration to another, rather than through a slow and gradual evolution involv-ing continual adaptation and change. A single major change can maintain internal consistency and may be more efficient, even though the organization will appear out of keeping with the external world.

Success depends on the right mix of these fac-tors at the right time. Each individual has their own feel or preference for a particular style or cul-ture. It is becoming increasingly important for individuals to get the right match with different organizational cultures in order to make progress through their careers. The success of the organiza-tion is directly related to the success of the people in the organization. Individuals, whatever their own personal preference, function best where they are acknowledged and valued for their contribution.

Table 6.4 Successful organizations

Environment	Management	Structure	Human resources
Customer oriented	Needs effective leadership	Simple in structure	Trusted and trusting
Proàctive	Designed for doing rather than talking	Allows responsible autonomy for staff	Takes a long-term view
Clear business or service focus		Allows control, enables flexibility	Achieve through consensus

Table 6.5 Organizations with narrow and wide spans

| Narrow span | | Wide span | |
Advantages	Disadvantages	Advantages	Disadvantages
Close supervision Close control Fast communication between subordinates and superiors	Superiors tend to get too involved in subordinates' work Many levels of management High costs owing to many levels of management Excessive distance between lowest level and top level	Superiors forced to delegate Clear policies have to be made Subordinates must be carefully selected	Tendency of overloaded superiors to become decision bottlenecks Danger of superior's loss of control Requires exceptional quality of manager

Learning activity 6.4

A successful organization is likely to take positive steps to promote sexual health. The rights (RCN 1996) identified as themes throughout this book provide a means of assessing the success of your organization (see Reflection point 6.1).

Copy the diagram below and rate your organization on each of these five rights with a mark out of 10. Plot these marks on to each of the spokes in the wheel, which represent the five rights. The full circle represents the potential shape of sexual health within the organization.

What sort of shape is your organization in? How successful would you say it is? What are the implications for clients, customers and patients? What measures could you suggest to improve the score for each of the rights in order to contribute to an overall improvement in the sexual health of your organization?

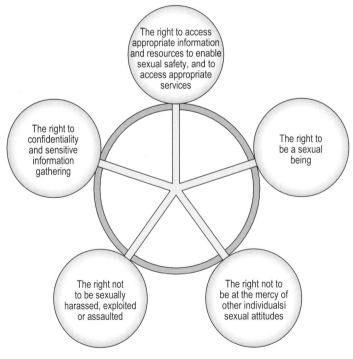

Fig. 6.1 The organizational wheel of sexual health.

EXCLUSION

Most, if not all, of the different types of culture described above exclude women in a variety of ways. Exclusion underpins many workplace behaviours, for example behaviours involving sexual harassment, bullying and some forms of sex discrimination. In order to promote sexual health in the workplace we need to understand the concept of exclusion in relation to these behaviours. Lemert's notion of the dynamics of exclusion is described here as it offers a means of understanding these complex organizational behaviours.

Lemert (1969) approaches the process of exclusion from the perspective of the paranoid person, and the development of paranoid relationships within organizations. Paranoid reactions, paranoid states, and paranoid personality encapsulate a diverse range of behaviours, including suspicion, envy, jealousy, antagonism, stubbornness, hostility and aggression through to delusions – fixed false beliefs – and ideas of reference, where some personal significance is identified in distant events or actions. Paranoid behaviours vary: there is no precise definition.

The paranoid person attributes to others negative attitudes and beliefs that he or she holds towards him or herself. This process of attribution becomes generalized, so that these cognitions organize the way the paranoid person views the world. This way of seeing the world is not accessible to others and cannot be shared. The paranoid person will experience this as active contradiction by others – further evidence that they are united against him or her.

Paranoid relationships

Rather than see paranoia solely as an attribute of a disturbed individual, Lemert (1969) focuses on paranoid behaviour as a function of a social relationship, in particular as a social process of exclusion. He refers to a paranoid relationship involving *reciprocating behaviours* between the individual and others. In this instance 'others' includes another individual or group within the same social environment as the paranoid person. These reciprocating behaviours are a central fea-

ture of this relationship. They are also characteristic of other complex forms of organizational behaviour.

Different perspectives

Reciprocating behaviours are seen from one of two different perspectives:

1. The individual's behaviour as perceived by others. This involves:
   ◆ 'a disregard for the values and norms of the primary group, revealed by giving priority to verbally definable values over those which are implicit, a lack of loyalty in return for confidences, and victimising and intimidating persons in positions of weakness'
   ◆ 'a disregard for the implicit structure of groups, revealed by presuming to privileges not accorded him (or her), and the threat or actual resort to formal means for achieving his (or her) goals.'
2. The behaviour of others as perceived by the individual. The individual will experience the spurious quality of the interaction between others and himself (or herself) or between others interacting in their presence; interactions and general communication will involve:
   ◆ the overt avoidance of himself (or herself) by others
   ◆ the structured exclusion of himself (or herself) from interaction.

The process begins with interpersonal difficulties associated with the threat or actual loss of status for the individual. These reciprocating behaviours and lack of mutually perceived trust characterize the disruptive process of exclusion which leads to the paranoid relationship.

Spurious interaction

Lemert (1969) describes a chain of interactions that are part of a transformation from inclusion to exclusion. The perception others have of an individual's behaviour changes from a variation of normal, routine or expected behaviour to behaviour characteristic of a spurious relationship. This relationship is false, deceptive, deceitful, phoney, fictitious or feigned. Interactions are characterized by patronizing, evasion, guarding reactions, increased silences, intimidation, threat, marginalization and put-downs. All of these behaviours decrease the level and quality of interaction within the relationship. Lemert asserts that 'this kind of spurious interaction is one of the most difficult for an adult in our society to cope with, because it complicates or makes decisions impossible for him (or her) and also because it is morally invidious'.

Interactions restrict access to individual and group values, and may have a protective function at the same time as an excluding function. Perceptual reorientation is brought about through continuous interaction and new biographical information. Vacillation may be common: both parties may feel guilt and anxiety as a result of their behaviour.

The dynamics of exclusion

Exclusion involves a distortion in the balance of social relationships, which become redefined, through the manipulation of norms of reciprocity, in terms of perpetrator self-interest. There is no single nor simple way out, no 'win–win' solution, because of the multiplicity of factors involved.

The excluding group forms a coalition to oppose the individual. Group cohesion has a conspiratorial nature based on loyalty, solidarity, secrecy, manipulation and misrepresentation. The group will take active measures to gain consensus for their view, which may include isolating and silencing those who do not share this view, presenting the appearance of unanimity, developing contingency plans for a range of possible eventualities, introducing rules to restrict behaviour, changing dates and times of meetings, and not passing on messages. This may be maintained over a considerable period of time, and is likely to escalate into an intolerable situation where something must be done. The reciprocating behaviours of the individual and the group may raise intolerable anxieties, leaving no choice but to take action: the group may take action against the individual; the individual or group may go to a higher authority, or to an authority outside the organ-

ization. The escalation of these behaviours and events may lead to an organizational crisis.

The process of exclusion is common with sexual harassment, sex discrimination and bullying. Each is a form of organizational behaviour that results from a process of exclusion where individuals and groups are caught up in a series of reciprocal behaviours and spurious relationships. These behaviours are not clear or distinct types, nor are they mutually exclusive: for instance, bullying is often a component of sex discrimination and sexual harassment. Harlow et al. (1996) address the use of silence as a form of bullying and sexual harassment, e.g. men refusing to acknowledge women in the corridor, or respond to their greetings. It hard to complain that someone will not speak to you. Depending on the context, this may be reported as sex discrimination, sexual harassment or bullying.

SEXUAL HARASSMENT

Sexual harassment is usually addressed in terms of unwanted heterosexual advances by men towards women. Although this is the most frequently encountered situation, sexual harassment is not restricted to this pattern: the perpetrator may be female, the victim male; and both men and women may experience homosexual advances (Schneider, 1982).

Identification and definition

The nature and extent of experiences associated with sexual harassment are difficult to assess. There is no generally accepted shared terminology nor means of categorization for the experience of harassment. However, definitions of harassment and their interpretation in practice are usually set in terms of equal opportunities, organizational policy and employment law. Lay and feminist definitions of sexual harassment usually view it as an exclusively male behaviour, but legislation and policy protocols may not stipulate the sex of either the perpetrator or the victim of harassment.

Courts define sexual harassment at work as 'any unwelcome sexually oriented behaviour, demand, comment, or physical contact, initiated by an individual at the workplace, that is a term or condition of employment, a basis for employment decisions, or that interferes with the employee's work or creates a hostile or offensive working environment' (Lloyd 1991, p. 7).

The focus is on the specific incident or behaviour, and not on the past history, behaviour or relationship between the parties. What constitutes 'unwelcome sexual behaviour' is often quite subjective and dependent on the perception of the individual recipient or victim.

Different perceptions

Studies of sexual harassment address the perception of behaviours in terms of how they come to be labelled as particular types. For example, differences in the way men and women perceive behaviours associated with sexual harassment have been identified. Men are less likely to report instances of sexual harassment than women, as they perceive situations as being less sexually harassing than do women (Gutek et al. 1983, Pryor 1985). Gutek et al. (1983) used scenarios or hypothetical situations in a survey of sexual harassment and found that sexual advances from a woman to a man are seen as less disturbing by both sexes than the same advances from a man to a woman.

Studies also report conflicting results. Some suggest that the greater the difference in power between the perpetrator and victim, the greater the likelihood that the behaviour will be described as harassment (Reilly et al. 1982, Gutek et al. 1983). Others suggest that the perpetrator is more likely to be the victim's peer and colleague than their superior (Gutek and Morasch 1982). However, any previous relationship between the perpetrator and the victim, and any suggestive or 'encouraging' behaviour on the part of the victim or recipient, reduces the likelihood that the perpetrator's behaviour will be seen as sexual harassment (Reilly et al. 1982).

Pryor and Day (1988) look at the attribution of causality in sexual harassment. They hypothesize that the cause of the key actor's behaviour, whether they are the perpetrator or the victim, will be attributed to characteristics of the other party. They report that judgements of sexual harassment are influenced strongly by the perspective taken, whether this is perspective of the perpetrator or that of the victim. Subjects tend to empathize with one individual, seeing this individual's behaviour in terms of the situation and circumstances, rather than attributing the cause of the behaviour to any personal characteristics or disposition of that individual. However, the behaviour of the other is attributed to their personal disposition and characteristics.

Both men and women are more likely to interpret the perpetrator's social sexual behaviour as harassment if it is attributed to enduring negative intentions and factors, including hostility, insensitivity or callousness toward the victim (Pryor and Day 1988).

Williams and Cyr (1992) report that men appear more likely to interpret ambiguous friendly behaviours as sexual, whereas women may be more likely to see a male's ambiguous sexual behaviours as provocative but harmless or friendly. They argue that it is precisely these divergent interpretations that facilitate and perpetuate instances of sexual harassment. Both male and female parties wrongly assume they share a common understanding and perspective on their relationship. From this initial ambiguity develops the relationship between the male perpetrator and the female victim. There are similarities between the ambiguity of the relationship between perpetrator and victim in sexual harassment and the spurious relationship described in Lemert's account of paranoia. The emphasis on the different perspectives of the victim and the perpetrator in sexual harassment (Pryor and Day 1988) reflects the different perspectives taken by the individual and others in the excluding relationship described by Lemert (1969). The perpetrator may be excluded from the victim's perspective, as is the victim from the perpetrator's perspective.

The cycle of sexual harassment

Sexual harassment has been described both in terms of the development of social relationship and in terms of specific behaviours that constitute sexual harassment. Williams and Cyr (1992) address the social relationship. Using different scenarios of sexual harassment, they report how escalating negative relationships between male perpetrator and female target or victim are associated with an increasing commitment to the relationship on the part of the target. These factors illustrate the process of exclusion within a cycle where sexual harassment involves reciprocating behaviours in an increasingly negative and spurious relationship, the development of which may be described in terms of three phases:

Phase 1: the victim experiences persistent exposure to mild innocuous sexual innuendoes. They adjust by tolerating this continued exposure in order to maintain the relationship. The perpetrator interprets this 'doing nothing' as the victim's willingness to continue the relationship.

Phase 2: The perpetrator's sexual behaviours intensify but lack any obvious negative intentions. The victim is uncomfortable with this behaviour but adjusts, gradually complying with and accepting the situation in order to maintain the social relationship. They may not define the behaviour in terms of sexual harassment, being able to maintain a consistent view of the relationship, for example by discounting the perpetrator's behaviour as something provoked by the victim's own behaviour, or by emphasizing the benefits of maintaining the relationship against the costs of leaving it. In maintaining the relationship the victim may inadvertently be encouraging the perpetrator and colluding with their belief that their behaviour is appropriate and justified.

Phase 3: The relationship develops into a self-perpetuating cycle, a vicious circle from which it is difficult for the victim to withdraw without blame for the consequences of the perpetrator's actions. Having accepted the perpetrator's behaviour in the past it becomes more difficult for the victim to decline advances of increasing intensity without the situation reaching a crisis.

TYPES OF SEXUAL HARASSMENT

The lack of agreed definition for behaviours involved in sexual harassment contributes to the

---

> **Box 6.2** Sexual harassment behaviours
>
> I Verbal requests
>   Sexual bribery
>   Sexual advances
>   Relational advances
>   Subtle advances/pressures
> I: Sexual remarks/comments
>   Personal remarks
>   Subjective objectification
>   Sexual categorical remarks
> III Non-verbal displays
>   Sexual assault
>   Sexual touching
>   Sexual posturing
>   Sexual materials

complexity of the problem. Gruber (1992) describes a classification system for sexual harassment behaviours based on a content analysis of material, including surveys, personal accounts, court decisions and equal opportunities guidelines. Three general forms (see Box 6.2) are identified:

◆ Requests, which have relationship-oriented goals
◆ Remarks, which are expressions of sexual interest/humiliation of the victim
◆ Non-verbal displays of behaviour.

These three forms incorporate 11 distinct categories of sexual harassment behaviour, identified in terms of increasing severity. The severity of the experience increases as the perpetrator's behaviour takes a more personal and sexual focus on the recipient.

Verbal requests

Sexual bribery

This is the most severe form of request: the promise of reward in exchange for sex and/or threat of punishment for refusing sex – an overt 'quid pro quo'. Punishment may include the withholding of information or training essential for performance of the work role. Rewards may include money or promotion. This is the clearest examples of sexual harassment. Differences in power and status between perpetrator and victim are evident.

Sexual advances

The perpetrator solicits or demands a sexual relationship. This usually involves a single request or repeated requests through the use of romantic symbolism, threatening or intimate sexual language. Requests may be crude and direct, or romantic and humorous. Each request breaches sexual privacy and the usual social relationships. This does not involve the 'quid pro quo' described above.

Relational advances

These are not directly sexual, but may be more harassing in that they are persistent and frequent. They are unlikely to be regarded as harassment unless repeated, e.g. face-to-face contact, telephone calls, letters. The perpetrator's goal is a social encounter with the victim. The intrusive nature of these advances may be masked as routine and acceptable within social norms.

Subtle advances/pressures

The goal or target is not stated by the perpetrator. Requests are subtle, implied rather than direct, e.g. double entendres, innuendo, humorous comments, questions, comments and assumptions about sexual behaviour.

Sexual remarks/comments

Personal remarks

Remarks made to a woman which are offensive or embarrassing or demeaning and humiliating, for example sexual jokes, personal questions, teasing. Comments may focus on the woman's sexuality or appearance. They may be humorous, thoughtless, inconsiderate jokes or direct insults.

Subjective objectification

As above, but these comments are made about a woman, rather than directly to her. The woman is discussed by others in her presence, or sexual rumours about her are spread about the workplace. The woman is effectively excluded – treated as if invisible or a non-person.

Sexual categorical remarks

Non-personal misogynist statements degrading women generally, or comments that objectify women, are directed at an individual woman. Such comments may be made to the victim about other groups of women or individual women, and include comments about female anatomy. They differ from sexist comments in that they are directed at an individual.

Non-verbal displays

Sexual assault

The most severe form of behaviour in this group includes all actions of a sexual nature involving physical force, aggression and coercion. Examples include actual or attempted sexual intercourse, or groping of the victim's sexual anatomy.

Sexual touching

Physical contact with the sexual anatomy or sexualized contact, e.g. offensive touches on the arms, legs, back; hugs and 'friendly' embraces. The context as experienced by the victim is important in this category.

Sexual posturing

Gestures or behaviours of a sexual nature not involving physical contact but carried out in the presence of a woman. They constitute an invasion of personal space and are oriented towards the victim. Non-contact harassment includes looks, stares, gestures, following, cornering and feigned contact in relation to the victim. Non-contact sexual posturing may also include the woman as a 'bystander' in the sexual harassment of others.

Sexual materials

May be non-personal but have an enduring presence in the work environment, e.g. sexual graffiti and pornographic pictures. They may be directed personally at an individual woman, e.g. being shown pornographic material, or being described in sexual graffiti.

Case study 6.1

A female staff nurse based on a surgical ward dealing with cardiothoracic illness reports her experience of sexual harassment at work.

'I was used to being in charge most weekends when the ward was run on a skeleton crew. There was one registrar who worked on the unit and was known as a bit of a slimeball. He would do things like hold his body close to mine when I needed to check a patient's prescription. It really was unnecessary. He would lean across me while I was writing notes – to reach for the phone or something – but he would press himself against me. It was disgusting. He would always read things into what you said – seeing a double meaning – sexual innuendo – where clearly none was intended. You know the sort of thing: I'd be describing a patient with a large swollen area around their wound and he would say, 'I bet you like them large and swollen – you know I've got a big one just for you' – really gross behaviour. Another time he commented on my perfume and how sexy he found it, using it as an excuse to stand in really close to me. He would leer at me and make as if he was going to kiss me.

'I thought it was important not to let on that it bothered me, and hoped he would go away. I tried to keep cool about it. It did make me nervous though, and sometimes I felt apprehensive about going to work. I never changed my shifts though, but some of my colleagues would try to swap if they knew he was covering the unit. It seemed to happen to everyone. Anyway, one evening I was invited over to a barbecue at the doctors' mess by a couple of the female doctors. He was there and came and sat in the same comfy chair as*

me. He put his arms around me and licked the side of my face. It was horrible. The more I tried to stop him the more it seemed to egg him on. He somehow got me on to the ground and was sat on top of me. By this stage my friends, who had been in the kitchen, came outside and realized things were getting out of hand. They pulled him off. I told him that if he ever did anything like that again I would report him. They supported me, saying that they would be my witnesses. He never bothered me again but he still has a bad reputation.'

Here the perpetrator's behaviour may have been encouraged by the victim's determination to 'keep cool' and not show it bothered her. Both have quite different perspectives on the behaviour, which included personal remarks on the perfume and presumed sexual preferences of the victim, sexual posturing, sexual touching and sexual comments. The relationship develops through the different phases described in the text, finishing in a crisis situation experienced by the victim as physical sexual assault. The threat of being reported and the weight of the corroborative witness evidence finally breaks the cycle of harassment.

Reflection point 6.2

Think about whether or not you have had any similar experience to the one in Case study 6.1. What phases were involved in your experience and how did you deal with it? At what point were you able to break into the sexual harassment cycle, and were you alone in doing this or did you get help? After considering the case study and your own personal experience of sexual harassment, how might you manage this experience differently in the future?

BULLYING

Bullying may be distinguished from sexual harassment and sex discrimination. This distinction may be clear when the behaviour is associated with individuals and groups of the same sex, or where the behaviours are not sexualized to a great extent; however, bullying may also include sexual harassment between parties of the same or opposite sex. It may also include sex discrimination. The commonalties include behaviours where the perpetrator holds enduring negative intentions and shows hostility, insensitivity and callousness toward the victim.

Bullying involves an abuse of power and status, leading to the active exclusion of an individual by another individual or group. The perpetrator may hold a position of power, having a higher status and greater formal authority over the target or victim. They may be a colleague, peer or co-worker who asserts power and authority over the victim, and may be a single individual or a group.

Envy, fear or threat are possible motivating factors for the perpetrator, who may see the victim as a threat, either too confident, too successful, too promising, too popular or too able. The perpetrator's behaviour is calculated to keep the victim or recipient in his or her place, or worse, to humiliate and degrade them by exploiting weakness in others. Bullying behaviour patterns may be well established in the perpetrator. Whatever the individual motives and perceptions, bullying is seldom as simple as one individual abusing another: many people may be involved, wittingly or unwittingly being caught up in a web of deceit and collusion.

The effects may be serious both for the individuals involved and for the organization as a whole. Bullying can reduce otherwise competent and able people to a level where they lack self-confidence, lose motivation and lose interest in work. The results include stress, poor performance, absenteeism, increased illness, disturbed sleep and increased anxiety. In addition to the intense psychological trauma, victims of workplace bullying may have to contend with the effects of sickness, redundancy, redeployment and transfer. They easily become disadvantaged through lost career opportunities, and may suffer from the consequences of bullying for a long time after the event. However, it is possible for them to build up their self-confidence again, although this takes time and effort. They may become more assertive and intolerant of workplace bullying among managers, peers and subordinates in their future careers.

Identification and definition

Bullying is usually identified in terms of interpersonal relationships rather than as an organizational characteristic. However, organizations can create environments that are hostile and intimidating, for example the bullying of the 'barrack yard' culture described by Parkin and Maddock (1995). Bullying behaviour is a threat to individual and organizational values, it blocks and undermines routine work practices, and breaches acceptable behaviour. It may lead to a situation best described in terms of psychological warfare and organizational crisis.

Organizations and employers are becoming increasingly aware of the problems associated with bullying and their responsibilities towards employees. The Manufacturing, Science and Finance Union (MSF) defines bullying as 'persistent, offensive, abusive, intimidating, malicious or insulting behaviour, abuse of power or unfair penal sanctions, which makes the recipient feel upset, threatened, humiliated or vulnerable, which undermines their self-confidence and which may cause them to suffer stress'.

Adams (1992) defines bullying as 'the persistent demeaning and downgrading of human beings through vicious words and cruel unseen acts which gradually undermine their [the victim] confidence and self-esteem'. Definitions emphasize the effect of the behaviour on the victim while identifying the behaviour of the perpetrator or perpetrators in broad terms.

Under regulations of the Health and Safety at Work Act 1974 employers have a duty to provide a safe working environment. A breach of this legislation can result in criminal prosecution and be costly in terms of damages awarded to individuals. If employers fail to intervene and deal with the problem they may breach the implied duty of mutual trust and confidence. For example, failure to follow up an employee's complaint about bullying could result in civil proceedings on grounds of stress, personal injury and unfair constructive dismissal.

Different perceptions

Bullying behaviours need to be viewed in the context of the relationship between the victim or recipient, the perpetrator and others. The behaviours may result in the victim being sidelined, put down in meetings or being set up to fail. The bullying relationship takes on elements of the paranoid relationship described earlier. The victim is likely to become preoccupied with the relationship, and may develop an acute awareness of the significance and meaning of the behaviour which appears out of proportion to the actual behaviour. Any action by the victim to avoid or limit the bullying behaviour may be seen by others as further evidence of paranoia. This in turn increases the victim's sense of paranoia. The reciprocating behaviours develop into a spurious relationship and the victim is excluded. This can be perceived as having similarities to situations of sexual harassment.

The vacillation described by Lemert (1969) is common. The victim may feel angry about how they are being treated and guilty that they are to blame for the perpetrator's behaviour, or that they should do something about it.

Others' perception of the behaviour will, like the perception of sexual harassment, be dependent on the perspective taken, i.e. that of the victim or that of the perpetrator. Those taking the perpetrator perspective may become embroiled in conspiracy or collusion; others may be aware of the situation but withdraw from it, excluding themselves in order not to become involved.

TYPES OF BULLYING BEHAVIOUR

It may be difficult to identify bullying behaviour, as a behaviour perceived by others as socially acceptable may be experienced as harassment or bullying by the recipient or victim. The behaviour itself may appear ordinary, inoffensive and innocuous. Sometimes subtle and intangible, bullying may go unrecognized and unreported. However, it is persistent and persecutory. A chronic social relationship may develop between perpetrator and victim.

Bullying behaviour includes aggression, rudeness, being abrupt, cutting short, sarcastic comments, shouting, highlighting shortcomings in front of others, taking away responsibility, ignoring or devaluing success and achievements, changing goalposts, denying a sense of achievement, general putting down, destructive criticism and actual physical abuse.

Insulting, arrogant and presumptuous behaviours may be confined to interactions with the victim. In the company of others the behaviour may be acceptable and usual: to others the bullying person may appear courteous, kind and considerate.

Some of the behaviours described by Gruber (1992) in relation to sexual harassment and sex discrimination include behaviours involved in bullying. Certain categories from this framework are helpful in identifying types of bullying behaviour. Five different categories under two general forms of the sexual harassment typology are applicable to bullying behaviour.

1. Remarks/comments
   ◆ Personal remarks
   ◆ Subjective objectification
   ◆ Categorical remarks
2. Non-verbal displays
   ◆ Assault
   ◆ Posturing.

Remarks/Comments

Personal remarks

These are directed at the victim and include personal digs and 'nit-picking', subtle expressions, innuendo, humorous comments, taunts, comments and assumptions about the victim's behaviour. Remarks may be calculated to publicly offend or embarrass; they may be demeaning and humiliating. They may be humorous, thoughtless, inconsiderate jokes or direct insults. For example, in Brearley v WM Morrisons Supermarkets plc (COIT 3073/168B) a manager called the individual 'brain dead' and 'illiterate' in front of subordinates.

Often these personal remarks will be made to test the victim. The perpetrator may focus on an insignificant personal detail, for instance perhaps finding fault in the way a brooch is pinned or a tie knotted. This may have the effect of demeaning the victim but give poor grounds for complaint. If they do complain about such an insignificant issue they risk laying themselves open to further humiliation.

Subjective objectification

These behaviours are not aimed directly at the victim, for example comments made to others about the victim. The victim is discussed by others in his or her presence or malicious rumours about them are spread about the workplace. The victim is excluded: treated as if they were not there, or as if they do not matter. This disruption of the work environment may also involve, for example, increasing noise levels in the office or rearranging furniture.

Categorical remarks

Again, these are non-personal statements that degrade a social group or activity with which the victim is involved. Comments are directed at the victim and may be associated with their sexual identity, their role models or their achievements. For example, a perpetrator described a professional journal as not worth the paper it was written on, a week after the victim's article was published.

Non-verbal displays

Assault

The most severe form of behaviour in this group includes any action involving physical force, aggression or coercion. For example, in Hatrick *v* City Fax (COIT 3041/138H) the victim had her hair forcibly cut by colleagues. Other cases report a series of physical assaults, including cleaning fluid being added to the victim's tea (Brearley *v* WM Morrisons Supermarkets plc, COIT 3073/168B), scalding and burns through deliberate and malicious intervention, grease being added to the victim's sandwiches, their car being tampered with, personal possessions being covered in paint, physical assault with a weapon, and hospitalization of the victim (Evans *v* Sawley Packaging Co. Ltd, COIT 2916/185E).

Posturing

Of a threatening and aggressive nature, not involving physical contact but carried out in the presence of the victim. This constitutes an invasion of personal space and is oriented towards the victim. Non-contact gestures or behaviours include certain looks and glances, e.g. aggressively narrowing the eyes, staring, gestures, the victim being followed, being unacknowledged and ignored, and threats of physical violence to the victim.

THE JOHARI WINDOW

The Johari window (Luft and Ingham 1977) is a useful tool for analysing interpersonal interactions between oneself and others. It is particularly useful in developing an understanding of difficult situations involving conflict, including sexual harassment and bullying. Such an understanding may raise awareness of the effect of one's own behaviour and the behaviour of others, and contribute towards the effective reduction or containment of conflict.

The 'window' has four cells in a two by two arrangement (Fig. 6.2).

	Known to others about self	Not known to others about self
Known to self about self	Open self	Closed self
Not known to self about self	Blind self	Undiscovered self

Fig. 6.2 The Johari window.

Open self Here knowledge about yourself is known by you and by others. Openness relates to personal awareness and trusting relationships. In this situation there is little conflict in relations with others.

Blind self Here you are unaware of how others see you and your behaviour. Conflict may arise through your own lack of awareness of how others see you, or how you or your behaviour come across to others.

Closed self Here you have knowledge about yourself that is not known to others. This remains undisclosed. You may be concealing information or waiting for a more appropriate time to disclose it. It is possible that true feelings and desires are being concealed, for whatever reason. This could lead to personal conflict, perhaps embarrassment, misunderstandings and misinterpretations.

Undiscovered self This covers areas which are not known to you about yourself, or to others about yourself. It is an area of potential, experiences yet to be lived.

Learning activity 6.5

Think of a situation where you have experienced some conflict at work and try to analyse it using the Johari window as a framework. Are you able to identify your 'closed' self in operation, for example? After completing the analysis, suggest ways in which you might have adapted your behaviour in order to elicit a more appropriate response from others.

Case study 6.2

The following personal account highlights the experience of a male victim bullied by a female colleague.

'She is very clever and gets others to do her dirty work. She makes the bullets and he fires them. You cannot pin anything on her. I don't think even he realizes what is going on. They appear as nice as pie to others. It makes my complaints all the more unlikely. Like the week I did a case presentation to the team. It's quite a big thing – the patient is there and the consultant and managers from different units. I was really pleased with how it went and had some good feedback. Its quite something to get asked to do it. Anyway, later that week I heard her talking to the others, saying that they hadn't missed anything and had been better off sorting out the patients' notes. And just as*

I feel I am getting somewhere, you know, more confident with myself, it all goes sour again.

'My boss was totally unsympathetic, said I had to sort it out myself. Well I really didn't see how I could but felt I had no choice. I tried confronting her [the bully]. She laughed at me, continued to put me down, saying I was too sensitive, imagining things and paranoid. She said no-one likes me, and that I didn't contribute anything to the team.

'At the worst times I feel I am losing my grip on reality – I cannot judge whether I am making rational judgements or not. Sometimes I get really upset and quite angry – how dare they do this to me! You do feel driven to do something desperate – murderous even. But there is nowhere for all that to go and you end up feeling even worse. It all just sounds so stupid and petty when you actually list what they do.'

The victim reported increased anxiety, for example constantly checking and double-checking his work, having lost confidence in his own ability. Fear and intimidation played a key role. He believed that the perpetrator would notice any little mistake and use it against him. Over a period of about 6 months he suffered from disturbed sleep, increased alcohol intake, loss of motivation and constant anxiety. He feared going to work, considered going off sick for weeks at a time, and felt a drain and a burden on his family. He contacted the personnel office at work and, through his trade union, arranged to see a counsellor away from the organization. However, relationships at work seemed beyond repair, and he decided the best option was to leave. He was successful in obtaining another, more senior and responsible position in a different organization.

POSSIBLE SOLUTIONS TO SEXUAL HARASSMENT AND BULLYING

Any solution must provide a means of breaking out of the cycle of exclusion. There is no single or simple solution: by the time the situation has been defined in terms of bullying, sexual harassment or discrimination it is likely to be complex, involving a matrix of negative relationships caught up in a vicious circle, a web of deception across the organization. Effective solutions may involve radical changes and interventions.

Confronting the perpetrator may be considered as an initial reaction to the situation. The perpetrator may be confronted by their superior, which may be effective if appropriate sanctions can be imposed. The superior needs to have an understanding of the nature and extent of the problem. However, this approach may be ineffective in the long term, as the situation is likely to consist of more than a direct relationship between perpetrator and victim, or cause and effect. As the case study suggests, confrontation of the perpetrator by the victim may make matters worse, as the perpetrator can use the situation to further humiliate the victim. Lemert (1969) describes three types of solution for the management of the paranoid individual: transfer, encapsulation, discharge and forced resignation. In cases of bullying, sexual harassment and sex discrimination these solutions may be considered as possible outcomes for either the perpetrator or the victim, depending on the circumstances.

Transfer

The individual (and the problem) is moved to another department or section within the organization. In order for this to happen the individual must be persuaded to make the change and must be accepted by the other department. Factors that need to be considered include the size of the organization and the reputation of the employee, and the future reputation of the transferring department.

Encapsulation

This involves a reorganization and redefinition of the individual's status, effectively isolating him from the rest of the organization. They are made directly accountable to one superior, who intermediates for the organization. This solution is most effective if material rewards associated with status are apparent, for example a nominal promotion

without additional responsibilities, the removal of onerous responsibilities, or the creation of a special status. This is a form of collusion where the individual is offered formal recognition by the organization and their intense commitment to status is rewarded. It requires an appropriate superior.

Discharge and forced resignation, non-renewal of appointment

This may be associated with a 'critical incident', for example formal disciplinary proceedings for disreputable conduct, or be marked by nothing other than the end of the individual's contracted period of employment.

For the victim of bullying and harassment the outcome may involve transfer from the department or resignation from the organization. However, this outcome may be achieved through the development of an action plan based on rational decision making and a realistic timeframe. The components of such an action plan are identified below. The process of achieving this goal offers the victim direction and purpose: it can increase their sense of control, self-worth, confidence and achievement.

In order for the victim to take action it is necessary to focus on the distressing events and circumstances. The following measures may be helpful and supportive. Each should be considered carefully in terms of likely consequences, as it is possible to exacerbate the problem, particularly when other people from within the organization are involved. For example, are individuals being put in positions where they have little choice but to take a certain course of action?

Some of the following options may help in cases of sexual harassment, sex discrimination and bullying.

1. Keep a journal of critical incidents. Record dates, times, people involved. Include incidents that cause distress, are undermining, and attacks on character, personal integrity and competence.

2. Write down any thoughts linked to these events.

3. Write down any feelings associated with these events.

4. Keep records of any relevant correspondence, e.g. letters and memos from the perpetrator.

5. Check work responsibilities, e.g. ensure that job descriptions are up to date, collect copies of any performance reviews and appraisals. Plan work in a way that avoids unnecessary contact with the perpetrator, for example plan meetings and visits elsewhere. Be prepared to change routine.

6. Try to identify how the bullying and harassment is affecting work.

7. Keep a record of personal achievements, successes and interests at work.

8. Identify someone who will provide constructive and positive feedback, perhaps from another department.

9. Identify and maintain outside work interests.

10. Find someone to talk to away from usual work and home life – a counsellor, GP or mental health nurse. This avoids overloading family and friends.

11. Contact a more senior manager in the organization.

12. Speak to peers/colleagues – some may be having or may have had similar experiences.

13. Identify and mobilize other sources of help, e.g. seek advice from a trade union representative, personnel, equal opportunities adviser, occupational health staff.

GOOD ORGANIZATIONAL PRACTICE

Several organizations have introduced antibullying and harassment measures. For example, British Rail has a code of practice designed to address bullying at work, and MSF (Manufacturing, Science and Finance Union) campaigns to raise awareness of bullying at work. Others, for example The Bethlem and Maudsley NHS Trust, have introduced policies on bullying and harassment in the workplace. Antibullying and harassment policies should include an assurance of confidentiality, a complaints procedure, formal and informal means of support, counselling from an independent source, recourse to external investigation or enquiry, and reinforcing

the conviction that disciplinary proceedings will be applied to perpetrators.

Policies alone will not overcome bullying and harassment: the culture of the organization needs to reinforce the notion that they will not be tolerated. This message must be clearly communicated through all managers, from board level down, across the organization. Investing in education and training will help to change attitudes. Dissemination of information about sexual harassment and assertiveness training for employees are measures that will help raise awareness and provide effective skills among the workforce to prevent the escalation of bullying and harassment.

 Learning activity 6.6

Pick out three or four job adverts of interest from the national or professional press and send off for information. What does the information tell you about the organization's commitment to sexual health? What does it say about equal opportunities, policies on sexual health, sex discrimination, sexual harassment and bullying? Is further information available?

 Learning activity 6.7

Stakeholders are any group, person or organization that can make a claim on an organization's output. They have influence and power that can shape the sexual health of the organization in ways that are overt or covert, positive or negative. Identify all the stakeholders in your organization.

◆ Develop a profile of the stakeholders.

◆ Compile information on, for example, gender, race and ethnicity.

◆ Are there issues of representation and non-representation? Which groups are conspicuous by their absence? Who has a voice and who does not have a voice?

◆ Identify key stakeholders in terms of their influence, power and authority on strategic plans relating to sexual health.

◆ How do stakeholders measure the sexual health of the organization?

◆ What is their key means of influence?

◆ Do you have any influence or control over these measures?

◆ What are the implications for future practice developments around sexual health?

CONCLUSION

This chapter contributes to a sexual health agenda for the organization. It outlines different ways of seeing the organization and different types of organizational culture. Traditional or popular conceptions of organizational culture are outlined, and ways of seeing organizations in terms of sexual health and gender cultures are introduced.

Bullying, sexual harassment and sex discrimination are addressed within an organizational context, with reference to the organizational culture, social and sexual relationships. They are viewed as complex organizational behaviours that affect functioning at an individual and organizational level. The cumulative effect of sexual harassment and bullying is often devastating for the victim or recipient and may lead to psychological and organizational crises for all those involved. Lemert's (1969) conception of paranoia as a social attribute maintained by particular patterns of reciprocating behaviours enhances our understanding of these complex behaviours, and provides an organizational context for social relationships based on exclusion.

Ways and means of identifying and understanding these behaviours are described. The activities identified throughout the chapter aim to help readers examine their own organizations in terms of how the issues addressed may affect sexual health policy and practice.

RESOURCES AND ANNOTATED FURTHER READING

The Andrea Adams Trust Shalimar House,

24 Derek Avenue, Hove, East Sussex BN3 4PF. Tel/Fax: 01273 417850

UK National Workplace Bullying Advice Line: Tel: 01235 212286
http://www.successunlimited.co.uk/

Campaign Against Workplace Bullying (CAWB)
http://www.bullybusters.org

Institute of Personnel and Development, IPD House, Camp Road, London SW19 4UX. Tel: 020 8971 9000; Fax: 020 8263 3333

Commission for Racial Equality, Elliot House, 10–12 Allington Street, London SW1E 5EH. Tel: 020 7828 7022; Fax: 020 7630 7605

Sexual harassment (information pack) Equal Opportunities Commission, Overseas House, Quay Street, Manchester M3 3HN. Tel: 0161 833 9244; Fax: 0161 835 1657

Department of Employment. Sexual harassment in the workplace: a guide for employers. Department of Employment, London, 1992 (10pp) (PL 923)

Equal Opportunities Commission for Northern Ireland. Sexual harassment at work: guidance on prevention and procedures for dealing with the problem (1993) (ISBN 0906646316). Sexual harassment at work: a guide for employees (1993) (ISBN 0906646308). Equal Opportunities Commission for Northern Ireland, Belfast

Hearn J, Sheppard D L, Tancred-Sheriff P, Burrell D (eds) 1989 The sexuality of organizations. Sage, London

This book brings together a range of topics on gender issues and sexuality from an international group of contributors. Topics addressed in detail include sexuality and the labour process, social research and organizational practice, private and public service organizations, sexual harassment, men's sexuality, lesbians in organizations, reports of women managers and secretaries.

Itzin C, Newman J 1996 Gender, culture and organizational change: putting theory into practice. Routledge, London

This book addresses organizational change and the management of change in terms of gender issues and sexuality. The content is arranged under two broad headings of gendering organizational culture and strategies for organizational change. Topics include gender cultures and organizational typologies, men and power, gendered ageism, gendered noise, welfare organizations, racism, social service organizations, women chief executives in local government and trade unions.

Royal College of Nursing Lesbian and
Gay Nursing Issues Group,
20 Cavendish Square, London W1M 0AB.
Tel: 020 7409 3333

Rubenstein M. Preventing and remedying sexual harassment at work: a resource manual. Industrial Relations Service, London, 1989. 52pp (ISBN 180771044)

Trades Union Congress. Sexual harassment at work: TUC guidelines. London Trades Union Congress, 1991. 13pp.
Trades Union Congress, Congress House, 23–28 Great Russell Street, London WC1B 3LS.
Tel: 020 7636 4030; Fax: 020 7636 0632

REFERENCES

Adams A 1992 Bullying at work. Virago, London

Gruber J E 1992 A typology of personal and environmental sexual harassment: research and policy implications for the 1990s. Sex Roles 26 (11/12): 447–463

Gutek B A, Morasch B 1982 Sex ratios, sex role spillover and sexual harassment of women at work. Journal of Social Issues 38(4): 55–74

Gutek B A, Morasch B, Cohen A 1983 Interpreting social sexual behaviour in the work setting. Journal of Vocational behaviour 22(1): 30–48

Handy C 1985 Understanding organisations. Penguin, Harmondsworth

Handy C 1988 Understanding voluntary organisations. Penguin, Harmondsworth

Handy C 1990 Understanding voluntary organisations. Penguin, Harmondsworth

Harlow E, Hearn J Parkin W 1996 Gendered noise: organisations and the silence and din of domination. In: Itzin C, Newman J (eds) Gender culture and organizational change. Routledge, London, pp 91–107

Itzin C 1995 The gender culture in oganizations. In: Itzin C, Newman J (eds) Gender culture and organizational change. Routledge, London, pp 30–53

Kanter R M 1989 When giants learn to dance. Simon & Schuster, New York

Kanter R M 1975 Women in organizations: sex roles, group dynamics, and change strategies. In: Sargent A (ed) Beyond sex roles. West, St Paul, MN

Lemert E M 1969 Paranoia and the dynamics of exclusion. In: Spitzer S P, Denzin N K (eds) The mental patient: studies in the sociology of deviance. McGraw-Hill, New York, pp 68–84

Lloyd K L 1991 Sexual harassment: how to keep your company out of court. Panel Publishers, New York

Luft J, Ingham H 1977 The Johari window. In: Luthans F (ed) Organisational behaviour. McGraw-Hill, p 395

Maccoby R 1976 The gamesman: the new corporate leaders. Simon & Schuster, New York

Mintzberg H 1989 Mintzberg on management. Free Press, New York

Newman J 1996 Gender and cultural change. In: Itzin C, Newman J (eds) Gender culture and organizational change. Routledge, London, pp 11–29

Parkin D, Maddock S 1995 A gender typology of organizational culture. In: Itzin C, Newman J (eds) Gender culture and organizational change. Routledge, London, pp 68–80

Pryor J B 1985 The lay person's understanding of sexual harassment. Sex Roles 13(5/6): 273–286

Pryor J B, Day J D 1988 Interpretations of sexual harassment: an attributional analysis. Sex Roles 18(7/8): 405–417

Reilly T, Carpenter S, Dull V, Bartlett K 1982 The factorial survey technique: an approach to defining sexual harassment on campus. Journal of Social Issues 38: 99–110

Royal College of Nursing 1996 Sexual health: key issues within mental health services – a position paper. RCN, London

Schneider B E 1982 Consciousness about sexual harassment among heterosexual and lesbian women workers. Journal of Social Issues 38: 75–98

Williams K B, Cyr R R 1992 Escalating commitment to a relationship: the sexual harassment trap. Sex Roles 27(1/2): 47–71

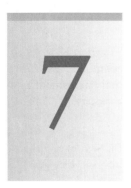

7

Sex and the statutory bodies

Heather Wilson

| *'I can resist anything, except temptation.'*   (Oscar Wilde)

KEY ISSUES/CONCEPTS

◆ Sexual health-care practice

◆ Sex and the law

◆ What is lawful?

◆ Sources, courts, types and sites of law

◆ Classification of crimes

◆ The law and sexual activity

◆ Code of professional conduct and sexual health care

◆ Gender identity disorder and sexual health

OVERVIEW

Chapter 7, *Sex and the statutory bodies*, starts by looking at British law and goes on to explore some of the legislation that permits or prevents certain acts related to sexual behaviour. This is followed by a review of professional regulation as prescribed by the statutory bodies, and examples of how it affects sexual health practice. The final section presents a range of sexually related activities which have legal, moral and/or ethical implications with which the reader may be confronted at some point in their personal or professional life.

INTRODUCTION

There is a well known popular book called *The joy of sex* (Comfort 1996); perhaps there should also be a book called *The trouble with sex*. The trouble with sex is that it can be funny, offensive, illegal, exciting, painful, harmful, embarrassing, damaging, enlightening, invigorating and much, much more.

Sexual health and sexuality lie on a very broad spectrum of activities and have their own language, politics, culture and even industry. One could almost describe sexual health as being in a world of its own. Values and beliefs regarding sexual behaviour vary so widely that sexual freedom for some creates problems and dilemmas for others. In order to maintain appropriate levels of protection without unduly prohibiting freedom, there has to be some kind of management and order. Sexual activity is governed by a series of rules, which impinge on aspects of care, protection and the education of clients.

Some of these rules are legal and binding (legislation) and **must** be obeyed. Some are principles for guidance (regulation) and **should** be obeyed. Some rules are personal and based on specific sets of beliefs and value systems (morals and ethics), and **probably** will be obeyed. This chapter concentrates on legislation (Acts of Parliament) and professional regulation (United Kingdom Central Council for Nursing, Midwifery and Health Visiting (UKCC) Code of Professional Conduct) and how it affects personal rules in relation to sexual health practice.

SEXUAL HEALTH-CARE PRACTICE

Sexual health-care practice in nursing covers the spectrum from human embryology and conception, to the care of people dying from sexually transmitted diseases. It is encyclopaedic in its scope, and in order to comprehend its range look at Learning activity 7.1.

Learning activity 7.1

In pairs or small groups brainstorm the number of words or phrases that link up with the words 'sex' or 'sexual'.

See if you can group the phrases that you come up with into specific headings, such as health related, social or personal activities. (This has probably just confirmed what you knew already about the breadth of topics associated with sex and/or sexual health.) You will probably need to undertake a literature search in the library, on the Internet or on CD-ROM. Limit your search when you put in the word sex or sexual, otherwise you will be offered a greater range of publications or information than you can cope with. Try to be more specific by adding another word or words to your keyword.

The *Wordsworth Dictionary of Sex* (Goldenson and Anderson 1987) has 290 pages with an average of 18 entries per page, and covers all aspects of sex from the scientific to folklore. The scope and range of sex-related activities are matched only by the scope and range of their complexity.

Equally complex are British attitudes to sex (Wellings and Bradshaw 1994), which are as diverse as people themselves. Everyone views sexuality and sexual health from their own personal perspective, using a cultural, probably gender-related, framework. Different societies and cultures have different views on sex-related activities. One only has to look at the press to see the spectrum of views on sex in contemporary Britain.

Some individual sexual choices and preferences can and do offend or harm other people. Some people view certain sexual preferences as immoral (for example the laws on homosexuality and the age of consent), whereas others lobby hard to increase freedom for sexual choice. Some sexual activity is illegal even when those involved are consenting and caring. One person's legislation is another person's restriction.

In order to provide some clarity the examples of legislation that relate to sexual health have been broken down into three categories:

◆ Legislation associated with offences against public morals and public policy (see Box 7.1)
◆ Legislation associated with professional and employment issues (see Box 7.2)
◆ Legislation associated with aspects of sexual health care and the protection and/or education of clients (see Box 7.3).

Familiarity with the structure and function of law as outlined in this chapter will help you to identify specific sex-related examples in the public domain which have a bearing on the protection of the public and order in society.

There are over 600 000 registered nurses in the UK, and as a group they probably represent the range of views shared by the rest of contemporary Britain. Their spectrum of values, beliefs, emotions, prejudices and sexual preferences are con-

Box 7.1 Legislation associated with offences against public morals and public policy

Children Act

Criminal justice

Criminal injuries

Criminal Law Act

Marriage Act

Obscene publications

Sexual offences

Street offences

Vagrancy Act

ceivably very similar. Nursing, like many other professions, is regulated by its own unique rules in the shape of the Code of Professional Conduct (UKCC 1992a). Later in the chapter there will be a section on professional accountability and the laws that form the basis of statutory authority in professional nursing (see Box 7.2).

The final part of this chapter looks at employment law and considers the ways in which one group of individuals face discrimination because of their sexuality and gender.

Chapter 1 gave a list of sexual health-related national surveys and described the different perspectives of health held by people in society, i.e.:

◆ Professional versus lay
◆ Positive versus negative
◆ Subjective versus objective
◆ Biomedical versus holistic
◆ Public versus private.

These perspectives show the scope and range of sexually related behaviours, attitudes, practices,

study, experience etc., and reinforce the complexity of this particular sphere of health care.

In nursing, some areas of practice and care are specifically related to sexual health, for example genitourinary medicine, reproductive health care, sexual abuse and gender reassignment. In other areas maintenance and respect for clients' sexuality is less specific, but equally important to the client.

Box 7.3 shows examples of some of the legislation associated with aspects of sexual health care, protection and/or the education of clients.

Sometimes, nurses may find themselves caring for clients whose sexual activity or behaviour confronts their own personal beliefs and values. They may have conscientious objections, or feel that the client's lifestyle is morally wrong. For example, homophobia, like racism, is not restricted to the public: nor is contempt for clients undergoing gender reassignment. Abhorrence of child sexual abuse may create moral dilemmas for nurses treating clients who are known sex offenders. Equally, nurses continue to be removed from the professional register because they sexually abuse their clients (UKCC 1992b). The purpose of the law and professional regulation is to underpin all health practice, including sexual health, in order to protect the client and improve the quality of health care and education.

 Reflection point 7.1

Consider your professional development so far; in general terms:

◆ Which laws are you aware of that control or regulate your professional life?

◆ Can you recall any incidents with clients where your personal feelings have been influenced by the client's behaviour or particular lifestyle?

◆ Have you ever been in a situation where colleagues or clients have openly expressed negative views about other clients because of their lifestyle or behaviour? How did you respond?

◆ Have you ever expressed negative views yourself?

◆ Consider the above questions again, but this time try to relate them to a sexual health context.

SEX AND THE LAW

There is not the scope or the space in this chapter to deal with the law in any depth, other than a general introduction. However, if you are not familiar with the basics of English law and want to know more, Learning activity 7.2 will be a useful exercise to help you to identify sources of information.

What is and what is not lawful?

To some extent one knows almost instinctively what is and what is not lawful. Sometimes there are signs which forbid certain things, such as driving over 30 mph, buying alcohol when under the age of 18, travelling on the underground without buying a ticket, dropping litter, trespassing etc. However, mostly there are no such signs and individuals have to learn that they are prohibited from doing certain things, and need to obey laws, rules and regulations. Whether or not they do so is related to personality, culture, circumstances and society. Hopefully, people learn respect for others and the environment from their family, friends and school.

One of the earliest authorities to set down a series of rules relating to behaviour did so by forbidding the use of bad language, murder, idolatry, stealing, lying, coveting and overworking, and also commanded people to respect their parents (*Exodus* Ch. 20).

Even without laws, the majority of people know that certain acts are morally or ethically wrong, but this does not mean people are not capable of doing them anyway. Indeed, some companies have made a commercial success out of this and have invented games and television programmes to demonstrate how people know they have done something 'wrong', but will react against their principles in certain situations.

A dictionary definition of the law is . . . '*a rule established by authority*'. Dimond (1990) states

that . . . '*the law and ethics overlap, but is each both wider and narrower than the other*'. Salmond (1993, cited in Jenkins) defines it as . . . '*the body of principles recognised and applied by the state in the administration of justice*'. Jenkins (1995) suggests that '*we all know what the law is*'.

Whereas there is an expectation by society that people should have a clear idea of what is right and wrong, it may not always be clear to what extent something is actually defined as an offence or crime by an authority.

Sources, courts and types of law

Sources of law

There are two sources of law in this country: *statutory sources*, which are derived from Acts of Parliament, and the *common law*, which comes from custom and general agreement and is based on decisions taken by judges, who use previous case evidence.

Courts of law

Cases of law are tried in different courts according to their type:

◆ House of Lords
◆ Court of Appeal
◆ High Court
◆ Family Division
◆ Crown Court
◆ County Court
◆ Magistrate and Youth Courts
◆ Coroner's Court
◆ Occasional Court.

Types of law

There are two types of law in this country:

◆ *Civil law*, which is actionable in civil courts (and not necessarily a crime)
◆ *Criminal law*, which can lead to prosecution in criminal courts.

Civil law is related to offences against the person, property or issue of contracts and tort (civil wrongs). Civil law is tried by a judge alone and may lead to the award of damages. In criminal law the defendant is prosecuted by the state for the Crown, and is tried by a judge and jury, which can lead to punishment.

Crimes are described as public wrongs and the action is brought by the State, represented by the Crown. It is interesting that the House of Lords cannot agree on a statutory definition of crime, as it is regarded as '*not possible to discover a legal definition of crime which can be of value for English law*'.

However, Redmond and Shears (1993) define a crime as '*a public wrong whose commission will result in criminal proceedings which may in turn result in the punishment of the wrongdoer*'.

The fact that the Lords found it impossible to discover a definition helps the layperson to understand the culture of the law to some extent. There are other areas in the statute where clear definitions have not been used. For example, the term *gross indecency* is used in the Sexual Offences Act 1967, but has no definition in law.

Classification of crimes

Between 1870 and 1967, under the scheme for the classification of offences, crime was either a felony (those actions which put good order in jeopardy, including murder and rape) or a misdemeanour.

The Criminal Law Act 1967 abolished felonies and misdemeanours and characterized the seriousness of the offence according to whether it was (a) arrestable or (b) indictable. This system has now been incorporated into the Police and Criminal Evidence Act 1984 (PACE), and arrestable offences are now defined as those where:

◆ there is a penalty fixed by law (e.g. murder)
◆ offenders under 21 years may be sentenced to over 5 years or more
◆ the offence is one of the named offences, including sexual offences.

The law and sexual activity

Table 7.1 lists a selection of some of the laws pertaining to sex-related activities.

You may be interested to explore a specific aspect of the law in relation to client care or professional

Table 7.1 Table of statutes

Abortion Act	1967
AIDS Control Act	1987
Children and Young Persons (Harmful Publications) Act	1955
Children Act	1989
Criminal Injuries Compensation Act	1995
Criminal Law Act	1977
Criminal Justice Act	1988
Criminal Justice and Public Order Act	1994
Education Act	1988
Education Reform Act	1993
Human Fertilization and Embryology Act	1990
Indecency With Children Act	1960
Indecent Displays (Control) Act	1981
Local Government Act	1986
Marriage Act	1983
Mental Health Act	1959
Mental Health Act	1983
Mental Health Amendment Act	1982
Obscene Publications Act	1959
Obscene Publications Act	1964
Offences Against the Person Act	1861
Police and Criminal Evidence Act	1984
Post Office Act	1969
Prohibition of Female Circumcision Act	1985
Protection of Children Act	1978
Sexual Offences Act	1956
Sexual Offences Act	1967
Sexual Offences Act	1985
Sexual Offences Act	1992
Sexual Offences (Amendment) Act	1992
Sexual Offences (Conspiracy and Incitement) Act	1996
Street Offences Act	1959
Vagrancy Act	1924

conduct. If you do not know which law you want, or whether there is an actual law relating to the area you are exploring, start by trying the reference section of your library. The local public library should keep all the reference books you need.

SEX AND THE STATUTORY BODIES

A nursing journal once asked its readers what they thought a statutory body was, and gave them a choice of:

Learning activity 7.2

Here are some hints on how to find up-to-date information on current laws, rules and Acts of Parliament at your local library.

A good start would always be to *ask the librarian*, who will probably point you towards the reference section and something like the Reader's Digest *You and your rights* guide. This provides an alphabetical and understandable source of information on your rights and is supported by further sources of advice and information. This will give you an indication of what kind of offence is involved.

You will need to check that the information is up to date, but it would help to get you started when looking for specific information.

The next reference could then be the *Citizen's Advice Notes Service: digest of social legislation* – (*CANS Trust 1999*). Simply known as *CANS,* it should be held and up to date in the reference section of your local library, and you can use the index to identify a particular law in relation to a specific Act of Parliament and obtain further details.

Stone's Justices Manual (Draycott and Carr 1996) is an annual publication giving detailed information on any amendments to Acts of Parliament, changes in the law, the actual offences and types of punishment, as well as detailed information on court sessions and what is happening in the legal world.

If you know exactly which Act and the year it was enacted, use the *Public General Acts and General Synod Measures* (HMSO 1996), also in the reference section, to find the complete statutory instrument.

◆ A person in charge?
◆ A stationary body?
◆ An organization?

They also asked what readers would they do if they were handed a statutory instrument; would they:

◆ clean it?
◆ boil it for 20 minutes?
◆ use it as an essential reference document?

Despite the humour in the question, it raises an important point about the level of understanding about statutory bodies in the nursing profession. Practitioners sometimes express confusion about the difference between statutory bodies, governmental, departmental and professional organizations.

Whereas the statutory bodies ensure that standards are being met to uphold the Nurses, Midwives and Health Visitors Act, the Department of Health (DoH) is responsible for the implementation of government policy. National Health Service Executive (NHSE) regional offices are responsible for ensuring the most effective use of health service resources. There are also several professional nursing organizations (for example the Royal College of Nursing, the Community Nursing and Health Visitors Association) that promote the development of the profession and which, with other unions, represent the employment rights of health-care professionals. Because the department, statutory and professional organizations provide a range of services and are involved in sometimes similar activities, there is often a degree of confusion as to their specific roles and responsibilities.

Some might argue that this lack of knowledge is due to the image of the statutory bodies themselves, whereas others may feel that nurses have a responsibility and an obligation to ensure that they are well informed about organizations that support and regulate the profession. Whatever the reason, actual physical contact with the statutory bodies, because of their size and locations, is to some extent limited to the 600 000 registered nurses in the UK. What is not limited is communication of information in the form of publications, newsletters, electronic mail and websites (for addresses see end of chapter).

A statutory body is an organization which has responsibilities set out by law. The 1979 Nurses, Midwives and Health Visitors Act established five statutory bodies for nursing, midwifery and health visiting in the UK. The present arrangements for nursing regulation have recently been reviewed and new legislation will soon be in place to develop a new regulatory framework for nursing, midwifery and health visiting.

The statutory bodies are responsible for protecting the interests of the public. They set the standards for education, training and professional conduct for registered nurses, midwives and health visitors. The new Central Council for Nursing, Midwifery and Health Visiting will still maintain the Professional Register of Nurses, Midwives and Health Visitors and will continue to determine the standards of entry for the register and decide when the right to practice should be removed from an individual.

The code of professional conduct

The current central council for nursing, the United Kingdom Central Council for Nursing, Midwifery and Health Visiting (UKCC) Coat of Arms motto reads: '*Care, protect and honour*'. Unfortunately, there are instances where patients do not receive care or protection from some members of the nursing profession. The UKCC is responsible for the standards of professional nursing and requires that its members practise and conduct themselves within the framework provided by the Code of Professional Conduct (1992a), i.e: '*Care in a way that reflects the Code of Conduct . . . Protection of patients and clients . . . Honour the responsibility of being a registered practitioner . . .*'. The mechanisms, processes and guidelines of the UKCC all relate to ensuring that nurses are accountable for their own practice, and that they fully understand the consequences of omissions.

The code highlights points of principle in relation to professional conduct, and these must be adhered to in order to ensure that nurses are accountable for their own practice. Briefly, these relate to:

◆ safeguarding patients' wellbeing
◆ causing them no harm
◆ fostering patients' independence
◆ involving clients' families and carers in the care process
◆ maintaining professional knowledge

◆ assisting others in their professional development
◆ acknowledging own limitations
◆ raising conscientious objections
◆ avoiding abuse of privileged position
◆ refusing gifts/favours which could exert influence to obtain preferential consideration
◆ ensuring professional judgement is not influenced by commercial considerations
◆ working in a collaborative and cooperative manner with others
◆ reporting jeopardized standards, unsafe/ inappropriate care, health and safety risks (Fig. 7.1).

Code of professional conduct and sexual health

The code is written in universal terms to be applied to all areas of practice by every member of the nursing profession; however, when working in a sexual health-related area certain clauses have significant importance for practitioners and clients. Examples are:

◆ **Clause 7:** 'Recognize and respect the uniqueness and dignity of each patient and client and respond to their need for care, irrespective of their ethnic origins, religious beliefs, personal attributes and the nature of their health problems or any other factor.'

◆ **Clause 10:** 'Protect all confidential information concerning patients and clients obtained in the course of professional practice and make disclosures only with consent where required by the order of a court or where you can justify disclosure in the wider public interest.'

 Reflection point 7.2

Consider Clause 7 and the issues raised in relation to clients who wish to undergo or have undergone gender reassignment. Anecdotal evidence suggests that, far from their 'uniqueness and dignity' being respected, transsexual individuals suffer humiliation and

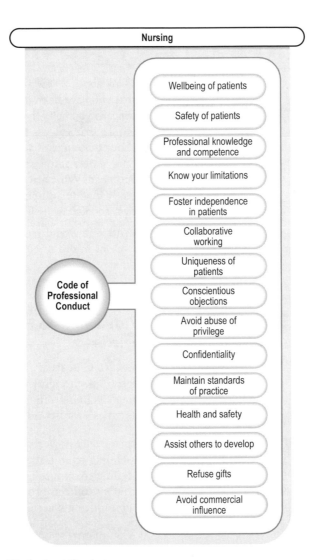

Fig. 7.1 The nursing Code of Professional Conduct.

trauma at the hands of some health-care professionals and receive different standards of care because of their uniqueness.

What arrangements are made in your area of practice to ensure that a transgendered individual would be respected and cared for? What issues do you think might arise when nursing someone who has formerly been a male or female in a new and different gender environment?

Reflection point 7.3

Consider Clause 10 and the issues raised in relation to clients who attend a sexually transmitted diseases clinic. What steps are taken to ensure that confidentiality is maintained? How does the clinic protect and offer care to others who may have been in contact with the person and still maintain confidentiality?

Professional conduct and accountability

Dimond (1990) states that: '. . . accountability of the nurse is concerned with how far the nurse can be held in law to be accountable for her actions'. Dimond outlines four areas of accountability:

◆ Public – criminal law
◆ Professional – UKCC Professional Conduct Committee
◆ Patient – civil law
◆ Employer – contract of employment/industrial tribunal.

In all four areas there has been and continues to be an astonishing rate of change. The UKCC recognizes this and acknowledges that 'practice is taking place in a context of continuing change and development and must therefore be sensitive, relevant and responsive to the needs of individual patients and clients and have the capacity to adjust where and when appropriate to changing circumstances'.

Before 1992 nurses undertaking any new intervention or activity that could be seen as an extension to their role were given official and certified recognition; however, it became clear that, rather than collecting certificates, the development of new skills in practice should be underpinned by sound principles. Consequently, the UKCC developed the Scope of Professional Practice (1992c), which was designed to ensure that practitioners:

◆ serve the needs of the client and the wider society
◆ are supported by appropriate education and training
◆ know their own limits
◆ do not compromise existing aspects of care
◆ ensure personal accountability
◆ enhance trust and confidence and promote collaborative working.

In essence, practitioners are accountable for their own actions at all times, whether engaged in current practice or not, and whether on or off duty. The interests of the public and the patient must predominate over those of the practitioner.

Reflection point 7.4

Think about a new area of sexual health practice that you have been involved in. How did you prepare yourself for your new role? How do you ensure that you are practising safely? Think about the range of skills you apply for the first time in new settings: what new knowledge do you need? What are the resources available to you? How do you demonstrate and test your own accountability in practice?

What else would you need to do if you were working in the area of sexual health for the first time?

With a view to removal from the register

The UKCC deals with cases of misconduct which are serious enough to justify removing the practitioner's name from the register (UKCC 1996a). The types of misconduct include:

◆ physically or verbally abusing patients
◆ stealing from patients
◆ failing to care for patients properly
◆ failing to keep proper records
◆ committing a serious criminal offence.

Complaints about professional conduct are investigated and considered by a committee of the UKCC, which goes through a process of considering evidence and responses from the practitioner before deciding to take action. This can result in the committee administering a caution or removing the practitioner from the register.

Professional conduct: summary

The role of the statutory body is to protect the public, to ensure that in the pursuance of their profession nurses do the patient no harm. The UKCC sets the standards for the profession of nursing; its function is to:

◆ safeguard and promote the interests of individual patients and clients
◆ serve the interests of society
◆ justify public trust and confidence
◆ uphold and enhance the good standing and reputation of the professions.

These principles apply equally across all areas of care, but in sexual health complicated legal, ethical and moral issues abound. In some cases practitioners' own personal value systems and beliefs can be threatened by the behaviour or attitudes of clients, in the same way that the clients' value systems and beliefs can also be threatened by the behaviour or attitudes of the 'caring' professions.

Learning activity 7.3

In *A guide for students of nursing and midwifery* (UKCC 1998) there is advice on the following areas.

The stages of clinical experience:

◆ Observer

◆ Participant observer

◆ Participant

◆ Identifying yourself, informing patients and clients about your role and respecting their wishes

◆ Accepting responsibility

◆ Respecting confidence

◆ Making records

◆ Dealing with compliants

◆ Accountability.

Choose a specific area of sexual health practice, for example STD or family planning clinic.
Prepare an induction pack for student nurses or new members of staff working in that area.

What information would you provide?

What support should be given?

How would you ensure appropriate supervision for each stage of clinical experience?

The scope of sexual health care, protection and education

Think about the range of sex-related issues that affect sexual health care and promotion. Learning activity 7.4 provides a framework for a resource directory for sexual health-care practice. All of these topics have either legal, ethical or moral implications for practice. It is no accident that 26 topics have been selected and presented in alphabetical order: this has been done to reinforce once again the breadth and scope of sexual health issues. In this instance, depth of subject has been deliberately sacrificed. Further details can be obtained by researching in the library or accessing resources highlighted in the information points.

LEGISLATION AND GENDER IDENTITY

Although the laws on employment and sex discrimination have been developed to provide equity and fairness in the workplace, transsexuals have been marginalized, discriminated against and even criminalized both in society and in the workplace. Toleration of such discrimination is tantamount to a failure to respect the dignity and freedom to which all are entitled. Until the legislation is set in place to provide clear guidelines on equal opportunities and employment for transsexual individuals, discrimination will continue. What is required is a better understanding of the issues surrounding this inequality, in order to promote good workplace practice to ensure that those who wish to undergo or have undergone gender reassignment can find employment, make relationships, integrate with the larger community and live a fulfilling life (Reid 1996).

Gender dysphoria: definitions

Gender dysphoria or transsexualism has been defined as:

> ... *A gender identity disorder* in which there is a *strong and ongoing cross-gender identification*, i.e. a *desire to live and be*

Learning activity 7.4

Using the sexual health directory below as a starting point, draw up a directory of definitions, statutory instruments, resources and references for your own area of practice in sexual health. As you read through this list, try to identify ways in which these topics and issues affect your practice and how the issues related to sexual offences challenge the way in which you uphold your own code of professional conduct.

SEXUAL HEALTH DIRECTORY

Term	Definition/explanation	Information point
Abortion	Justified medical abortion was legalized by the Abortion Act in 1967. Previously abortion was illegal and procured by the use of 'poison or noxious thing, instrument or other means whatever' as described in the Offences Against The Person Act of 1861	See Guidelines for Professional Practice (UKCC 1996b), p. 24, for advice on conscientious objection
Buggery	(From the French bougre), is defined in the Sexual Offences Act 1956 as intercourse (penetration to the slightest degree) per anus by a man with a man or a man with a woman (this is also known as sodomy). Buggery also consists of anal or vaginal intercourse by men or women with animals, which is also known as bestiality. Section 1(1) of the Sexual Offences Act 1967 was amended by the Criminal Justice and Public Order Act 1994, lowering the age for consenting adults from 21 to 18 years	Stonewall is a national civil rights group working for legal equality and social justice for lesbians, gay men and bisexuals. Website: http://www.stonewall.org.uk
Children Act (1989)	Set out the need for courts and authorities to take into account the physical, emotional and educational needs of children according to their age, sex and background, and to consider any harm the child has suffered or is at risk of suffering	See www.nds.gov.uk/coi for government plans to fight child abuse
Depravity	Defined as making morally bad, to pervert to debase or corrupt morally; a term used in relation to sexual offences acts. Sometimes it is just used to express a view about a type of behaviour which is not tolerated because it is different. Frequently it is used with the term 'evil', particularly in relation to child abuse	See Home Office publications on: www.nds.coi.gov.uk/coi
Equal opportunities	In 1970 the Equal Pay Act meant that men and women who were employed in like work should receive the same pay. Subsequently the Sex Discrimination Act 1975 made it generally unlawful for an employer to discriminate on grounds of sex or marriage; currently the laws are being challenged when people are being discriminated against because of sexuality	see COI Website www.nds.coi.gov.uk/coi
Family Planning Association	Provides expert and accessible information in order to increase confidence about sexual health	Website: www.fpa.org.uk

Gross indecency	Although this term has not been defined either by statute or by common law, the Wolfendon Committee agreed that it usually takes one of three forms: mutual masturbation, intercrural contact or orogenital contact, and is still an offence under the 1994 Act. Nurses have been removed from the register by the courts and the UKCC following conviction for gross indecency with patients	Wolfendon Committee 1957 published a report which partially decriminalized homosexuality and set the age of consent for consenting adults in private places at 21. It is anticipated that the age of consent will be lowered to 16, when the Home Secretary uses the Parliament Act to push through the final legislation
Harassment	An employment and health issue caused by unwanted sexual attentions	COI Website Department of Education and Employment for details
Incest	It is an offence under the 1956 Sexual Offences Act for a man to have incestuous sexual intercourse. In English law incest is sexual intercourse between a male aged 14 or over and a female whom the man knows to be his daughter, granddaughter, mother or sister or half sister. If the female is under 13 the crime carries a possible sentence of life, the same as for rape. If she is over 13, 7 years is the maximum sentence	Section 54 Criminal Law Act 1977
Jorgenson	Christine, the female name taken by one of the first people to undergo pioneering sex change in the 1960s. Involved in the first compilation study of transsexualism	The Gender Trust e-mail: gentrust@mistral.co.uk. Website: http://www3.mistral.co.uk/gentrust
Kerb crawling	It is an offence for a man to kerb crawl to persistently solicit prostitutes to have sex	Sexual Offences Act 1985
Learning disability	People with learning disabilities have sexual health needs that require appropriate and sensitive support. Contentious issues such as informed consent, sterilization and termination create many ethical and legal dilemmas for clients, their families and health-care professionals	Mental Health Acts deal with the sexual conduct of patients and staff for the protection of people with mental health or learning disability problems
Mental health	Discriminatory attitudes towards lesbians, gay and bisexual men and women cause considerable stress, leading to isolation and loss of emotional support	Sexual orientation and mental health guidance for nurses, RCN (Issues in nursing no 48)
Necrophilia	A severe but rare sexual disorder in which sexual excitement is derived from contact with corpses removed from graves. Necromania is pathological desire for sexual relations with a corpse	There are a range of sexual dysfunctions and deviations that require behavioural psychotherapy
Obscene telephone calls	Illegal under the Post Office Act of 1969. This forbids sending by means of public telecommunication a message grossly offensive or of an indecent, obscene or menacing character	Purge on phone box pests announced by Home Office May 1999
Psychoanalytical theories	Freud's theories suggest that neurotic symptomatology is a result of unresolved childhood experiences; he outlined theories of psychosexual development	Freud Erikson Jung
Rape	Unlawful sexual intercourse with a woman who at the time does not consent to it. Rape also occurs within marriage and, for clients with learning disability, may bring into question their consent to intercourse within marriage	1956 Sexual Offences (Amendment) Act

Soliciting	The offence of inviting, enticing or making appeals or requests to another person for the purposes of sex	Section 3 Vagrancy Act 1824 (Females) Section 32 Sexual Offences Act 1956 (Males)
Tourist sex	Since October 1996 it has been possible to try in an English or Welsh court any person who has conspired with or incited others to commit any of the sexual tourist offences anywhere in the world	Home Office supports UK action to combat child sex exploitation. Sex Offenders Act 1977
Unconsummated marriage	Reasons for unconsummated marriage may be social, emotional or physical	Relate offers advice and counselling to couples, whether married or single
Venereal disease	Sexually transmitted diseases, chlamydia being the most common	Expert advisory group established to consider practical implications of screening programmes 1998
Whore	From the Latin word *carus*, meaning dear, beloved. Used as a term for prostitutes since 12th century. Defined for the purposes of the Street Offences Act 1959 it refers only to a woman who is a prostitute; however, men can solicit for immoral purposes under Sexual Offences Acts and can be described as male prostitutes	Child prostitution guidance: Home Office www.homeoffice.gov.uk
Young people	Teenage pregnancies and contraceptive advice	Office for National Statistics 1998 Conceptions in England and Wales 1996
X-rated material	Used to be the certification for films, which are now regulated by age. If the materials have the effect of depraving and corrupting persons who are likely to read, see or hear them	Offence under section 160 Criminal Justice Act 1988 possession of indecent photographs of children
Zina	A Muslim category for all forbidden sex acts, including bestiality, prostitution, anal sex and lesbianism. The penalty for Zina is death	Consider the importance of different ethnic cultures and religious beliefs on sexual behaviour and tolerance

accepted as a member of the opposite sex. There is a persistent discomfort with his or her anatomical sex and a sense of inappropriateness in the gender role of that sex. There is a wish to have hormonal treatment and surgery to make one's body as *congruent as possible with one's psychological sex* (Reid 1996).

The Gender Trust, which provides advice and support for transsexuals and transvestites, describes transsexuals as follows:

'... *transsexuals feel that they have been born with the wrong physical anatomy for the gender which they "are" psychologically, and feel they have always been inside. They want to change their physical body to fit their psychological gender. This means that they will require hormone treatment and gender reassignment surgery after careful counselling and a trial period of living in role, usually of 1–2 years.'*

The Beaumont Society estimate that 1 in 30 000 men and 1 in 100 000 women experience gender dysphoria, and that there are approximately 35 000 transsexuals living in Britain. Whereas Schutzer (1998) refers to one's basic self as a male or female, it is usually assumed that there is congruence between biological sex and gender identity. Where discrepancies exist, either mild or severe, individuals may experience feelings of gender dysphoria. Money and Ambinder (1955) developed the term *gender role* to signify that which is 'anything a person says or does to indicate the self to others as his/her status being male/female or ambiguous'.

Individuals who are experiencing gender dysphoria will have a particular *gender direction*, either from male to female or from female to male.

Their *gender status* may be described as not seeking surgery, not yet referred, referred for surgery (preoperative), surgery completed (postoperative), not decided, or transgenderist, i.e. wishing to live in other role without undergoing surgery. Their *social status* could be one of three things: still living in original role; living full time in adopted role; or living part time in adopted role.

Diagnostic process

For those who are undergoing a diagnostic process, there are two phases: psychodiagnostic assessment, and the 2-year *real life test*, where the individual has been undergoing clinical assessment and intervention for at least 6 months and has had a successful cross-living test over a 1-year period.

Under UK law an acquired sexual identity (whether or not involving gender reassignment) can be given some official recognition, e.g. passports and National Insurance numbers can be issued in the new name, which can be changed by deed poll. However, marriage is not allowed, the details on a birth certificate cannot be changed, and the age of receipt of pension cannot be altered.

Services and organizations relating to gender dysphoria

The Gender Trust is an organization that provides confidential help for those who feel themselves to be gender dysphoric and those who are close to them emotionally. They also provide information for professionals in the field of care for transsexuals.

Press for Change provides information and speakers and training sessions, and is a political lobbying and educational organization that campaigns to achieve civil rights and liberties for all transsexual people in the UK through legislation and social change. Affiliated to the National Council for Civil Liberties, Press for Change supporters include politicians, public figures and church leaders.

The Gender Identity Development Service is a specialist service that provides help for children, adolescents and their families who are experiencing difficulties in the development of gender identity.

The International Gender Dysphoria Association provides guidance for gender identity clinics, such as that at Charing Cross Hospital or the Tavistock Clinic, but for many patients undergoing treatment their contact with health services will be general practice professionals, psychiatric or mental health services, obstetrics and gynaecology, genitourinary departments, plastic surgery units or general surgical departments.

TASK: Transsexual Awareness and Self-Knowledge is a voluntary group that works on a consultancy basis to provide training and information to public service agencies and holds support meetings for members. TASK has produced a video on the issues surrounding transsexualism and equal opportunities in the workplace.

Equal opportunity issues

Since the 1950s, when Dr Harry Benjamin first introduced the syndrome and advocated compassionate treatment, there have been over 70 evaluation studies conducted to investigate the therapeutic effectiveness of gender reassignment surgery, many of which use employment as one of their objective criteria for effectiveness. Many transsexual individuals experience discrimination, marginalization and even criminalization. This has been recognized by the European Parliament, which called on the member states to enact provisions on transsexuals' rights to change sex by endocrinological, plastic surgery and cosmetic treatment in order to ensure that human dignity and personal rights include the right to live according to one's sexual identity.

The range of problems encountered may be social, political and/or legal. One case in particular (P *v* S (1995) and Cornwall County Council) has been used to highlight issues relating to equal opportunities in the workplace for those who have undergone gender reassignment or wish to do so.

In the case of P *v* S, P stated the intention to undergo surgery in order to change her biological sex to suit her sexual identity, and was dismissed from her employment on that account. In the judgement on this case the European Court of Justice determined that transsexuals do not constitute a 'third sex' and considered it a matter of principle that they are covered by the EEC Equal Opportunities Directive, which states that equal treatment for male and female workers constitutes one of the objectives of the Community.

The judgement interpreted the Directive as precluding the dismissal of a transsexual on account of change of sex. Subsequently, the judgement of the Court, 30 April 1996, stated that discrimination is based essentially if not exclusively on the sex of the person concerned. Where a person is dismissed on the grounds that he or she intends to undergo, or has undergone, gender reassignment, he or she is treated unfavourably compared to persons of the sex to which he or she was deemed to belong before undergoing gender reassignment.

It was stated at this time that toleration of such discrimination would be tantamount to a failure to respect the dignity and freedom to which the person is entitled, and which the Court has a duty to safeguard.

Sex discrimination

Following on from this specific case, the Department of Education and Employment put out a consultation paper in January 1998 on legislation regarding discrimination on grounds of transsexualism in employment. The purpose of the consultation process was to ensure that the Equal Opportunities Commission and the review of the Sex Discrimination Act would make provision in the fields of recruitment, employment, terms and conditions of work, training, promotion, dismissal and mistreatment, such as harassment at work.

The government sought views on whether gender reassignment gives rise to some circumstances when it might be considered reasonable to allow employers to treat transsexuals differently from other staff, if only temporarily.

The DOE sought views on the following areas and posed a series of questions and views for consultation, including the following:

What comparator?
In sex discrimination the basis for comparison is between men and women: should this continue to be the case for transsexuals?

What defines the individual who needs protection?
Should the point at which a specific request for medical intervention is made mark the appropriate point at which a person is regarded as transsexual, and should this be formally recorded?
What exceptions?
The Sex Discrimination Act 1975 and Race Relations Act 1976 allow certain narrowly defined circumstances to reject individuals on grounds of sex or race, where authenticity is required.
Restrictions to working with children?
The government sought views on whether there should be a specific objection for jobs which involve working with children.

In the consultation document, the government also proposed that:

During the process of gender reassignment it will be lawful for the employer to specify that the transsexual individual must use particular facilities for that period (e.g. male or female toilets).
During the period and for 1 year afterwards it will be lawful to exclude individuals from activities that involve intimate contact or close personal interaction.
During the period and for 6 months afterwards it will be lawful to exclude individuals from jobs involving contact with members of the public or customers who are changing.
After the gender reassignment the government intention is to treat individuals as belonging to the reassigned sex for the purpose of employment and education, and as having the protection of the Sex Discrimination Act in that new sexual identity, apart from the following:

◆ *Where employment has to comply with an organized religion*
◆ *Where a transsexual seeks to return to the same employer and activity and to work with same people (e.g. patients) who were of an unusually vulnerable nature and could be disturbed by the fact of gender reassignment in someone they know*
◆ *In rare cases where someone has been through the process of gender reassignment and was in a job is restricted to either sex (e.g. a single-*

sex hospital), the regulations would make it lawful to dismiss a transsexual from such a post.

The consultation paper also raised a series of questions for employers, as follows:

Issues for employers
Whereas it is clear that it is an offence to discriminate against an individual on grounds of sex, what is not clear is how individual organizations/employers should support individuals experiencing gender dysphoria. The consultation paper highlights employment issues encountered, but provides only a series of questions to be answered. These include:

Harassment
Employers have duties to prevent harassment of staff about undergoing gender reassignment. How can this be prevented using the same basis as sexual harassment?

Confidentiality
Is it always right or practical to maintain a transsexual's confidentiality at work, or is it a matter for consideration depending on the particular circumstances?

Dress code
What special arrangements might be needed for individuals who work in a uniform?

Changing rooms and toilets
What consideration might be given as to whether special and appropriate working arrangements might be necessary for the individual?

Offering alternative work
The employer should offer alternative work at the same pay if possible; if not, at a lower rate. Unpaid leave may be appropriate until a vacancy arises. Dismissal should be the last resort.

Jobs with 'vulnerable' individuals
Where the gender of the person is irrelevant, how might this affect vulnerable persons adversely where an individual changes gender?

The new Regulations

Despite recognizing the difficulties of dealing with this issue in areas where individuals have close or intimate contact with clients or patients, some of the proposals appear to go against the philosophy of equal rights and opportunities and almost deny

individuals the support and help they need to be able to achieve their own required outcomes from reassignment. Despite this, the legislation was passed, and the new Sex Discrimination (Gender Reassignment) Regulations 1999 clarify British law relating to gender reassignment. They are a measure to prevent discrimination against transsexual people on the grounds of sex in pay and treatment in employment and vocational training. (For more details, see the Press for Change website.)

The Guide to the Sex Discrimination (Gender Reassignment) Regulations 1999 (Department for Education and Employment, 1999) has no special legal status and is not intended to equate with a Code of Practice. Its purpose is to provide guidance in relation to the application of the Regulations, and to suggest some aspects of good practice for employers and employees on the issues that might be encountered in accommodating an individual for whom gender reassignment grounds exist in the workplace.

In terms of respecting human dignity and equal rights, a 'quality of life' model could be applied in employment practice. This is the model used for measuring the effectiveness of patient care, and includes the ability of the gender reassignment patient to:

◆ find employment
◆ make relationships
◆ integrate with a larger community
◆ live a fulfilling life.

Reflection point 7.5

Several publications make it clear that the current legal status of people who have undergone or wish to undergo gender reassignment has prevented them from achieving these goals, and that the force for change and improvement lies with members of society who are willing to tackle these issues in a fair and open way.

◆ How tolerant do you think society is of issues such as these?

◆ How do you feel personally and professionally?

◆ What can you do as a member of society to tackle these issues?

Definitions (Press for Change Website*)

Gender
Gender is expressed in terms of masculinity and femininity. It is how people perceive themselves and how they expect others to behave. It is largely culturally determined.

Gender dysphoria or gender identity disorder
Refers to the dissatisfaction with one's gender (masculinity or femininity), which is in conflict with one's physical sex. The term is usually, but not always, restricted to those who seek medical and surgical assistance to resolve their difficulty.

Gender identity
The gender to which one feels one belongs.

Gender role
To interact with society as a member of a specific gender (i.e. as a man or woman) by following arbitrary rules assigned by society that define what clothing, behaviours, thoughts, feelings, relationships etc. are considered appropriate and inappropriate for members of each sex. What is considered masculine, feminine or gender neutral varies according to location, class, occasion, time in history, and numerous other factors.

Physical sex
To what sex does the body match, i.e. male, female, hermaphrodite or neuter?

Hermaphroditism and intersexuality
Where the physiological sex is ambiguous. The condition may or may not be accompanied by various degrees of gender dysphoria, and may be due to chromosomal complexes, such as Turner's or Klinefelter's syndromes, congenital errors of metabolism such as androgen insensitivity syndrome, and adrenogenital syndrome. There may also be effects from the hormone balance in the fetus or the placenta.

Transvestite
The clinical name for a cross-dresser, a person who dresses in the clothing of the opposite sex. Generally these persons do not alter their body.

Transsexual person
A person who feels a consistent and overwhelming desire for transition and to fulfil their lives as members of the opposite gender. Most transsexual persons actively desire and complete gender-reassignment surgery.

Transgender
A term used to include transsexual persons, transvestites and cross-dressers. It can also represent a person who, like a transsexual, transitions, sometimes with the help of hormone therapy and/or cosmetic surgery, to live in the gender role of choice, but who has not undergone, and generally does not intend to undergo, gender reassignment surgery.

CONCLUSION

Legislation and policy are only as effective as the interpretation and implementation they are given. In all aspects of health care, education or employment, the legal, ethical and moral aspects must be considered and put alongside the client's needs, yet practitioners continue to abuse their position or ignore inappropriate practice.

It is important to be familiar with legislation relating to practice, and to develop an awareness of sexual politics and the law.

Information and advice can be obtained from a range of statutory, professional and voluntary organizations to ensure that all individuals have

---

* Source: Press for Change Website at http://www.pfc.org.uk. Reproduced by kind permission of Press for Change.

equitable access to quality health care without undue harassment, and that confidentiality is assured.

RESOURCES

Stonewall, 16 Clerkenwell Close, London EC1R 0AN. Tel: 020 7336 8860. Website: http://www. stonewall.org.uk/

The Gender Trust, BM Gentrust, London WC1N 3XX. Tel: 0303 269 2222. Email: gentrust @mistral.co.uk. Website: http://www3.mistral.co. uk/gentrust

Sex and Race Equality Division, Department for Education and Employment, Caxton House, 6–12 Tothill Street, London SWIH 9NE. Tel: 020 7925 5000. Public Enquiry Unit. Email: info@dfee.gov.uk

NHS Equal Opportunities Unit, Quarry House, Quarry Hill, Leeds LS2 7UE

FTM Network, BM Network, London WC1N 3XX. Tel: 0161 432915

Offers free and confidential advice for female to male transsexuals

Mermaids, BM Mermaids, London WC1N 3XX. Website: http://www.geocities.com/ WestHollywood/Village/2671/mermaids.html

Offers support and advice for parents of children with gender identity problems

The Beaumont Society, 27 Old Gloucester Road, London WC1N 3XX. Information line, Tel: 01582 412220

Offers free and confidential advice and support for transvestites

Press for Change, BM Network, London WC1N 3XX. Website: http://www.pfc.org.uk/employ/ index.htm

A political campaigning group for equal civil rights for transgendered people, *providing legal help advice, information and speakers*

Gender Identity Development Service, Portman Clinic, 8 Fitzjohns Avenue, London NW3 5NA. Tel: 020 7794 8262

United Kingdom Central Council National for Nursing, Midwifery and Health Visiting, 23 Portland Place, London W1N 3AF

English National board for Nursing, Midwifery and Health Visiting, 170 Tottenham Court Road, London W1P 0HA

National Board for Nursing, Midwifery and Health Visiting for Scotland, 22 Queen Street, Edinburgh EH2 IJX

Welsh National Board for Nursing, Midwifery and Health Visiting, Floor 13, Pearl Assurance House, Greyfriars Road, Cardiff CF1 3AG

National Board for Nursing, Midwifery and Health Visiting for Northern Ireland, RAC House, 79 Chichester Street, Belfast BT1 4JE

FURTHER READING

Bromham D, Pearson R 1996 The pharmacological treatment of transsexuals. British Journal of Sexual Medicine Sept/Oct

Dimond B 1990 Legal aspects of nursing. Prentice Hall, London

Jenkins R 1995 The law and the midwife. Blackwell Science, Oxford

Redmond P W D, Shears P 1993 General principles of English law, 7th edn. The M & E Handbook series. Pitman, London

Zhous J J, Hofman M A, Gooren J G, Swaab D F 1995 A sex difference in the human brain and its relation to transsexuality. Nature 378: 2 November

For a useful list of publications on transsexualism and transgenderism, see the Gender Trust Website at http://www3.mistral.co.uk/gentrust/gt_pubs.htm

REFERENCES

CANS Trust 1999 CANS digest of social legislation. September. Citizens Advice Notes Service Trust, London

Comfort A 1996 The joy of sex. Updated edn. Mitchell Beazley, London

Department for Education and Employment 1999 Guide to the Sex Discrimination (Gender Reassignment) Regulations 1999. Department for Education and Employment, London

Dimond B 1990 Legal aspects of nursing. Prentice Hall, London

Draycott A T, Carr A P 1996 Stone's Justices Manual. Shaw & Sons and Butterworths, London, vols 1, 2 and 3

Goldenson, R, Anderson K 1987 The Wordsworth Dictionary of Sex. Wordsworth Reference, London

HMSO 1996 Public general acts and general synod measures. HMSO, London

Jenkins R 1995 The law and the midwife. Blackwell Science, Oxford

Money J, Ambinder R 1955 Two year real-life diagnostic test: rehabilitation versus cure. In: Brady J P, Brodie H K H (eds) 1978 Controversy in psychiatry. Saunders, Philadelphia, p. 833

Reader's Digest 1991 You and your rights. Reader's Digest, London

Redmond P W D, Shears P 1993 General principles of English law, 7th edn. The M & E Handbook Series. Pitman, London

Reid R 1996 Transsexualism: The current medical viewpoint. Press for Change, London

Schutzer N 1998 Transsexualism, its social, legal and medical aspects in European society with comparisons to American and Canadian cultures with associated suggestions for English legislation. Unpublished

United Kingdom Central Council for Nursing 1992a Code of professional conduct. United Kingdom Central Council for Nursing, Midwifery and Health Visiting, London

United Kingdom Central Council 1992b Professional conduct – occasional report on selected cases 1 April 1991 to 31 March 1992. United Kingdom Central Council for Nursing, Midwifery and Health Visiting, London

United Kingdom Central Council for Nursing 1992c The scope of professional practice. United Kingdom Central Council for Nursing, Midwifery and Health Visiting, London

United Kingdom Central Council for Nursing 1996a Reporting misconduct – information for employers and managers. United Kingdom Central Council for Nursing, Midwifery and Health Visiting, London

United Kingdom Central Council for Nursing 1996b Guidelines for professional practice. United Kingdom Central Council for Nursing, Midwifery and Health Visiting, London

United Kingdom Central Council for Nursing 1998 A UKCC guide for students of nursing and midwifery. United Kingdom Central Council for Nursing, Midwifery and Health Visiting, London

Wellings K, Bradshaw S 1994 Sexual behaviour in Britain: the national survey of sexual attitudes and lifestyles. Penguin Books, London

3

Part Three
Developing practice – issues and ideas

8

Sexual health and the service user

Ian Hicken

> *'It's unwise to pay too much, but it's unwise to pay too little. When you pay too much you lose a little money. That is all. When you pay too little you sometimes lose everything because the thing you bought was incapable of doing the thing you bought it to do. The common law of business balance prohibits paying a little and getting a lot. It can't be done. If you deal with the lowest bidder it's well to add something for the risk you run. And if you do that, you will have enough to pay for something better.'*
> (John Ruskin 1819–1900)

KEY ISSUES/CONCEPTS

◆ Consumers and consumer audit

◆ Health policy

◆ Professional practice

◆ Society

OVERVIEW

Chapter 8, *Sexual health and the service user*, explores the relationship between consumers and consumer audit, health policy, professional practice and society, and examines the issues raised. It aims to enable the reader to become aware of factors that influence the development of their own skills and abilities in sexual health. The terms consumer and consumer audit will be discussed in relation to quality of care, and activities and reflection points will be used to enable the reader to identify what is needed to ensure the sexual health needs of individuals and communities can be met within a culturally sensitive climate.

INTRODUCTION

The past two decades have seen a rise in the notion of consumerism and the importance of engaging the consumer in quality assurance processes. For a long time consumerism has been central to the survival of business, commerce industry and the private sector. This has been reflected in the public sector, with the views of service users increasingly being taken into account when new services are being developed. However, political and social change has brought about a move to introduce the concept of consumerism in the public arena. The general public now has greater expectations of public service, creating the need for health-care professionals to ensure that their health needs are being appropriately met. To ensure appropriateness of health service delivery the statutory bodies require health-care professionals to engage in high levels of care and accountable practice. The introduction of quality assurance mechanisms (clinical audit, clinical supervision, clinical governance) will provide a strategy for health-care effectiveness.

CONSUMERISM IN HEALTH CARE

The consumer

What do we actually mean when we talk about the consumer? The term is increasingly used in health-care circles, and in some circumstances has replaced the traditional labels of patient, carer, resident etc. Borrowed from the commercial retail sector, the term consumer, in relation to health care, has come to mean any individual or group that has used or that currently uses health services. Perhaps one reason for the growth in popularity of this term is the changing organization and management of health-care provision, which has resulted in a market culture where products and services are purchased from providers and where there is increasing accountability for those products and services. It has been suggested that health-care workers, including nurses, midwives and health visitors, are also consumers, not only of the services but also of the policies, procedures, professional relationships and information and communication strategies that shape and direct their professional practice (Hicken and Butterworth 1995). For the purpose of this chapter the term 'consumer' will denote service users, carers, patients' advocates and health-care professionals.

The use of the label consumer in health care is potentially problematic, one reason being that, by definition, a consumer is someone who uses a product or service. In many areas of health care this can exclude individuals and groups who may have a need for a service or product but where that service or product is not available or not widely known about and therefore not used by those who are in need. For example, in relation to sexual health it is likely (although not guaranteed) that most people are aware that family planning clinics, breast screening clinics and departments of genitourinary medicine or sexually transmitted disease clinics exist, i.e. specialist services that are explicitly about sex, sexuality and sexual health. However, is it as likely that those people are also aware that other services or products may be available in other health-care settings, such as advice on sexual relationships following surgery, safer sex and contra-

ception, or counselling on sexually related issues? Unless a person has had specific experience of such services or products, or knows someone who has, then it is very likely that most would feel unsure about raising such issues or seeking information about worries and concerns relating to sexual health. It might be more useful to identify two target groups, current and potential consumers.

It could be argued that health-care workers have a duty to ensure that consumers are aware that such services and products exist; however, in the main, guidelines for professional practice are not always readily available and professional education on sexual health-related matters is often inadequate, leaving the health-care worker without clearly defined protocols or boundaries for their work and without a sound knowledge base on which to base practice (Few et al. 1996), and without specific practices or services to promote.

Learning activity 8.1

Spend 5 minutes listing the sexual health-related services that are available (a) in your organization, (b) in your district, (c) in your region, and (d) on your current unit or ward.

Feedback on Learning activity 8.1

You may wish to keep this list as the basis for a directory of services: perhaps you could add contact names, addresses, telephone numbers, hours of opening, method of referral and scope of services offered. You may have found it difficult to think of sexual health-related services that are offered on your current unit or ward: if so, try to identify whether there is scope to develop such services or practices.

Consumer audit

The term 'consumer audit' was first used in a health-care context by Michael Young, President of the College of Health, in a report on a pilot study that observed communications between consultants and their patients (College of Health 1994).

Consumer audit has been defined as 'a qualitative approach to obtaining feedback from patients about health-care services. It aims to look at the health service from the patient's point of view, emphasizing emotional as well as physical well-being, and also the quality and clarity of information and communication with patients' (College of Health 1994). The report goes on to suggest that consumer audit should aim to 'help define standards of care that patients wish to receive and give providers and purchasers of health services the information they need to make positive change and make services more patient centred'. Involving local people in the consultation process has been demonstrated to have a direct impact on purchasing plans and/or contracts (NHSE 1994a). Ham (1992) suggests that consumer groups are in a weak position, as they are heavily dependent on the quality of their arguments and the willingness of ministers and civil servants to listen to what they have to say. He goes on to suggest that the interests of consumers may be compromised by producer groups who 'are well able to promote and defend their interests'.

As part of an audit cycle, consumer audit techniques can benefit both purchasers and providers by providing a framework for future monitoring of the quality of services, identifying how services work together, pinpointing weaknesses and gaps, identifying issues for professional education, helping to set clinical standards, identifying good practice, and by complementing other forms of quality monitoring, such as clinical and medical audit, thereby completing the audit cycle (College of Health 1994).

In simple terms, consumer audit is a mechanism that will help us in our capacity as health-care professionals, in partnership with service users, to deliver the services we are responsible for developing, operating and evaluating.

Reflection point 8.1

The growth of consumerism and consumer audit in health care has brought about a greater need to consult with those groups and individuals that use services. What problems do you envisage with this process? You may wish to consider the following issues:

◆ Who are the consumers of sexual health-related services?

◆ What mechanisms exist to consult with 'hard to reach' individuals and/or groups?

◆ What is it we are currently trying to achieve in relation to the sexual health of consumers?

◆ Are there any obvious gaps in this service provision?

Link between consumer audit and quality

Since the early 1980s welcome advances have been made in raising the quality of health-care services, as well as in raising health-care workers' awareness of quality and its impact on health outcomes. Quality of care has been defined as 'the degree to which health services for individuals and populations increase the likelihood of desired health outcomes and are consistent with professional knowledge' (Lohr 1990). Peters (1993) states that 'traditional quality assurance has relied on the routine, systematic collection of data retroactively to determine if certain standards were met'. She goes on to say that 'the new paradigm toward total quality management and a focus on outcomes recognise that quality is no longer simply an attribute of a technically correct product or service; it is also dependent on relationships'.

Total quality management is a phrase increasingly used in health care to describe a comprehensive and continuous process for assessing and responding to need and for ongoing evaluation of services. Collard et al. (1990) define total quality management as 'a cost-effective system for integrating the continuous improvement efforts of people at all levels in an organisation to deliver products and services which ensure customer satisfaction'.

The growth of consumerism in health care has without doubt validated the work of many health-care professionals who, for many years, have striven to develop high-quality patient-led services. Consumerism in health care is not a new concept: health-care workers have long sought the views of their patients in an attempt to ensure that the services they provide are relevant and user friendly and more likely to be used. There are many excellent examples of consumer audit in relation to sexual health-related services, but in the main these relate to established sexual health-specific service provision and rarely take account of health issues that fall outside planning and priorities guidance, established public health issues or sexual health in generic health care.

The growth of consumerism in health care

In a speech on 'Purchasing for health' at a national purchasing conference in Birmingham (NHSE 1994b), Dr Brian Mawhinney MP (Minister for Health) reiterated the need for every health authority 'to demonstrate that it was taking systematic action to seek and act on the views of community health councils, voluntary bodies, the wider public and their representatives'. The emphasis of his speech was on the need to canvass the views of those who use services to ensure that purchasing arrangements deliver high-quality strategically planned value-for-money services. Dr Mawhinney's speech encapsulated the concept, highlighted in various government publications and initiatives, that consultation with consumer groups is fundamental to the process of planning and delivering services based on local need.

Successive documents such as *Working for patients* and *Caring for people* (Secretary of State for Health 1989a, b), *Local voices: the views of local people in purchasing for health* (NHSME 1992), *The patients' charter* (DoH 1991) and *The health of the nation* (DoH 1993a) have laid down a framework that emphasizes the need to consult with consumers and clearly identify their needs in relation to service provision.

Central government planning and priorities guidance in relation to greater involvement from consumers is to be welcomed; however, it could be argued that those most vocal and/or empowered are more likely to be heard than those who do not know how to influence the development of services.

SEXUAL HEALTH NEEDS OF CONSUMERS

The introduction of consumerism in sexual health care is problematic and makes two basic assumptions: first, that consumers know what they want from a product or service and therefore voice an opinion on the subject, and secondly that consumers see sexual health as a public issue. Clare (1986) comments that 'part of the appeal of the western-style nuclear family, with its emphasis on individual choice and romantic love, may lie in the fact that personal and sexual relations within such a model appear to be the concern of the people involved and nobody else'. He goes on to say that seemingly private matters, such as how we experience and express our sexuality, whether we marry and, if we do, to whom and at what age, whether we remain faithful, divorce or have children, are all personal decisions embedded in the 'larger human network of custom, tradition and law'.

Reflection point 8.2

Clare (1986) suggests that our personal decisions about sex and sexuality are all 'embedded in the larger human network of custom, tradition and law'. The law element of his supposition is clear, i.e. that there are laws governing what is permissible and acceptable in relation to sex, sexuality and sexual health (see Chapter 7, Sex and the statutory bodies).

◆ What influence do custom and tradition have on our personal decisions relating to sex and sexuality?

◆ Do these influences reinforce sex and sexuality as a private matter, or do they bring them into the public arena?

One of the fundamental problems relating to the development of practice incorporating sexual health-related issues is that the debate on what is private and what is public in relation to sex and sexuality has never really taken place in health care. The result is that as a profession we remain unclear about what we are trying to provide for our 'customers'. Should we only address issues that are clearly defined by law? Should public health be the driving force behind the development of services and scope of practice, or should we aim to develop services and practice that take account of the diverse and ever-changing sexual health needs and wishes of a multicultural society?

Case study 8.1

Julie is a third-year student nurse currently working on an acute medical admission ward in a busy district general hospital. The ward uses the Activities of Living Model for Nursing (Roper et al. 1985) as a basis for nursing practice. A 47-year-old man with chest pain has arrived on the ward following referral from his general practitioner. Julie has been given responsibility for undertaking the initial nursing assessment of the patient, and proceeds to work through the routine admission procedure. While gathering the basic data, Julie comes to the section on the patient assessment form that states Sexuality. After a few embarrassed seconds she looks skyward and asks: 'and are you sexually healthy Mr Hopkins?' Somewhat bewildered by the question, Mr Hopkins replies 'um yes!' Julie writes 'Sexually healthy – expresses sexuality without difficulty'. Sexuality or sexual health was never discussed again throughout Mr Hopkin's stay in hospital.

How would you respond if you were asked the same question during a consultation with a nurse or doctor?

Case study 8.2

Carl is a staff nurse on a busy surgical ward. While admitting a patient (Mr King) for surgery he suspects that the gentleman is homosexual – he doesn't know why, but 'there is something about him'. Mr King has previously given as his next of kin 'Steven Jones at the same address – relationship: friend'. Carl continues with the admission and is trying to find a way of asking the patient if Steven Jones is his partner/lover. On the patient assessment form there is a section marked Expressing Sexuality. Of the categories listed, Carl ticks 'Divorced' and 'No children at home'. For the remainder of Mr King's stay in hospital rumour that he is gay is rife within the ward team, but no one manages to talk openly with Mr King about his sexuality, and find talking to him 'slightly awkward'.

Was it appropriate for Carl to make further enquiries about Mr King's sexuality and his relationship with Steven Jones? If it was, why? If not, why not? What views do you hold on people with differing sexuality from your own? How might this affect your relationship with patients?

Feedback on Case studies 8.1 and 8.2

Both of these case histories clearly demonstrate that the inclusion of sexuality and sexual health as assessment criteria is problematic, especially where the practitioner is unprepared for such lines of inquiry. In Case study 1 Julie has worked her way systematically through the assessment sheets and has chosen to take a literal interpretation of the section marked 'Sexual health'. It is clear that Julie has had limited guidance on sexual health, and that she does not fully understand her role or remit in the assessment process in relation to Mr Hopkin's sexual health. In Case study 2 Carl was limited in his assessment of Mr King, owing partly to lack of expertise and lack of confidence in facing the issue of sexuality, and partly to the constraints of the assessment form. On the form the section Expressing Sexuality contained several statements from which he could choose to apply to Mr King's circumstances and appearance. These were:

◆ *Children at home*
◆ *No children at home*

◆ *Single*

◆ *Married*

◆ *Widowed*

◆ *Divorced*

◆ *Lives with common-law husband*

◆ *Lives with common-law wife*

◆ *Separated*

◆ *Well groomed*

◆ *Slight neglect*

◆ *Unkempt*

◆ *Likes to wear makeup*

◆ *Wears a wig/hairpiece*

◆ *Wears contact lenses*

◆ *Mastectomy/prosthesis*

Clearly the listed criteria do have an effect on an individual's expression of their sexuality; however, in the main they are indicators of social circumstances and self-esteem, and not primarily related to the explicit expression of sexuality or indicators of sexual health. Carl clearly felt uncomfortable about raising the issue of sexuality with Mr King, resulting in their relationship feeling strained and difficult at times.

Savage (1989) comments that 'sexuality is woven into the structure and practice of nursing itself and until it is made explicit we cannot expect nurses to come to terms with promoting sexual health care'. Perhaps there is a need to examine the use of the terms sexuality and sexual health within health care. All too often these terms are used inappropriately, which results in health-care workers determining the need for sexual health-related interventions on the basis of an individual's expression of their sexuality, or misinterpreting concerns about sexual health as problems relating to the individual's sexuality.

Preparing to meet consumers' needs

Throughout this book you will have read various definitions of sexuality and/or sexual health. The

terms 'sexuality' and 'sexual health' continue to appear in nursing and medical literature, and have done so, to varying degrees, since the early 1900s; however, it has only been since research on nursing practice related to sexuality began in the late 1960s and early 1970s that real progress has been made in these areas (Waterhouse 1996). In 1973, the World Health Organization (WHO) proposed that information on sexuality be offered in medical and nursing schools (Mace et al 1974). Research findings in the mid-1970s demonstrated that nurses had very limited knowledge on issues pertaining to sexuality and sexual health (Fontaine 1976), a finding that has been replicated many times since (Bond 1989, Akinsanya and Rouse 1991, McHaffie 1993).

In response to a growing awareness that professional education on sexual health was inadequate, in 1994 the English National Board for Nursing, Midwifery and Health Visiting (ENB) developed guidelines: *Sexual health education and training: guidelines for good practice in the teaching of nurses, midwives and health visitors.* The publication of these guidelines was intended to:

◆ highlight the need for a systematic and rigorous approach to sexual health education and training

◆ provide guidelines for good practice by identifying the guiding principles that underpin quality in sexual health education and training

◆ provide an adaptable framework for sexual health education and training

◆ provide examples of how sexual health education and training have been successfully integrated into professional education

◆ serve as a resource for those involved in sexual health education and training.

Despite the efforts of nurse educators over recent years to ensure that nurses can address issues relating to sexuality and integrate aspects of sexual health into nursing practice, in the main this has had little demonstrable effect on the sexual health care, in generic health-care settings, of consumers generally. To date, anecdotal evidence suggests that as a profession we are 'playing the game but without a full deck'.

Since the mid-1980s sexual health has received a high profile in health care. In part this has been due to the advent of the human immunodeficiency virus (HIV), which has crystallized in the public's mind that sex can be dangerous, sexuality is diverse, and sexual health is a basic human right. There appears to be little doubt that HIV has got people talking about sex in a much more open and forthright manner. The mass media have seen an explosion of programmes and news items on issues relating to the sexual diversity of the general public. What used to happen only behind closed doors is now fully exposed in a way that we have never seen before. For the first time in recent social history, sex, sexuality and sexual health is a legitimate issue for all health and social care professionals, and not just for those who work in sexual health-specific areas. A significant consequence of this liberation of ideas has been that many professionals feel confused, ignorant and unskilled to address the implications for practice. By the same token, the general public feels confused and ignorant about a greater focus on sexual health-related issues in health care.

Reflection point 8.3

◆ Has your education and training prepared you adequately to address issues relating to sexuality and sexual health in health care?

◆ What are you trying to achieve in relation to the sexual health of patients?

◆ When is it appropriate to raise issues relating to sexual health?

◆ What guidelines are there to shape and direct your work in relation to sexual health?

Feedback on Reflection point 8.3

If the answer to the first question is no, then it is likely that you are struggling with the next two questions. Try making a list of issues you feel unsure about, or write down an account of a situation in which you felt inadequate or unskilled. This will be a good starting point for examining your professional development needs in sexual health, and for developing an action plan.

Sexuality or sexual health?

Sexuality and sexual health are not easy concepts to define and even harder on which to agree. To some sexuality remains a private and personal issue determined by the individual's biological sex, gender identity, their own frame of reference, personal ethics and moral code. To others, the 1990s media-led focus on sex, sexuality and sexual lifestyles has become a liberating experience that has helped to erode some of the taboos associated with discussions on these issues. The following quotes illustrate the diverse and personal opinions people have in relation to sexuality (Hicken and Butterworth 1995):

> *'My sexuality is nothing to do with anyone other than me and my partner; it really irritates me when people judge me for being a lesbian – after all, it is not as though I go around molesting other women all the time. People think that just because you're gay you automatically fancy every woman you come across.'* (A gay woman.)

> *'I do not mind them talking about other ways of having safer sex; I mean, fantasy is OK but what if it gets out of hand? What do you do if your partner asks you to do something really perverted? Where do you draw the line?'* (A gay man.)

> *'I can't see what all the fuss is about personally. If we encouraged more open and frank discussion about sex then we wouldn't be having the problems [a rise in STDs and teenage pregnancies] we've got.'* (A female health visitor.)

> *'In my day sexuality was gay or straight; nowadays they say that you can't exclude the fact that if the circumstances are right you might have a dabble. Complete rubbish if you ask me, I know what I am and I don't need some New Age trainer telling me that "I'm on a journey".'* (A male nurse.)

> *'I think that it would be a very sad day if we reverted to the days – like my parents'*

generation – when if you got pregnant and were unmarried, then you were the black sheep of the family and you were sent to stay with your great Aunt Nellie. (A heterosexual woman.)

Waterhouse (1996) suggests that nursing practice in the area of sexuality may include assessing sexuality, providing anticipatory guidance about sexual development, validating normality, educating about sexual health and disease prevention, counselling clients who must adapt to changes in their usual forms of sexual expression, providing intensive therapy for sexual problems, and referring clients to other health-care providers. She goes on to say that sexuality is an important aspect of nursing care in a variety of settings, with clients of all ages and most medical diagnoses. The examples she uses to illustrate her point include nurses teaching testicular self-examination; encouraging the discussion of sexual concerns related to living with changes following surgery; providing information on birth control and sexual behaviour to adolescents; and assessing all clients for concerns about sexuality. Waterhouse's article focuses on the need to strengthen sexuality-related nursing practice. It could be argued that using the term sexuality causes further confusion and undermines nurses' confidence in addressing sexual health-related issues. Of course sexuality is an integral part of sexual health, but it should not be the main 'hook' on which to base practice or policy development. Perhaps one reason why so many health-care workers feel reluctant to address the sexual health concerns of their clients is because their preparation for intervening has been based on intensive discussions about sexuality, rather than sexuality as a part of sexual health. This could also be true for consumers of services: for example, is it really necessary to question all patients about their sexuality, such as is indicated on many patient admission assessment forms? Surely a starting point should be to assess concerns about sexual health only if these are offered; further discussions on sexuality might then be required. For most people their sexuality is not in question; however, their sexual health might be.

SEXUAL HEALTH SERVICE USERS IN SOCIETY

This section explores sexual health as an issue for communities, families and individuals in British society. To help illustrate some of the issues involved, a scenario is set that describes the lifestyles and concerns of five 'families' living in a mid-England city in a small cul-de-sac on a medium-sized housing estate. It will examine sexual health as an issue for them as part of a community, as families and as individuals.

Scenario I Fairway Close

Place: Mid-England city, six average semi-detached houses in a small cul-de-sac on a medium-sized housing estate, Fairway Close.
Residents:
◆ No. 1. Mr and Mrs Harris: retired civil servants, no children, both active in local church group.
◆ No. 2. The Richards family: Terry (38), Zoe (35), Katy (11), Robin (17). Daily life revolves around work, school and the family.
◆ No. 3. Ms Susan Freeman (40) and daughters Lucy (10) and May (8): Susan works part-time and is a single mother.
◆ No. 4. The Cooper family: Heather (27), Hugh (26) and daughter Gillian (6 months).
◆ No. 5. Zahid Patel (24): cohabiting in a long-term relationship.
◆ No. 6. Empty property: why not become the new neighbour for the next part of this section?

Sexual health and the community

The residents of Fairway Close do not lead extraordinary lives: like most of us, they are average people leading average lives. Most of their time is taken up with the family, work and their homes. As part of a local community, sexual health is not really an issue. Recent press coverage about maternity services moving to a hospital further away at the other side of town, complaints about street prostitution near a local school and reports on a local rise in teenage conception rates has sparked some interest and has been the topic of several neighbourly exchanges, but on the whole nothing much changes. Through its research and reporting mechanisms, the local health authority has data on health issues that affect the local population. Several methods have been used to collect these data, including:

◆ information from the Office of Population Censuses and Surveys (OPCS)
◆ death rates: standardized mortality ratio, life expectancy and potential years of lost life, and morbidity (illness) rates
◆ demography
◆ research into specific health problems, focus groups with consumers (Krueger 1994)
◆ lifecycle framework (Department of Public Health Medicine 1990).

Other issues, such as socioeconomics, environment, ethnicity and culture, are also examined and considered to help identify and predict need so as to ensure appropriate resource allocation. The local health promotion department has run several campaigns on cervical cytology and breast screening, sexually transmitted infections and other health issues. Health promotion leaflets are generally available through healthcare centres, libraries and community centres, and there is an active sex education programme in local schools.

 Learning activity 8.2

As with most communities, sexual health is not really a priority. The issues currently facing these residents include the closure of local libraries, crime and vandalism, drugs, housing, education and unemployment.

What other organizations and/or initiatives on sexual health and related issues may be available in the community?

On a community level, how might health professionals raise the profile of sexual health and related issues?

Feedback on Learning activity 8.2

There are probably many organizations and initiatives available locally that address issues of sexual health; however, not all of these will be specifically promoted as being concerned with sexual health. Examples include Well Man and Well Woman clinics, which consider sexual health as a routine health issue; other health promotion clinics, such as 'Look after your heart', where information on sexual health may be available; voluntary, community and support groups set up to support individuals and their families who have specific health or social problems. These are often the best source of information on a specific problem, and it is likely that information on sexual health-related issues is available from the organization either locally or nationally.

Despite the best attempts of many health authorities and NHS Trusts to encourage local people to use services and take a more proactive role in health matters, in the main most people are busy with day-to-day life and it is only when a particular health issue arises that it becomes a priority. In some areas community development workers have been employed who work within the community's priorities and to assist people in what they perceive to be their immediate needs, which are often different from the professionals' defined need. There may be scope for health professionals to work collaboratively with other organizations to raise the profile of sexual health (Department of Health 1993b).

Sexual health and the family

The residents of Fairway Close represent a small cross-section of their local community. Each household has a nuclear and extended family that is unique and which does not readily fit the stereotypical heterosexual two-parent family model. Whall (1990) defines the family as 'a self-identified group of two or more individuals whose association is characterized by special terms, who may or may not be related by bloodlines, but who function in such a way that they consider themselves to be a family'. For all the families in Fairway Close sexual health is not an issue, although they do have their own views and opinions about sex, sexuality, morality and health. Mr and Mrs Harris are appalled at the sex education in schools initiative, as they believe that 'teaching children about sex only encourages immoral behaviour'. Susan Freeman believes that sex education from an early age is 'crucial in this day and age'. She does not want her daughters to grow up ignorant of the facts. The Coopers cannot have children of their own and have just recently adopted their daughter Gillian. Zahid Patel has a long-term girlfriend who is not accepted by his family, as they had planned for him to marry into an Asian family. The Richards family is very 'easy going' about sex and sexuality: Uncle Robin is gay and has spent a lot of time with the Richards – their philosophy is to live and let live.

Like most families, the residents of Fairway Close have their own cultural and religious beliefs, which have developed over the years and have been inherited, adapted and adopted from their families, friends, experiences and life events. Their views on issues such as sex and sexuality are ever changing and evolving. The media and television have played an important role in bringing to their attention information and misinformation on sexual lifestyles, sexual health matters and sexual dysfunction. Some of the families find the television programmes and magazine articles of great interest, some find great entertainment value in them, and some find them totally unnecessary. There is a certain amount of censorship in some households, and sex, sexuality and sexual health are discussed to varying degrees, usually during a programme, after reading a magazine article, or at work and school the following day. Most of the time their new-found 'knowledge' is pushed to the back of their minds fairly quickly, and only brought into conscious thought when an issue arises. Most of the families find talking about other people's sex lives and sexuality acceptable, but see their own as something private and not to be discussed outside the security of their personal and intimate relationships.

Learning activity 8.3

Consider your own situation and personal development. Take a few minutes to think about your family and your family's culture.

◆ What influences have shaped your beliefs about sex, sexuality and sexual lifestyles?

◆ How do your beliefs and opinions differ from those of other members of your family and other members of your community?

◆ As a health professional, how might your beliefs and opinions affect your practice in relation to sexual health-related interventions?

Feedback on Learning activity 8.3

You may have found that the most significant influences contributing to your beliefs about sex, sexuality and sexual lifestyles stem from your own life experiences, such as relationships from childhood to adulthood, exposure to different cultures and lifestyles, and health and wellbeing. It is likely that exposure to these issues via the television or media has either strengthened your existing beliefs, confirmed what you already know, made you 'hungry' for more information, or feel that they have got it all wrong. If you repeat this exercise in 6 months' time you will probably find that your views, beliefs and opinions on some issues have changed or shifted.

Your views and opinions are probably very different from those of your family and neighbours, although there may be some core values that are very similar. You may find that your differing beliefs are 'at odds' with members of your family or community, and as a consequence you keep them to yourself or only share them with people you know have similar beliefs.

As a health professional it is sometimes very hard to differentiate between what is personal and what is professional. The boundaries are often blurred, and our beliefs do influence the way we interact with our patients. In extreme cases this can put health-care professionals in a very vulnerable position. For example, during a clinical supervision session Darren (a newly qualified staff nurse) admitted that he did not like nursing Mr Smith because he was vulgar and abusive towards female members of staff (something Darren finds hard to understand or tolerate). This had resulted in Darren finding it very difficult to treat Mr Smith as he would other patients. He preferred to keep out of his way in case he lost his temper and said something he might regret. As a consequence, Mr Smith did not always receive the care he required.

Sexual health and the individual

Resident no. 1: Mr and Mrs Harris. Mrs Harris has always regretted not having children. Mr Harris had a brief affair at work 10 years ago but ended it after a lot of emotional turmoil and feelings that he could never leave Mrs Harris. He made the decision to 'try to make the relationship work'. They have sexual intercourse rarely and consider themselves to be companions rather than in love. Mrs Harris attends regular breast screening clinics following the discovery of a benign lump several years ago. Mr Harris is troubled by frequent trips to the toilet during the night.

Resident no. 2: The Richards family. Terry works extremely long hours to earn enough money to take the family on holiday at least once a year. His libido is low and he feels physically tired most of the time. Zoe is a working mother who juggles her time to look after the family and see to the house. She never seems to have the time to attend the Well Woman clinic – the opening hours clash with life generally, but feels she has no need to as everything seems OK. Katy is attending regular sex education sessions at school and often asks Mum about things she has not properly understood. Robin is a moody teenager who has lots of monogamous relationships. Testicular self-examination means absolutely nothing to him.

Resident no. 3: Susan Freeman has not had a sexual partner for the past 8 years and feels old and frumpy most of the time. She is thinking about trying the lonely-hearts column, but is worried about meeting someone and having 'to do all that safer sex stuff'. Her daughter Lucy has been seeing the doctor with obesity problems.

Resident no. 4: The Cooper family. Heather is extremely happy since adopting Gillian. Hugh is finding it difficult adapting his routine, but feels generally happy. He has accepted the fact that Heather cannot have children but is angry that fertility treatment was not available. Gillian is worried that her father is drinking again and being physically abusive to her mother. Hugh thinks it is none of her business and that she should keep out of it.

Resident no. 5: Zahid Malik. Zahid's mother had told him when she last visited that she had some 'women's' problems. She had seen her GP and the practice nurse had given her some leaflets to read. The problem was that they were in English and she could not read them. Zahid has still not told his parents that he wants to marry his long-term white girlfriend.

Resident no. 6: What about you?

 Learning activity 8.4

Review the brief case histories of the residents. Taking into consideration their individual and family circumstances, make a list of any sexual health-related issues/problems they are experiencing.

Feedback to Learning activity 8.4

You have probably identified a list of ongoing and potential problems and issues. It is likely that they can be categorized into physical problems; emotional and mental health problems; behavioural problems.

Sexual health will remain a low priority for most people, and as a result it will be difficult to engage the general public in constructive and meaningful discussion about their needs. In the main, only those who have been affected by dysfunctional sexual health issues will be motivated to become involved in change. The pressures and pleasures of everyday life will continue to dictate our involvement in the change process. For most, sexual health is an abstract, multifaceted concept that only comes into question when it begins to significantly threaten health or personal stability. The involvement of consumers in health-care planning, professional education and clinical audit will undoubtedly only involve a minority of people who see themselves qualified (through experience) to contribute to such processes, or who are seen by others to have the necessary skills and experience. The caution must be that we are in danger of excluding by default all those who to date have not had a perceived need, either personal or professional, for services.

Learning activity 8.5

Consider the following definition offered by the World Health Organization in 1974.

Sexual health is defined as:

◆ a freedom to enjoy and control sexual and reproductive health in accordance with a social and personal ethic

◆ freedom from fear, shame, guilt, false beliefs and other psychological factors inhibiting sexual response and impairing sexual relationships

◆ freedom from organic disorders, diseases and deficiencies that interfere with sexual and reproductive functions (Mace et al. 1974).

Comparing your list of residents' issues and problems with the above definition, take a few moments to consider the following points:

◆ What problems and issues are appropriate for intervention by the health-care team? Make a list of the criteria you would use to assess these.

◆ If any problems and issues do not meet your criteria, provide a rationale.

◆ What would prompt the residents of Fairway Close to seek help, advice or support with these problems/issues?

◆ What steps should be taken by local health providers to ensure that services are better promoted and accessible to local residents?

Feedback on Learning activity 8.5

The definition of sexual health is ambitious and it is clear that it is unrealistic in terms of both resources and the time that health services can actively spend on seeking out such a range of problems and offering intervention. Part of the criteria for assessing a need for intervention must be the motivation of the individual or family concerned. From the case histories it is clear that for many of our residents their problems are ongoing, part of everyday life, multifaceted and dynamic. It is usually only when there is a crisis or when circumstances dictate that we need to do something about a problem, that we actively seek help, advice or support. Several theories have attempted to explain the influence of different variables on an individual's health-related behaviour (Naidoo and Wills 1994). These include: the Health Belief Model (Becker 1974); the Theory of Reasoned Action (Ajzen and Fishbein 1980); the Health Action Model (Tones et al. 1990); the Stages of Change Model (Prochaska and DiClemente 1984) (all cited by Naidoo and Wills 1994).

CONCLUSION

The growth of consumerism in health care will inevitably mean that consumers want a greater involvement in their care and treatment choices. As people become better informed about sex, sexual lifestyles and sexuality, their expectations of their own sexual health will rise and bring with them a need for skilled, sensitive and compassionate practitioners. This chapter has introduced four factors that directly affect service users and which will continue to influence the importance of sexual health as an issue. Increasingly, health policy requires us to develop services, in partnership with consumers, to ensure that high-quality cost-effective and appropriate care and treatment is offered. With regard to sexual health there is still a long way to go before we are in a position to negotiate and collaborate in such a way. As a society we know very little about the sexual lifestyles of communities. Little reliable information has been available on the sexual behaviour of the general public (Wellings et al. 1994), and the information that has shaped our thinking about sexual health has been based on random probability samples or on the results of studies prompted by the threat of increasing HIV infection.

As health-care providers we need further discussion and debate on what it is we are trying to achieve in relation to sexual health, and to refine our understanding of the differences between assessing sexuality and assessing sexual health. Working definitions of sexual health present many challenges for health-care professionals, not least acknowledgement that limited resources will inevitably define our criteria for intervention. It seems unrealistic to suggest that we aim to offer a comprehensive, open-door policy on sexual health matters for all people from all cultures, when in reality the development of sexual health-related practice is embryonic.

Perhaps in time our consumers will be better placed to demand that we give permission to raise such issues: until then we will no doubt continue to struggle with this dynamic and complex topic.

RESOURCES AND ANNOTATED FURTHER READING

SPOD, (Association to aid the sexual and personal relationships of people with a disability), 286 Camden Road, London N7 0BJ. Tel: 020 7607 8851

Organization that provides a useful information and counselling service for people who are physically or learning disabled, their partners and carers.

Lesbian and Gay Switchboard, BM Switchboard, London WC1N 3XX. Tel: 020 7837 7324

Operates a 24-hour phone line offering support and information to lesbians, gay men and bisexuals.

Women's Health, 52 Featherstone Street, London EC1Y 8RT. Tel: 020/7251 6580

A voluntary organization that operates an enquiry and information service on women's sexual and reproductive health issues.

http://www.equip.ac.uk/issue3/sex quiz.htm

A short and informative quiz on sexual health prepared by Dr Mary Cooper, Consultant in Public Health medicine, originally designed and presented to people attending the World AIDS Day Conference in Harlow 'One World – One Hope', answers given.

http://www.bmaids.demon.co.uk/

A useful site from the BMA Foundation for AIDS promoting specialized education about AIDS, HIV and sexual health for professional groups and policy makers.

http://www.healthcentre.org.uk/hc/clinic/websites/men.htm

A site index to UK websites covering issues relating to men's health, and offering information and other resources for patients, families and carers.

http://www.ppa.co.uk/tmap/research.htm

A report from Kaye Wellings, Department of Public Health and Policy, London School of Hygiene and Tropical Medicine: The Role of Teenage Magazines in the Sexual Health of Young People.

Few C, Hicken I, Butterworth T 1996 Principles and practices of sexual health and sex education in schools – a framework for developing professional education and training

A framework designed to help educators improve the quality of professional education and training available to health and education professionals who work as sex educators for children and young people in schools.

Available from The School of Nursing, Midwifery and Health Visiting, University of Manchester,

Coupland 3, Oxford Road, Manchester M13 9PL. Tel: 0161 275 5333.

College of Health 1994 Consumer audit guidelines

These guidelines provide an insight into how some of the key consumer audit methods can be used and give training guidance on the processes involved. There is a useful discussion of the setting in which consumer audit approaches may be appropriate.

College of Health 1995 Consumer Involvement Initiatives in Clinical Audit and Outcomes: a review of developments and issues in the identification of good practice

The Department of Health's Clinical Outcomes Group commissioned this report. Consumer involvement initiatives are discussed from a number of perspectives, including the fundamentals of consumer involvement and promoting good practice.

ENB 1996 Learning from each other: the involvement of people who use services and their carers in education and training. English National Board for Nursing, Midwifery and Health Visiting, London

A useful publication for those involved in teaching and curriculum development.

REFERENCES

Akinsanya J, Rouse P 1991 Who will care? A survey of knowledge and attitudes of hospital nurses to people with HIV/AIDS. Faculty of Health and Social Work, Anglia Polytechnic University

Bond S 1989 A national study of HIV infection, AIDS and community nursing staff in England. A report. Healthcare Research Unit, University of Newcastle upon Tyne

Clare A 1986 Lovelaw: love, sex and marriage around the world. BBC Publications, London

Collard R, Sivyer G, Deloitte L 1990 Total quality. Personnel Management 29 May

College of Health 1994 Consumer audit guidelines. College of Health, London

Department of Health 1991 The patients' charter. HMSO, London

Department of Health 1993a Working together for better health: the health of the nation. HMSO, London

Department of Health 1993b The health of the nation: HIV/AIDS and sexual health: key area handbook. HMSO, London

Department of Public Health Medicine 1990 Assessment of health need using the life cycle framework: an information toolbox. Department of Public Health Medicine, Newcastle upon Tyne

Few C, Hicken I S, Butterworth C A 1996 Principles and practice of sexual health and sex education in schools: a framework for developing professional education and training. University of Manchester, Manchester

Fontaine K L 1976 Human sexuality: faculty knowledge and attitudes. Nursing Outlook 24: 174–176

Ham C 1992 Health policy in Britain: the politics and organisation of the National Health Service, 3rd edn. Macmillan, London

Hicken I S, Butterworth C A 1995 Focus on quality: AIDS and community nursing. University of Manchester, Manchester

Krueger R 1994 Focus groups: a practical guide for applied research, 2nd edn. Sage, London

Lohr K N (ed) 1990 Medicare: a strategy for quality assurance. National Academy Press, Washington DC

Mace D R, Bannerman R H, Burton J 1974 The teaching of human sexuality in schools for health professionals. World Health Organization, Geneva

McHaffie H 1993 The care of patients with HIV and AIDS: a survey of nurse education in the UK. A report. Institute of Medical Ethics, University of Edinburgh

Naidoo J, Wills J 1994 Health promotion: foundations for practice. Baillière Tindall, London

National Health Service Executive 1994a Involving local people: examples of good practice. NHSE, Leeds

National Health Service Executive 1994b Purchasing for health: involving local people. A speech by Dr B Mawhinney MP, Minister for Health, National Purchasing Conference, Birmingham, 13 April 1994. NHSE, Leeds

National Health Service Management Executive 1992 Local voices: the views of local people in purchasing for health. HMSO, London

Peters D A 1993 Improving quality requires consumer input: using focus groups. Journal of Nursing Care Quality 23: 34–41

Roper N, Logan W W, Tierney A J 1985 The elements of nursing, 2nd edn. Churchill Livingstone, Edinburgh

Savage J 1989 An uninvited guest. Nursing Times 85(5): 25–27

Secretary of State for Health et al. 1989a Working for patients. HMSO, London

Secretary of State for Health et al. 1989b Caring for people. HMSO, London

Waterhouse J 1996 Nursing practice related to sexuality: a review and recommendations. NT Research 1(6): 412–418

Wellings K, Field J, Johnson A M, Wadsworth J 1994 Sexual behaviour in Britain: the national survey of sexual attitudes and lifestyles. Penguin, London

Whall A 1990 The family as the unit of care in nursing. In: Ismeurt R, Arnold E, Carson V (eds) Concepts fundamental to nursing. Stringhouses, Pennsylvania, pp. 52–57

9

Sexual health and you

Gordon Evans

'In the early days those of us with HIV saw ourselves as the super elite. It was like being a member of an exclusive club. The price of our membership was our lives.' (John Mordaunt)

KEY ISSUES/CONCEPTS

◆ Sexual health – implications for practice
◆ Intimacy and body boundaries
◆ Aspects of good practice
◆ Framework for continuing personal education and development

OVERVIEW

Chapter 9, *Sexual health and you*, enables the reader to explore how their personal attitudes and value frameworks might impinge upon professional practice.

INTRODUCTION

So much has been learnt from those origins of HIV, not only about ourselves but also about society at large. HIV and AIDS has made individuals think about themselves, their lifestyle and attitudes. Clearly much has been learnt through providing care and support for those with HIV that is transferable into other areas of personal and professional lives, and in particular opening up the arena of sexual health.

SEXUAL HEALTH AND ITS IMPLICATIONS FOR PRACTICE

Addressing sexual health needs raises a wide range of issues for clinical practice, presenting a variety of challenges for practitioners. There is a need for practitioners to review what has influenced their perceptions of sexuality and sexual health, and how these values affect their practice.

Over the last few years enormous efforts have been made to push back the boundaries relating to sexuality. There have also been attempts to develop a greater understanding of the true meaning of the concept of sexual health, which include greater appreciation of its wider implications when providing care (Hicken 1994).

Sexuality

Sexuality is viewed as inner beliefs and values based upon personal prejudices which in turn are influenced by culture and human development to date (Caplan 1991). Although the ways in which the concept of sexuality is addressed have changed over time, and there is an increased focus on issues of a sexual nature, it remains taboo for some practitioners. Their understanding of sexuality remains unclear and they often find themselves challenged when having to meet the sexual health needs of their clients. It is only when personal prejudice is identified, acknowledged and eliminated that the provision of effective care will be guaranteed.

By deliberately including sexual health within the framework of health-care delivery, the practitioner begins to address the issues central to the individual client's sexual health needs.

Familiar definitions of sexuality and sexual health relate to earlier work of the World Health Organization (WHO 1986). The key elements of the WHO definition include:

1. the capacity to enjoy and control sexual and reproductive behaviour in accordance with social and personal ethics

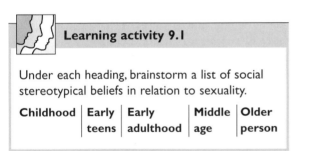

Learning activity 9.1

Under each heading, brainstorm a list of social stereotypical beliefs in relation to sexuality.

Childhood	Early teens	Early adulthood	Middle age	Older person

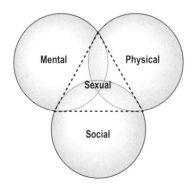

Fig. 9.1 Concept of health.

2. freedom from fear, shame, guilt, false beliefs and other psychological factors inhibiting sexual responses

3. freedom from organic disorder, disease and deficiencies that interfere with sexual and reproductive function.

These definitions have been in use for some time, and although they are seen as clear and all-encompassing, they present challenges for contemporary clinical practice which are only now being addressed (Webb 1994).

Applying definitions in practice

The key elements of the WHO (1986) definitions can be interpreted into practice in some of the following ways:

Key element 1
◆ Providing discharge advice to clients that includes sexual health
◆ Local policies for contraception services for under-16-year-olds
◆ Advice and support for women with unplanned pregnancies
◆ Unbiased sexual health education provision
◆ Anti-ageist policies and practice which challenge and prevent discrimination against older people
◆ Protection of vulnerable adults and children
◆ Respect for the right to make personal choices about parenthood.

Key element 2
◆ Maintenance of privacy and dignity for clients and carers
◆ Respecting individuals' values, beliefs and behaviour in relation to sexuality
◆ Understanding and accepting the wide range of sexual health terminology
◆ Providing clients with opportunities to express their specific sexual health needs
◆ Giving psychological support through access to appropriate information and sources of help and advice.

Key element 3

◆ Including appropriate sexual health assessment within the admission process

◆ Inclusion of sexual health needs in care planning

◆ Health promotion literature that includes advice on sexual health issues

◆ Provision of information about illness, therapies and drug treatments that may affect sexual health.

Reflection point 9.1

◆ The definition of sexual health offered by the World Health Organization focuses upon three key elements. Reflect on your area of clinical practice and determine how you meet each element.

◆ In order to check how consistent your practice is, it may be helpful to consider a small number of specific clients from differing ages/cultures/ sexual orientations.

Challenging practice

Historically, emphasis was placed firmly upon promoting the asexuality of both nurse and client, and the strict avoidance of involvement at a human level. Hopefully, this situation is far removed from today's stance of promoting the concept of empathetic holistic care, which includes sexuality and sexual health as part of the provision of health and social care. Only when this has been fully achieved can a service based upon the principles of a truly holistic approach to care be ensured. With this move towards an increased emphasis on holistic care, Pearson (1988) warns that 'task allocation can be seen as defending the nurse; the new holistic approach may pose a personal challenge for practitioners'.

These developments cannot be achieved without support for practitioners. Time should also be taken to gain the client's confidence and develop opportunities to explore and discuss their feelings about sexuality.

In order to gain clients' confidence it is important for nurses to develop the knowledge and skills to provide an appropriate environment and develop opportunities for their clients to explore and discuss their feelings about their lives, including sexuality.

As can be seen from carrying out this activity, there is an inbuilt hierarchy of acceptability to the invasion of body zones, which is partly influenced by the situation. Nurses find themselves in a unique position where at times they are allowed and required to invade these boundaries. It might be that in some situations the nurse, for health-care provision reasons, has gone further than the client's loved ones along the continuum of intensity of feeling relating to which body zones have been touched. Savage (1995) describes the therapeutic potential of nurses in such a situation; however, it may at times lead to explicit information being sought and given by the client. Such openness is central to the development of closeness when providing care: creating a partnership of care alters the original nurse's power basis (Hugman 1991). This may well be a situation that the nurse has not been prepared by her training to handle: there is therefore a clear need to review the opportunities to develop the required responding skills.

Booth (1990) emphasizes the need to review and challenge practices that relate particularly to sexual health. Where sexual health advice is provided for adults who have undergone gynaecological surgery up to the age of 65, those over that age also have both a right and a need for such interventions. There is a need to challenge ageist sexuality beliefs. Macleod Clark (1983) found that nurses tended to be superficial in their communication and channelled conversations away from delicate topics, even when they had time to pursue them. With some clients they actively used strategies to block or discourage conversation. For example, a young nurse may

Learning activity 9.2

Consider the following situations that reflect various levels of contact between clients and members of staff. Some may be regarded as normal when considering communication as part of client care, particularly at times of tension and stress associated with life and care events. Consider the following interactions between staff and clients, paying particular attention to your reactions to some of these situations, in which you may already be involved as part of your normal care practices.

	Staff F/ Client F	Staff F/ Client M	Staff M/ Client M	Staff M/ Client F
Shake hands				
Arm around elbow				
Hold hands				
Hugging				
Kiss cheek				
Stroke hair				
Kiss mouth				
Stroke body				
Touch bottom				
Touch genitals				

How would you feel and respond in the above situations?

◆ Yes, no problems.

◆ No, this would not be acceptable.

◆ Possibly, given certain situations.

feel embarrassed about pursuing a conversation with an older man who has had cardiac surgery in order to obtain information about his sexual health.

Reflection point 9.2

Imagine you are watching a television programme with explicit sex scenes. In whose company would you feel comfortable watching this? Your friends, partner, parent, grandparent? If there are any differences when watching with these different people, try to explore what they are and where they might come from. Consider your own feelings about discussing sexual health issues with people older than yourself.

With what client age would you feel comfortable and confident, and when would you feel as though entering dangerous or uncomfortable territory? Can you draw on any other parallels with other age groups? What factors other than the client's actual age would influence your feelings?

Value framework

The care provided to clients may at times reflect personal views and attitudes on sexual health. There is a need to discuss care strategies and the actions to be taken when what can only be described as 'delicate situations' arise. Such pro-active discussions should be held with the strategist and, more particularly, those practitioners who find themselves at the sharp end of the care interface. A range of mixed responses by practitioners is often encountered and regrettably, anecdotal evidence does exist suggesting that not all responses are positive and supportive of the required client care. Professionally, nurses are required to uphold their Code of Professional Conduct (UKCC 1992), that is, to act in the best interests of clients at all times.

Where practitioners feel they do not have the competence to provide appropriate care, it is clearly their responsibility to take steps to rectify such personal shortcomings. Until the nurse is able to offer a competent service they should ensure that clients are referred to other appropriate resources that will meet their sexual health needs.

Reflection point 9.3

It is useful to review personal values and attitudes in relation to aspects of client care. Reflect on any incident where you felt that you or a colleague demonstrated strong views and beliefs about a certain client or client group.

Consider the following points in relation to this situation:

◆ How would you describe the client/group of clients who were the focus of these strong views?

◆ In what way were these views expressed?

◆ How were the biases detected in the care provided to clients from this group?

◆ Can you identify the mechanisms used by yourself or colleagues to hide such negative values?

Feedback on Reflection point 9.3

Marginalized groups that might be identified are:

◆ Children

◆ Older people

◆ Prostitutes

◆ Pregnant teenagers

◆ Intravenous drug users

◆ Paedophiles

◆ Rapists.

Expressions of feelings many include:

◆ Anger

◆ Emotional numbness

◆ Offhand behaviour

◆ Avoid providing care

◆ Rough in care delivery

◆ Verbal aggression

◆ Lack of sympathy

◆ Viewed as time wasters.

Mechanisms used to hide such views are:

◆ Over caring

◆ Talking down to the individual

◆ Lack of discretion.

If nurses are honest about their own deficiencies and offer clients choice, their sexual health needs are more likely to be met. The impact on client care of a practitioner's negative attitude is that the client may not confide in them, they may not feel confident in the care being given, and they might not be able to discuss health-care issues fully and openly. This would clearly lead to a situation where a client does not receive holistic care. It might be colleagues who first alert you to the fact that a client does not feel comfortable with the way in which you provide care. Alternatively, you may be aware that you are marginalizing certain groups, or individuals with specific illnesses. Through the process of clinical supervision personal attitudes can be explored and, where conflict arises, the practitioner is given space to examine how this can be handled without detriment to the client. Practitioners have a duty to ensure that clients do not receive a less than satisfactory level of care. Nurses should not lose sight of their responsibility to supervise health-care support workers, who will also need the time and space to explore personal values and beliefs.

Reflecting back on the text, consider the following case scenarios, think about the issues raised and answer the associated questions.

Case study 9.1

Fred, an 80-year-old man, has recently moved to a local nursing home owing to his growing dependency; his wife remains in their home. He is seen touching a number of female residents in a sexual manner, although he has successfully been rebuffed. His wife, on visiting, is appalled to find that he is taking an interest in residents of the opposite sex. She says he has always had an eye for the ladies and would flirt with other women. She says that they have not been sexually active for some time, as he is unable to get an erection, but they do cuddle up in bed.

When Fred is confronted about his behaviour he denies any wrongdoing, but agrees to behave himself. However, he continues in his previous behaviour when he thinks nobody is observing him.

◆ *What are your reactions to his behaviour?*

◆ *What do you think his real needs are?*

◆ *In what way might you manage this situation?*

◆ *Discuss the support his wife might require.*

A number of issues will be raised by this scenario, including:

◆ *local policies on individual choices and protecting vulnerable clients*

◆ *expectations of 'acceptable' behaviour*

◆ *the level of open discussion within your care team on such issues*

◆ *the range of ways in which comfort is obtained and sexual needs met*

◆ *open feelings of disgust; uncertainty about telling his wife*

◆ *appropriate space in a clinical environment to discuss such issues confidentially.*

Case study 9.2

Mr Williams is 40 years of age and has strict moral views, based partly on his religious and family upbringing. He entered the army, working his way through the ranks until he left 12 years later as a sergeant. His wife died 2 years ago and since then he has remained single, enjoying his independence. He is told by his son, who is 18 years old, that he is gay.

How would you help Mr Williams to cope with this news?

Identify the support networks in your area to support both Mr Williams and yourself.

This is an interesting scenario that will bring out a number of issues, including:

◆ *Mr Williams' potential shock and how he might react to the information*

◆ *his view, possibly coloured by his military background, that this is abnormal*

◆ *the need to handle such situations sensitively*

◆ *who breaks bad news within your work area*

◆ *local support for those who provide such services*

◆ *where you would turn to locally for support both within or outside your service area*

◆ *gay helplines to support the son through what might be unexpectedly difficult times.*

This all assumes that there is a problem: Mr Williams may be fully understanding and take the attitude 'so what?.'

There is also a clear need to consider a client's individual rights, taking account of their beliefs, lifestyle, race or age. The nurse should offer an equal service to all. To deviate from this will undoubtedly meet with both public and professional disapproval. Pratt (1995) highlights the potential difficulties of allowing both nurses and clients to choose each other for a care partnership. He goes on to state that those who show a reluctance to care for a particular client group should initially be counselled, given extra education, and only then, if their reluctance persists, dismissed. It can be argued that nurses who exhibit biased and prejudiced behaviour lose credibility within the profession and their judgement is seen as questionable. Such actions are noted by clients, however subtle the attempt to hide personal views, and this may lead to the client losing confidence in the practitioner.

Case study 9.3

Richard Smith is a 22-year-old man who has a profound learning disability. He has lived in a continuing care home for just over a year. He is amicable but quiet and does not mix much with other residents, but enjoys looking at the newspapers and watching the television. One day while sitting in the day area along with mainly female residents, he is seen to be masturbating while reading the newspaper. The other residents complain about him, calling him dirty. When staff attempt to discuss his behaviour with him, referring to his 'self abuse', he does not appear to know what they are referring to.

Discuss your reactions to Richard's behaviour.

Consider how you might manage such a situation.

Your reactions could be quite mixed, including:

◆ *shock*

◆ *disgust*

◆ *unclear about action to take*

◆ *unable to discuss with the care team*

◆ *avoidance of situation*

◆ *avoidance of client with a challenging behaviour.*

Your management action might be to:

◆ *raise awareness of sexuality within the team*

◆ *discuss this particular client openly at team meetings*

◆ *develop strategies/protocols within the team to cope and manage such situations*

◆ *specific care interventions with this client: remove him to a private area when he is carrying out this activity.*

Consider the care issues in the above scenarios, which both relate to situations that challenge the role of individuals as clients, as well as the perception of the role of the nurse.

Skills in preparing to meet the challenge

Self-assessment is important for personal development in relation to sexual health. At the annual individual personal review (IPR) sexual health should be included in the issues to be explored. Existing skills that might be transferable should be acknowledged, and careful consideration given to the skills and knowledge that are essential if the practitioner is to become competent and confident in meeting the sexual health needs of the clients. As previously discussed, not all practitioners will feel comfortable about addressing the sexual health needs of their clients. The level at which this takes place will vary depending on

Reflection point 9.4

There is a need for personal review. Great emphasis is placed on critical reflection acting as a basis for development. Review your current clinical work, identifying the actions you take that relate to direct discussions with clients regarding sexual health. Identify the skills you already have that could be transferable to this specific area of practice. Think about what formal and informal knowledge you have on the subject of human sexuality, and lastly, consider your experience to date and what you have learned from it. Next, write down your strengths and weaknesses in relation to your skills, knowledge and experience. From this, try to form an action plan you could use when you next meet with your manager.

knowledge of the topic, skill in exploring sensitive areas, previous experience, confidence and competence. However, during IPR managers should pay attention to the skill mix needed in order to offer holistic service.

PREPARATION AND APPLICATION

When attempting to create an environment that encompasses sexual health issues, the following action points may be worthy of consideration:

◆ How to develop client information systems
◆ Ways of refocusing care records
◆ Interrelating sexual health with health promotion
◆ Developing support networks.

Developing client information systems

A wide range of client-centred information already exists that relates to identifiable illnesses.

Time should be taken to review such material to determine its range and comprehensiveness. Where appropriate, time should be taken to consider and develop the sexual health components: this should be carried out in a user-friendly manner and the approach should not offend the recipients. Select each of the identified action points and review their appropriateness to your area of practice. What is already carried out? What might be developed? This should relate to sexual health within your specialist area of practice.

Refocus care records

Opportunity should also be taken to revisit existing care plans within clinical areas. Earlier nursing models that underpin practice and reflect the philosophy of nursing practice included sexuality as an area to be explicitly explored (Roper et al. 1983). Later models included sexuality as an implicit expectation, being an area to be explored and included in care packages appropriate to individual clients' perceived needs. On reflection, this latter move was a retrograde step as those who did not feel comfortable discussing this aspect of care could avoid it. The space allocated for sexual health on care plans is often limited and used for more general notes. Possibly one of the most negative aspects in this part of the care plan, although probably unintentionally, is where the client's sexuality is seen as not applicable. The writing of the care plan in relation to sexual health often tells you more about the author, as well as the organization that accepts such an attitude.

Interrelating sexual health with health promotion

Issues that relate to sexual health cannot be ignored. An early step is to review the care in which each practitioner is currently involved. This can include all age groups and a diverse range of ill health episodes. For some time now it has been accepted that health promotion and health education are an integral aspect of care. Practitioners

have taken the time and trouble to equip themselves with the appropriate skills and knowledge to meet such demands. The next step is to identify situations where such interaction takes place and add sexual health to the discussion. Sexual health clearly needs to become an integrated part of health promotion and health education.

Support networks

There are a number of ongoing debates in the area of sexual health, with information and literature being generated at local, national and international levels. Benefit would be gained from establishing or joining a local special interest group related to your own professional background and which meets the sexual health needs of your client group. This would act as a focus for debating sexual health issues as they relate to individual groups, as well as examining the strengths and weaknesses of emerging examples of best practice. Such groups can act as a catalyst by supporting individuals who have an interest in sexual health as a specialist area but who alone may lack the volition and drive to move forward and push back the boundaries of care for clients. Such groups might also act as initiators and supporters of clinical research, and activity could be directed towards further identifying and developing the sexual health component of illness seen in the different areas of practice.

BARRIERS AND SOLUTIONS

Sexual health and management agendas

Once action points that relate to your area of practice have been identified, the next challenge is to put them into practice, with the support of your managers and colleagues. Personal development is often discussed as part of the IPR, where the hopes and aspirations of the individual practitioner are matched against the targets of the organization, in this case the health-care employer, either a Trust, a health authority, a private employer etc. There may be tension where an employer's agenda is driven by meeting contractual targets focused perhaps upon providing acute care; and where sexual health is not specifically mentioned, and so might not be seen as important. There is a clear need to move the concept of sexual health higher up the manager's agenda, possibly writing in such issues as part of the quality specification. This would place sexual health firmly on the list of organizational objectives.

Prioritizing resources

The resources available for any aspect of health care are limited. For a number of years finance has been available for HIV/AIDS work, but this has been ring-fenced, thereby preventing its use for other purposes. In addition, special funding has been available for such initiatives as campaign work by health promotion services and various drug dependency-related projects. Against this backdrop of fixed, if not reduced, resources, claims for staff development and service provision demand that practitioners and managers work together effectively to ensure that holistic health care is delivered. This requires a strong evidence-based rationale as to why such services are fundamental to the improved health of the public.

Determining professional and personal development

The concept of determining level of involvement in the arena of HIV could be transferred to the wider issues of sexual health, based upon the specialist issues that might arise.

◆ **Level 1** would be the raising of awareness in all staff about sexual health and the way it applies to their sphere of practice. This should be done in such a way as to include all individuals in open discussion about why and how sexual health relates to their clients and their own professional responsibility to meet those clients' needs.

◆ **Level 2** focuses on the transfer of existing skills and their use in the area of sexual health.

This may include the taking of sexual histories, the identification of sexual health issues that are worrying to the client, and acting as a resource person in terms of helping the client access the most appropriate service.

◆ **Level 3** As the demand for a sexual health service grows and the knowledge base develops, individuals will be needed who can collate, generate and initiate work relating to aspects of sexual health. In other areas of nursing practice, at the clinical level, they are referred to as link nurses. Often seen as a key role for fellow staff and clients alike, such a movement would actually promote the development of specialist practitioners at the clinical interface. Such individuals could also take over the responsibility for care relating to the sexual health of clients; alternatively, their function could be to support and guide fellow practitioners who have responsibility for hands-on care delivery. Individual practitioners need to carry out a self-assessment of their role and function within the team as regards sexual health. Their level of involvement is important, as it will determine the amount of development to be made available for that individual. Such actions will assist the manager to target fixed resources and for practitioners to determine personal development based upon need rather than tradition and/or personal preference.

Learning activity 9.3

◆ Determine level: 1/2/3 in your sphere of practice.

◆ Identify areas for personal development.

◆ List the sexual health elements of client care that you currently provide.

Identify the sexual health care that your clients need but do not at present receive. Determine whether a fellow nurse is already carrying out work in this area. State areas of sexual health work in which you have an interest that is not currently satisfied.

There is a need to determine personal and professional needs: a clear understanding of your clinical work and a focus upon the needs of clients will determine the way forward. This must then transfer into management commitment, along with educational opportunity. Local education provision will vary; key questions are the availability of courses/study days/education pathways leading to specialist degrees and diplomas in sexual health care. There may well be an integrated sexuality and sexual health aspect in other specialist courses. A model of sexual health may underpin a curriculum thread that focuses upon sexuality and sexual health.

Resource planning

In many areas of clinical practice there is a need for a balance of individuals interested in the selected topic, in this instance sexual health. It would be inappropriate to have a large number of practitioners skilled in providing reproductive advice at teenage drop-in centres if the numbers attending did not warrant such involvement. Therefore, an early step for managers and practitioners alike would be a skills analysis of the staff in their areas to meet client needs. The basis for proposing new services would initially be by defining gaps in service provision, along with a proposal encompassing the financial implications of bridging such a gap. However, there is a clear need for self-reflection to determine personal needs and suitability, and the appropriateness of such development.

Education debate

The current situation in sexual health is not too different from that described by Pellow (1995) in the early years of HIV/AIDS. The information available is not generally held in one central point, and many issues are raised by and through the media. It is only now that nurses educators are reviewing the sexual health component of the approved pre- and post-registration courses (Hicken 1994). It is left to both educators and those directly involved in clinical practice to ensure that practitioners are prepared to deliver care to meet the sexual health needs of clients.

Another parallel with HIV is the early moves to medicalize the issue, later taken over in some areas by 'feely education'; however, it soon became evident that one cannot survive without the other. Many nurses in clinical practice do need information, a view that is reflected by managers preparing to send staff on courses. McHaffie (1993) found that many nurses had not explored sexuality adequately, particularly with regard to marginalized groups such as homosexuals. There is a need to learn from the early experiences of HIV when planning to meet the education needs of those requiring sexual health development. The content of courses and other events should have well focused and thought-through outcomes, allowing potential participants to select those events that will meet their predetermined needs.

Practitioners should also be taking the initiative and asking whether and how the sexual health needs of clients who are the focus of courses are to be met. Educational development may also be achieved through either work or project groups: this may assist individuals to work towards meeting outcomes in more practical ways. The latter are preferred by managers as they do not require time away from work. The other advantage is that a clinically biased view can be taken, producing a tangible change for managers in the workplace.

This issue might be borne in mind by course planners as a way to develop links between theory and practice. New commissioners of education are increasingly practitioners themselves, taking responsibility for their own development. As a result education is being made more flexible, with a move to include open learning and flexible attendance. To be successful the individual practitioner must see the importance of the differing topics. Therefore, sexual health needs to be highly profiled and its importance made clear as an area to review when planning personal development. All of the above issues should be considered when planning and preparing to attend courses. Practitioners who have identified their training needs now have some very pointed questions to ask when approaching educational establishments, to help meet the issues raised.

RESOURCES

There is both commonality and difference in relation to the sexual health needs of the public. In order to maximize opportunities for meeting sexual health needs, the model of a 'one-stop shop' could be utilized. This has clear benefits for clients, and offers support for staff working in these areas. When reviewing services and voluntary agencies involved in offering support or care on aspects of sexual health, such a move would place all such groups under one roof. This in time would also contribute to the normalization of the concept of sexual health, helping to remove stigma.

Learning activity 9.4

Select an aspect of your work which is a well defined illness presentation. Then attempt to determine the contact points, both nationally and locally, of agencies that offer support, and find out whether their material includes relevant sexual health information.

The topic chosen will depend upon your area of work, for example continence promotion:

- ◆ Local continence promotion service
- ◆ Physiotherapy centres
- ◆ Age Concern centres
- ◆ Bard UK
- ◆ Health promotion literature
- ◆ Disabled Living Foundation
- ◆ Continence promotion suppliers
- ◆ Urology clinics.

The enquiries in Learning activity 9.4 may encourage organizations to review the content of their material. This activity, if shared with others, could be the start of a local directory of sexual health matters related to specific illnesses. A major consideration for practitioners is in the nature of the model of a network for sexual health. It provides opportunities for practitioners to reflect upon differing lifestyles, where sexual language may be very different and specific. This can be seen when caring for an intravenous drug user in the middle of a busy medical ward who has been admitted with a dermatology problem. His overriding drug use may quickly become centre stage, although not the cause of his admission. Not to be attuned to his sexual orientation and associated issues may lose the practitioner vital opportunities for health promotion. Specialists in the field need to determine whether their approach will be that of hands-on caregiver or that of a consultant who advises others, only taking on direct care that is possibly complex. Either role has implications for the development needs of those who work elsewhere in the care arena. Sexual health is the latest challenge to be faced by health-care providers and practitioners at a personal level, and an opportunity not to be avoided if holistic care is to be provided for clients.

CONCLUSION

So that the most appropriate care can be provided for clients with sensitive sexual health needs, practitioners need to be aware of their own limitations and inhibitions. In some instances issues may be addressed in clinical supervision, but some areas may require additional training and education.

Where practitioners' personal views obstruct the delivery of quality professional care, it is their responsibility to recognize this and ensure that the client does not suffer.

ANNOTATED FURTHER READING

Aggleton P, Davies P, Hart G 1995 AIDS: safety, sexuality and risk. Taylor and Francis, Bristol

A collection of conference papers considering sexuality in a range of different settings. Well referenced and would act as a good source of material for other work.

Hicken I 1994 Sexual health education and training, guidelines for good practice for teaching nurses, midwives and health visitors. ENB, London

This should be considered compulsory reading for all those involved in curriculum design, as it contains a blueprint for including sexual health in a number of existing courses. Well focused comments.

Hunt P, Sendell B 1987 A personal approach to patient care. Macmillan, London

Chapter 2 outlines an interesting schema for profiling individual and societal differences.

Johnstone M J 1989 Bioethics: a nursing perspective. WB Saunders, Philadelphia

This has interesting debates that underpin current issues on advocacy and feminist moral philosophy.

Lee J A 1991 Gay midlife and maturity. Harrington Park Press, London

Breaks down the debates relating to stereotyping of the homosexual person's experiences: also highlights the additional stresses experienced as a result of their sexual orientation.

Pratt R 1995 HIV/AIDS – a strategy for nurses. Edward Arnold, London

What is now regarded as the set textbook for many courses of study on HIV/AIDS, considers many issues from the perspective of the medical model. A well brought-together commentary on the current debates that surround this topic.

Seedhouse D 1988 Ethics – the heart of health care. John Wiley, Chichester

An interesting base reader that provides referenced access to other related topics.

Webb C 1994 Living sexuality: issues for nursing and health. Scutari Press, London

An interestingly written text that looks more generally at sexuality. Contains an interesting chapter on historical perspectives, which is highly commended to readers.

Related reading will be obtained by conducting computerized library information searches.

REFERENCES

Booth B 1990 Does it really matter at that age? Nursing Times 86(3): 50–52

Caplan P 1991 The cultural construction of sexuality. Routledge, London

Hicken I 1994 Sexual health education and training: guidelines for good practice in teaching nurses, midwives and health visitors. ENB, London

Hugman R 1991 Power in the caring professions. Macmillan, Basingstoke

Macleod Clark J 1983 Nurse–patient communication – an analysis of conversations from cancer wards. In: Wilson Barnett J (ed) Nursing research: ten studies in patient care. John Wiley, Chichester, pp 25–56

McHaffie H 1993 Improving awareness. Nursing Times 89(18): 29–31

Pearson A 1988 Primary nursing. In: Primary nursing in the Burford and Oxford Nursing Development Units. Chapman & Hall, London

Pellow C 1995 The education debate. In: Faugier J, Hicken I (eds) AIDS and HIV: the nursing response. Chapman & Hall, London, pp 70–84

Pratt R 1995 HIV–AIDS: a strategy for nurses. Edward Arnold, London

Roper N, Logan W, Tierney A 1983 Using a model for nursing. Churchill Livingstone, Edinburgh

Savage J 1995 Nursing intimacy, an ethnographic approach to nurse–patient interaction. Scutari Press, London

United Kingdom Central Council 1992 Code of professional conduct for the nurse, midwife and health visitor, 3rd edn. UKCC, London

Webb C 1994 Living sexuality, issues for nursing and health. Scutari Press, London

World Health Organization 1986 Concepts for sexual health. WHO, Copenhagen

10

Skills for sensitivity

Anne McNall

| *'The only way to get rid of the fear of doing something, is to go out and do it.'* (Jeffers 1989)

KEY ISSUES/CONCEPTS

◆ Developing self-awareness

◆ Identifying personal stressors related to meeting sexual health needs

◆ Examining responses to stressors

◆ Considering the effectiveness of coping strategies

◆ Managing stress related to meeting sexual health needs

◆ Providing care sensitive to the sexual health needs of clients

OVERVIEW

Chapter 10, *Skills for sensitivity*, explores the personal and professional barriers to promoting or maintaining the sexual health of clients. It will require you to look critically at your sexual health practice and challenge your attitudes and beliefs as you look at ways in which you respond to sources of stress in a sexual health-care setting. It also focuses on the development of effective coping strategies to enhance your skills in sexual health-care practice.

INTRODUCTION

In the preceding chapters you started to explore your abilities in promoting sexual health, and indeed, what this actually means in relation to your practice area. As you are taking the time to read this book, it is likely that you are aware of the need to address sexual health in your work and would like to improve your practice. Wanting, however, is not the same as doing, and many nurses and other professionals have already indicated that, although they recognize the need for sexual health-care interventions with their clients, this does not occur in practice (Gamel et al. 1993), nor do they feel comfortable with it in their daily work (Waterhouse 1996).

'I agree that there is a place for assessing sexual health needs, but I feel so awkward bringing the subject up. What if they don't want to talk about it?' (Staff nurse, surgical ward.)

'I could never ask someone old enough to be my grandmother about sex!' Student nurse, (BSc/RGN.)

'I do try to include sexual health in my work, but if my client has got problems I don't know what to do next'. (Midwife.)

'We're always being urged to ask about sexuality, but inside I still think it's inappropriate for disabled people to be sexually active'. (Sister, rehabilitation unit.)

'I'm always afraid that my colleagues will think I'm breaching the boundaries of professional practice if I discuss sexual health needs – they don't seem to discuss such personal issues.' (Community psychiatric nurse.)

'It's easier to discuss sexual health in this context, but I feel unsure about how far my role goes: should I be dealing with the STD issues I'm confident with, or any sexual health problem the client has?' (Health adviser, genitourinary medicine.)

'I feel it's really important to help my clients with their sexual health needs, but I'd hate to get it wrong. After all, they are already vulnerable – I might make things worse.' (Enrolled nurse, learning disability.)

'Most of the patients I work with are really ill. I sometimes wonder how appropriate it is to discuss sexual issues with them'. (Oncology nurse.)

These are just some of the problems that practitioners have raised in discussions about sexual health and sexuality: the literature indicates that they are not alone. In her study, McHaffie (1993) found little evidence that the matter of clients' sexuality had been addressed adequately, and that nursing was paying lip service to delivering holistic care in this area.

Hott and Ryan-Merritt (1982) found that nurses were unequipped to deal with the effects of specific disorders upon sexual functioning, despite the incorporation of sexual material in basic nursing courses. Wall-Haas (1991) found that even though nurses recognized the importance of issues of sexuality for adolescents, and were theoretically capable of addressing these issues, they were uncomfortable incorporating them into their nursing practice.

Briggs (1994) reiterates the fact that sexuality is rarely addressed when clients are recovering from myocardial infarction, despite it being a common concern.

A review of the literature on nurses' provision of teaching and counselling on sexuality revealed that the majority of nurses recognized sexual health care as a component of nursing practice; however, specific teaching, supporting and/or counselling interventions aimed at managing the effects of illness and treatment on sexual function are not provided most of the time (Gamel et al. 1993).

It seems strange that although nurses can be very skilled in communication in some instances, giving practical help and referring clients to appropriate others, there is a stumbling block when it comes to sexual health. In previous chapters you explored some of the possible reasons for this. This chapter is intended to help you develop this theme, and more importantly, to assist you in developing skills that will help you deal with real live sexual health issues in the context of your practice area.

DEVELOPING SELF-AWARENESS

You may feel that the ability to deal with sensitive topics is inherent and that only some people possess it. Although this may be partly true, there is no doubt that some of the factors that help are skills that can be learned. Not many people are naturally good listeners, but this ability can be developed with training and practice. Drawing comparisons between death and sexual health demonstrates this point.

 Reflection point 10.1

Consider how nurses and other health professionals dealt with the subject of death, dying and the bereaved in the past. Look at your practice and experience and focus on your thoughts and feelings when confronted for the first time with death and dying. Even if you have not been involved with caring for a dying person, you will still have thoughts and emotions about the experience.

There is also a wealth of literature which suggests that death was a very taboo topic and was denied, particularly in modern health care, which focused on cure and saw death as a failure. Developments such as the hospice movement, which have brought improvements to the practice of caring for the dying, have come about because individuals recognized a need for change, confronted their fears and discomfort with the issues, and learned new skills or developed existing ones to help them in their work with others. This has resulted in one of the great taboos in society – death – being addressed with far greater sensitivity by enlightened professionals. As the other great taboo, sex could surely benefit from similar attention!

 Learning activity 10.1

It may be helpful to think about how you, or your colleagues, became more confident and able in dealing with the dying and bereaved.

First, make a list of things that helped this development.

Secondly, consider how your skills in this area have developed, or how professionals generally have become more able and willing to assist others with these sensitive issues. Finally, keep in mind the things that have worked for you in the past. Consider how you may use some or all of these methods to work for you again, helping you to develop the required skills and ability to promote sexual health and respond to client needs in this sensitive area.

Feedback on Learning activity 10.1

There are many ways of learning, but some people find particular methods are more effective than others. Did you include things such as:

◆ Watching others work and learning from their practice?

◆ Talking to others about death, dying and bereavement?

◆ Reading about good practice in this area?

◆ Attending study days or courses?

◆ Reflection on the care provided, alone or with others?

◆ Trying out things in practice?

◆ Personal experience of loss, or bereavement?

◆ Keeping a personal journal of development in this area?

Development in practice is not without problems, and an acknowledgement of the need for self-awareness is imperative in order to face and overcome some of these difficulties. It would be naive to expect any members of society to have escaped the general attitude that sex, sexuality and sexual health are taboo areas. It is therefore unrealistic to expect to be perfectly happy and adept at helping others with these aspects of their lives, without some education and help in developing the relevant skills.

Stressors

In order to facilitate the development of self-awareness it is important to explore the potential stressors and difficulties in managing issues of an overtly sexual or sensitive nature. It is essential to be able to relate these to your practice, and discuss ways of overcoming them by developing the relevant core competencies.

'Being stressed' is the term we often use when faced with difficult or uncomfortable things. Stress can be defined in different ways. Several theorists have discussed stress, resulting in three different but complementary types of stress theory in contemporary literature.

Stress can be seen as a response to an environmental 'stressor', that is, anything physical or psychological that makes a demand upon the body, requiring it to adapt. A series of physiological responses are apparent and, if the stress is prolonged, lead to symptoms such as an upset stomach, headache and irritability.

Stress can also be viewed as a stimulus that causes a disrupted response. In this theory, 'life changes', which can be large or small, such as moving house, changing jobs or having an argument with someone, place demands upon the individual to cope or adapt; this in turn produces a physiological response.

Transactional stress theories place more emphasis on cognitive appraisal, or how events or demands are viewed, and the belief in an ability to cope at any specific time. Whereas the first two theories see stress as a response or as a stimulus, the outcome is theoretically the same for everyone. For example, in stimulus theories, specific life events are classed as similarly stressful for every-one. In response theories all demands are viewed as stressors, with the potential to elicit a stress response in every individual. These theories could be problematic, as stress responses seem to occur in a much less uniform way in real life! For exam-ple, having a baby and going on holiday are both listed as situational stressors by Holmes and Rahe (1967), yet individual reactions to each event seem to be very variable, with some people enjoying the experience and others feeling stressed by it.

Where the third theory differs is that it recog-nizes perception as having a vital role. In other words, stress is in the eye of the beholder: what one individual finds stressful, another may posi-tively enjoy. Perception also affects belief in cop-ing ability, so an individual may view an event as potentially stressful but feel that they will be able to deal with it, thereby minimizing the discomfort felt.

Perception is very important. Viewing stressful events in a different way, and enhanced belief in coping ability, could theoretically reduce stress levels even in what others may still see as difficult circumstances. Shuman and Bohanick (1987) reported a significant positive relationship between perceived comfort with providing sexual health care as a component of the nurse's role and the actual provision of care. In other words, if what is being done feels right, it is more likely to get done.

'Coping' is a common term used here to refer to active efforts to master, reduce or tolerate the demands created by stress. There is often a com-mon assumption that if someone is coping with his or her problems, that they have handled them effectively. In reality, however, coping responses can be more or less beneficial: that is, some work better than others, and indeed some methods do not work at all. Dealing with the stress of post-Christmas debts and weight gain by going out for a slap-up meal and several drinks is not really very effective!

The physiological mechanisms of the stress response are well documented, and individuals have experience of how stress feels. What is also important to understand is how we personally respond to stress when it occurs. Understanding this can help in consciously selecting alternative ways to respond where appropriate.

Responses to stress

There is a wide range of responses to stress. Vari-ous authors have categorized them in different ways, under five main headings:

◆ Indulging ourselves
◆ Having a go at others
◆ Giving up
◆ Adopting defensive coping mechanisms
◆ Choosing constructive coping strategies.

Reflection point 10.2

Try to envisage your use of each of these types of coping responses. If possible, note an example of how and when you responded in that way. It may be that you use some methods often and others only occasionally.

Indulging ourselves

Stress can lead to treating ourselves, e.g. with food, alcohol, spending, smoking, using drugs and other pleasurable activities. When things are not going well in one area of life, it makes sense to compensate by looking for other forms of satis-faction. Mostly these things are reasonably acces-sible and give rapid gratification.

Having a go at others

When individuals are worried or frustrated they can respond by acting aggressively with others, even if they have nothing to do with the situation. How often have you taken out your frustration after a bad day on your partner, family or col-leagues? We are often encouraged to express feel-ings to help deal with stress, yet this type of aggressive reaction is not really beneficial as it tends to backfire. For example, picking a fight with your husband/partner may release some aggres-sion, but may lead to negative repercussions later.

Giving up

Sometimes when things become too difficult one response is simply to give up. Can you recall a situation where you were so stressed that you felt unable to cope and just withdrew from it? Seligman and Rosenhan (1984) studied this response in animals and humans, and found similarities: when subjected to stress that could not be dealt with they become apathetic and listless, and give up trying. People learn this passive behaviour when exposed to unpleasant events which they perceive as unavoidable. This is very interesting, as helplessness seems to occur when the events are believed to be outside one's control: belief in the ability to cope increases the likelihood of success.

Adopting defensive coping mechanisms

Although originally proposed by Freud (1975), many psychologists now agree on the concept of defence mechanisms, and many different defences have been identified. Basically, these are attitudes or actions that can be adopted as a shield from the unpleasant feelings associated with stress, such as anxiety, guilt, anger and sadness. Such mechanisms are used mainly at an unconscious level, to prevent bad feelings about a situation, and work through self-deception – being used to distort reality so that stressful events are less threatening.

Table 10.1 lists some examples of defence mechanisms and how they might be used.

Defence mechanisms are normal patterns of coping; however, they are generally avoidance strategies and rarely provide a long-term solution to the problem. They can also delay facing up to a problem, which may actually make it worse.

Choosing constructive coping strategies

These are ways of coping that tend to be more positive. These involve confronting reality and taking some constructive action to deal with the causes of stress, and stress responses. They are the only long-term solution in stress management.

Constructive coping requires:

◆ a realistic appraisal of the situation causing the stress and your coping resources at the time. Sometimes a little self-deception can boost self-esteem and help you accept situations, but generally being truthful about what is going on is more effective

◆ direct confrontation of the problem, considering the options and the help available, and taking action to resolve the problem. This usually involves effort and may be uncomfortable

◆ recognition of the emotional reactions to stress, and their appropriate expression.

Table 10.1 Defence mechanisms

Defence mechanism	Description	Example
Denial	Refusing to acknowledge something	Going out when you have an assignment deadline tomorrow
Rationalization	Justifying your own or others' actions to make it seem acceptable and believing it	'I only failed the exam because the teacher didn't like me'
Displacement	Choosing a substitute object for expressing your feelings	Kicking the cat instead of your boss
Isolation	Separating thoughts and emotions which usually go together, to avoid unpleasant feelings	Laughing in the middle of a serious occasion, such as when laying out a body
Sublimation	Finding a substitute activity to express unacceptable impulses	Playing rugby to rechannel aggressive impulses
Projection	Attributing own unwanted feelings and characteristics on to someone else	Instead of feeling 'I'm unkind to him because I dislike him', believing 'I'm unkind to him because he hates me'
Fantasy	Believing in imaginary achievements to prevent frustrated desires	Being socially inept, yet imagining yourself as the life and soul of the party

Self-disclosure has been found to reduce stress (Johnson 1979)

◆ when necessary, learning to control emotional reactions as they may actually prevent resolution of the situation. For example, if stress causes weeping and exhaustion, then this reduces the ability to concentrate on the task that is causing the stress

◆ seeking the help of others where required

◆ protecting the body from the negative effects of stress by keeping as healthy as possible, and planning time for work, relaxation and rest.

There are many ways of reacting to stressful situations. Although they are all normal, only some are effective in reducing stress in the long term. In the following case studies the individuals are experiencing stress. Read them, and try to answer the questions by making notes in your reflective journal.

Case study 10.1

Elaine is a community nurse in a large city. One of her current clients is John, a 34-year-old man whom she is visiting regularly following a road traffic accident. He lives alone. He has made enormous progress, but still has one-sided weakness and some pressure damage to his hip and heel. He is virtually independent in the activities of daily living, but has persisting urinary incontinence for which he intermittently self-catheterizes. John was particularly keen to do this, despite it being difficult for him, as he was very unhappy to have an indwelling catheter or other continence aid. During her last few visits Elaine has become aware that something is troubling John. When she asks him what is wrong, he says that it's a personal thing. Elaine has not pursued the matter. Today, he looks really down. The following interaction occurs:

Elaine *You look miserable today. What's wrong?*

John *Oh, nothing really. It's just that Helen's coming home tonight, and she's coming round for a meal, and a chat.*

Elaine *That sounds nice; why are you worried about it?*

John *She was my girlfriend, before she worked away.*

Elaine *So what is your relationship like now?*

John *I'm not sure really, I think she's hoping we'll pick up where we left off. I'd like to, but I'm not sure if I can.*

Elaine *Why not?*

John *Well, things aren't the same are they? I'm hardly the man she knew.*

Elaine *Are you so different?*

John *Not inside. But I look different, and the other side of our relationship is going to be a farce.*

Elaine *You look really well.*

John *Yeah, with my clothes on. I'd best stay like that.*

Elaine *It'll be lovely to see her and talk again – I'm sure you'll enjoy it. Gosh, look at the time, I'll have to get on.*

When Elaine returns to base she asks one of her colleagues if they could take over John's care for a while, as she is too busy and needs to spend more time with new clients.

Discussion

What do you think is causing Elaine stress in this situation?

How is Elaine reacting to the situation? (It may be helpful to look back at the section on responses to stress.)

Highlight the points in the conversation where Elaine could have had a more positive impact. Write down how she might have responded more effectively.

Feedback on Case study 10.1

Some of the things stressing Elaine could be:

◆ *that she recognizes John wants to talk about his former girlfriend, but suspects he wants to talk about the sexual side of their relationship*

◆ that she has little experience of discussing the practicalities of sexual activity with persisting disability, and is concerned that John might ask her for factual information she does not know, such as alternative sexual positions, or how to prevent urinary incontinence during sex

◆ that he seems concerned about his body image, but she is not sure how to deal with this

◆ that even if she knew the answers, she would have to discuss these intimate things with him in a professional way yet has little experience of how to do this

◆ that she might embarrass him or, worse still, be embarrassed herself

◆ that she has not expressed her anxieties about these issues.

Her reaction to stress seems to be:

◆ to use denial (a defence mechanism).

Did you note how she used a blocking technique to pick up only on his concern about how he looked, and told him that he looked fine. She did not follow up **his** perception of how he looked, or his other concern about the 'other side of the relationship', instead quickly changing the subject: by handing over his care to a colleague she effectively gave up. It could be argued that she was acknowledging her deficits and allowing another professional to meet John's needs, but she did not inform her colleague of John's problems, so it is likely that he would have to voice his concerns all over again if he felt able.

Elaine could have used any of John's last three statements to explore his concerns further. More effective intervention would have involved exploring John's need to discuss his sexual health more directly. Elaine would need to acknowledge her limited experience in this area: she could use clinical supervision to explore ways in which she could offer help to him. This could include referring John to a more appropriate agency while maintaining her support. However, John may have built up a relationship with Elaine where what he requires at the moment is the opportunity to disclose his concerns to her as a person whom he trusts.

Case study 10.2

In a busy medical ward, Alan, a middle-aged single man, is admitted for investigations of weight loss. He has been feeling unwell for some time. At the handover between nursing staff his case is being discussed. His named nurse, Adam, is explaining that he is to have a range of tests. A student nurse asks which tests will be done. Adam replies that it is not really decided as yet. Alan asks if they think he needs an HIV test. Adam says no, then makes a joke about it, asking what he's been up to. He moves on to discuss the preparation required for a barium enema.

When they move away from Alan's room, Adam tells the student nurse off for asking inappropriate questions and causing embarrassment to the patient.

Discussion

Who is stressed in this case study?

What are the sources of stress?

Can you recognize any coping mechanisms being used?

Feedback on Case study 10.2

Adam, Alan and the student could all be suffering stress. Things that could be causing Adam stress are:

◆ that he was put 'on the spot' about the relevance of an HIV test in this situation. He may not know whether Alan has put himself at risk of HIV infection, thereby warranting this investigation

◆ that he may be unsure about what information he needs to establish Alan's possible risk of HIV, or how to seek it

◆ that he is aware that Alan brought up the issue of HIV testing and might actually want a test, but is unclear about who would be responsible for pre- and post-test counselling

◆ that he may be uncomfortable with aspects of his or Alan's sexuality – perhaps he suspects that Alan is homosexual, but is unsure about how to discuss this

◆ that he is concerned about breaching confidentiality: should this have been discussed at handover? Perhaps he did not express his real feelings about the situation.

Alan may have brought up the issue because he perceived negative attitudes towards him and was confronting the staff, and this is creating stress for him. He may also be concerned that he is HIV positive or that he is unsure of his diagnosis, condition and potential outcome.

The student could be stressed because she perceived the client to be embarrassed, felt that Adam's response was inappropriate and was unsure of the effect on the client. The student may also be concerned about the client's HIV status and the implications this might have for her.

Adam's reaction to stress seems to be:

◆ to 'have a go' at the student for providing an opportunity for Alan to ask this question

◆ to use defence mechanisms, such as isolation (laughing even though it was not funny) and displacement, to blame the student nurse, when really he was annoyed at his lack of knowledge or handling of the situation.

Case study 10.3

Jean is a school nurse in a small town, and has a drop-in session at the only senior school. She knows most of the young people well, and many of their families. She is a little taken aback one day when Kirsten, a 14-year-old pupil and the local vicar's daughter, asks her for some condoms. She asks why she wants them; Kirsten explains that she has seen a documentary about chlamydia, and wants to protect herself from it. Although there are some condoms available, Jean tells Kirsten that she has none

and that she will need to see her GP to get family planning advice. She knows that the GP is a close friend of Kirsten's family, and that the only other source of condoms locally is the chemist, where Kirsten is well known. Jean reassures herself that by making it more difficult for Kirsten to get condoms, she will think twice about having sex at this age.

Discussion

How does Jean's personal knowledge affect her professional decision in this situation?

Identify potential stressors.

How is she reacting and what might be the implications of her reactions in this situation?

Feedback on Case study 10.3

Things that could be causing Jean stress are:

◆ that Kirsten may be sexually active under the legal age of consent, and her personal discomfort with this

◆ being unsure of the legal and ethical issues surrounding providing condoms to minors

◆ that Jean knows Kirsten's parents, and suspects they would oppose her being sexually active at this age

◆ that she did not give Kirsten the help that she asked for

◆ that she referred her to a source she was unlikely to use, and that she might therefore commence or continue sexual activity without any protection against sexually transmitted infections or pregnancy

◆ that Jean's knowledge of chlamydia might be limited, or she may be unhappy about her abilities to demonstrate condom use, and so feels unable to help Kirsten

◆ that she is unsure about her position on confidentiality, and how and where to document her actions if she provided the condoms requested

◆ that she did not express her real concerns about the situation.

Her reaction to stress seems to be: to use defence mechanisms such as rationalization to convince herself that her actions were appropriate in the circumstances.

The implications of this situation are that Kirsten may continue to have unprotected sexual intercourse, resulting in an unplanned pregnancy or sexually transmitted disease. She has also lost a source of support and information which she formerly thought was available to her, and she may avoid seeking professional help in the future.

In each of the case studies there were four main areas that caused stress to the individuals:

◆ *Lack of specific knowledge*

◆ *Lack of specific skills*

◆ *Difficulty with feelings about sex, sexuality and professional roles*

◆ *Inability to be open about this discomfort.*

Case study feedback

Compare your notes to the feedback and/or where possible with your colleagues. Did you recognize some of the potential stressors and reactions to them? If you found this difficult, reread the appropriate section and try to find someone to discuss it with.

Reflection point 10.3

Perhaps you have experienced similar situations in your practice? Even if this is not the case, take some time now to consider your likely reactions if you were the practitioner involved in each of these case studies.

IMPROVING YOUR PRACTICE

It is interesting to note that many adopt a 'head in the sand' stance when situations are difficult or uncomfortable. No-one likes to feel that they are not coping, or are unable to respond appropriately to a client's needs: this is a normal reaction and does not mean they are bad people, or no good at their jobs. They are merely protecting themselves from stress. However, if there is a firmly held belief in the concept of holistic care, and that striving to meet clients' needs wherever possible is most important, then issues that could benefit from sensitive intervention cannot be ignored.

It may be felt that it is inappropriate to intervene here. The use of rationalization (one of Freud's defence mechanisms) provides reassurance that clients would be embarrassed if their sexual health needs were addressed. However, Young (1987), in a study of hospitalized patients, found that 48% thought that their sexuality or sexual function was affected by their disorder, 92% thought that it was appropriate for nurses or doctors to discuss sexuality with them, yet only 30% had experienced this. There is some research-based evidence highlighting clients' expressed needs, and many studies to support the fact that nurses and other professionals do not provide quality care in this area (see Kautz et al. 1990, Gamel et al. 1993, Lewis and Bor 1994, Brogan 1996, Waterhouse 1996).

Critical incident analysis

By focusing on your practice you should be able to recall similar situations or dilemmas you have experienced in relation to assessing or meeting the sexual health needs of those you care for. Perhaps there have been some situations which stay in your memory because you experienced stress when they occurred.

A useful technique for learning from situations such as these is critical incident analysis. This helps reflection upon, and enables learning from, practice. Smith and Russell (1991) explain that a critical incident can be described as:

'Any incident which made an emotional impact. It may have been in your interaction with a client, relatives or colleagues. It could be an incident which:

(a) was a positive incident
(b) was particularly demanding emotionally

(c) you found difficult to handle, perhaps making you feel anxious or annoyed
(d) you feel that your (or another member of staff's) intervention made a significant difference to the outcome of care.'

Learning activity 10.2

Record a critical incident about meeting the sexual health needs of your clients in your reflective journal. (If you have never recorded a critical incident before, practise first by using any situation from your experience.) Imagine you are making an entry in your diary and try to include some background to the incident, such as where, when and with whom it occurred. Record how you felt at the time, what you did, and what was particularly demanding about the incident. Finally, consider what is important to reflect upon about the incident (based on Gordon and Benner 1984).

When you have been using critical incident analysis for some time it may be that you will notice issues cropping up more than once. You may be able to identify trends or themes to what you find stressful with regard to sexual health. Critical incident analysis can help you identify whether lack of knowledge and skills, or your feelings, seem to be causing you difficulty, and how you cope with stress. The analysis can demonstrate whether the methods you use most often are effective in reducing stress related to meeting sexual health needs, and whether they are constructive coping strategies.

Using critical incident analysis in practice

Further value can be gained from critical incident analysis when you are able to share your incidents with colleagues. Ask two of your colleagues to complete a critical incident analysis related to a sexual health issue. Once they have completed this, share the findings from your critical incidents with their findings. Compare their stresses and reactions to yours.

You may find areas of similarity when using critical incident analysis in practice. For example, you may feel that you lack the necessary communication skills pertinent to the promotion and maintenance of sexual health. This in turn reduces your confidence. It therefore makes sense to try to explore how you could address these difficulties together with your client.

You may also find areas of difference. If so, you may be able to use each other's strengths. For example, if someone feels confident about the effects of commonly used drugs on sexual functioning, because of a previous project they have done, then why not share that learning with others?

Try comparing others' coping strategies with your own. Have any of your colleagues done anything constructive about their stressors in sexual health-related practice? What did they do? Is it something that could work for you?

Reflection point 10.4

Note any further action points in your reflective journal, under the heading: 'Things that others have found effective to reduce stress, that may help me', to assist you with action planning later

As you may recall there are various components of constructive coping, which were listed earlier. They included looking realistically at the situation(s) causing the stress, the coping resources employed at that time, and recognizing your emotional reactions to stress.

If you have understood the learning activities and reflection points so far, you have taken the first and most important step in coping constructively with the stress associated with meeting sexual health needs, by identifying what has caused you stress in your work in the past, and how you have responded to it.

Using a framework for sexual health promotion

The next step involves:

◆ examining your feelings about including sexual health in your work
◆ developing skills in the routine assessment of sexual health needs
◆ developing the use of interpersonal skills in relation to sexual health care.

Feelings

There are times when it is easier to deal with stress. Personal abilities depend upon self-aware-ness and self-esteem, what else is going on in life, and how this is perceived. Are there other major stressful events, or a lot of minor 'hassles' to deal with at this time? The availability of, and access to, social support is also important. Only you can assess whether your coping resources are good at present. If they are not, then you are unlikely to be effective and it may be better to delay any devel-opment activity until you are feeling more able.

It may also be useful to consider your current goals in promoting the sexual health of your clients. Learning new knowledge and skills and exploring attitudes can be a long process; there-fore, setting yourself more realistic goals which are achievable in a shorter space of time can be helpful, as it allows you to monitor your progress and motivates you by helping you see that you have achieved something.

Raising sexual health concerns/talking about sexual health issues with clients can be a potential stressor, requiring you to:

◆ want to include sexual health care in your work
◆ assess sexual health needs routinely as part of your normal assessment process
◆ pick up on cues that clients give, and respond to them
◆ know which language to use, and feel happy using it.

Reflection point 10.5

If your stressors are related to these aspects, you could examine your feelings about including sexual health in your work. In your reflective journal complete the following sentences (adapted from McLaren 1991):

When I was growing up, the messages I received about my body were . . .

Talking about sexual behaviours makes me feel . . .

Sexual behaviours or expressions of sexuality that are different from mine make me feel . . .

When I first learned about sex I felt . . .

My religious and cultural beliefs tell me that sex is . . .

The things I most enjoy about my sexuality are . . .

The areas of my sexuality that cause me guilt are . . .

My attitudes and biases about sexuality are . . .

This affects my work with clients by . . .

The things I need to concentrate on are . . .

Routine assessment of sexual health needs

Sexual history-taking will be dealt with in more detail in a later chapter. However, in order to pro-vide an opening and gauge what sort of informa-tion to seek, there are several tactics you could adopt. They take heed of the concerns of practi-tioners that the client will be offended at being asked about sexual health, or worried about what the information will be used for. One of the pur-poses of an 'opener' is to enable clients to begin discussing issues important to them in an envi-ronment where they feel safe. In order to provide that environment, sometimes it is the practitioner who offers the client the opportunity to proceed. This is almost like giving permission to another person: by signalling that you are 'open' to dis-cussion on a sensitive issue you allow the client to choose to proceed further if they wish to. Ross and Channon-Little (1991) include some useful openers for many aspects of sexual health care. When you feel ready, try incorporating them in your normal assessment process (see Chapter 12 for further examples). If you intend to develop routine assessment of sexual health needs with all clients, a useful framework, which can be used at a therapeutic level, is the PLISSIT model proposed by Annon (1976). This incorporates four levels of intervention:

P = Permission giving: inviting the client to discuss their sexual health concerns
LI = Limited information: providing simple, basic information regarding the above
SS = Specific suggestions: offering problem-specific suggestions to assist the client
IT = Intensive therapy: recognizing the need for specialist help and referring appropriately.

This model offers a logical sequence for development activity in sexual health care. It facilitates discussion with clients about their sexual health concerns before addressing their needs. As the level of intervention increases, greater knowledge and skills are required.

Consider your assessment framework in your area of work. Where could you introduce this model? How could it be adapted to be appropriate to your work area?

Learning activity 10.3

Find a colleague you are happy to try something out with. Carry out a role-play situation based on a client you have worked with in practice where you act as the nurse making an assessment, using the PLISSIT model.

◆ Identify the 'permission-giving' statements used. How did they help the situation?

◆ What kind of 'limited information' was useful?

◆ Which 'specific suggestions' helped the client?

◆ Was 'intensive therapy' required and, if so, where would you have directed the client?

Improving interpersonal skills

The recognition of cues used by clients in conversation or interview is extremely important in developing effective helping strategies. Cues can give valuable insights into important issues for the client. In order to facilitate the use of cues it is important to use some open questions, so that the client can tell his or her story and be assured that their cue has been recognized. This can be done by:

◆ reflecting: saying an important keyword back to the client
◆ paraphrasing: restating what has been said in several words
◆ clarifying: checking with the client that they have been understood
◆ summarizing: committing to memory the crux of the conversation and closing the dialogue.

Learning activity 10.4

Consider the interaction in Case study 10.1. Note the interpersonal skills, such as open questions and responding skills used.

Elaine You look miserable today. What's wrong? (*Notices body language, asks an open question*)

John Oh, nothing really. It's just that Helen's coming home tonight, and she's coming round for a meal and a chat.

Elaine That sounds nice, why are you worried about it? (*Picks up on his feelings, asks another open question*)

John She was my girlfriend, before she worked away.

Elaine So what is your relationship like now? (*Uses an open question to explore*)

John I'm not sure really, I think she's hoping we'll pick up where we left off. I'd like to, but I'm not sure if I can.

Elaine Why not? (*Encourages him to go on*)

John Well, things aren't the same are they? I'm hardly the man she knew. (*Cue to real concern*)

Elaine Are you so different? (*Open question*)

John Not inside. But I look different, and the

other side of our relationship is going to be a farce. (*Repeats cue, introduces next concern*)

Elaine You look really well. (*Ignores his perception of the situation, gives her opinion*)

John Yeah, with my clothes on. I'd best stay like that. (*Repeats his second concern*)

Elaine It'll be lovely to see her and talk again – I'm sure you'll enjoy it. Gosh, look at the time, I'll have to get on. (*Ignores cues, changes the subject*)

Can you identify John's real concerns?

Here are some ways in which Elaine could have shown John that she recognized his cues.

John Not inside. But I look different, and the other side of our relationship is going to be a farce.

Elaine The other side of your relationship? (*Reflection – invites development on his part*)

Elaine You feel that although you are the same person inside, the other side of your relationship will be difficult? (*Paraphrasing – invites exploration*)

Elaine Are you worried about the sexual side of your relationship? (*Clarifying – requesting him to ensure you have understood correctly*)

Elaine So you're worried that the changes to your body are going to affect your sexual relationship with Helen. (*Summarizing – to round up the themes of the discussion*)

These responses are core communication skills you will have no doubt used before. *Refresh your memory by considering the possible responses Elaine could have used at the end of the interaction, after John said:*

Yeah with my clothes on. I'd best stay like that.

Reflective response

Paraphrased response

Clarifying response

Summarizing response

As you can see, even if you miss the first cue you can still pick up on the issues in an interaction: all that is needed is to listen carefully, question skilfully, and remember to use responses that encourage the client to expand. As with any skill, this ability improves with practice.

Sharing a common language

Many practitioners suggest that their barrier to exploring further at this stage is uncertainty about which words to use so that both they and their clients understand and are not embarrassed. This involves thinking about and practising a suitable vocabulary. To do this, you could develop a sexual health glossary (see Learning activity 10.5).

 Learning activity 10.5

Brainstorm or write down as many terms as possible for the following:

◆ Female genitalia
◆ Male genitalia
◆ Penetrative vaginal intercourse
◆ Anal intercourse
◆ Oral sex
◆ Orgasm
◆ Masturbation
◆ Others?

To do this, use your knowledge, listen to friends, clients, entertainers and any other source to get a wide range of words and phrases. (There are some references at the end of the chapter that may also be helpful.) Some may be new to you and need clarification. Consider which of these words you would use personally, and which you feel are suitable to use with clients.

It may seem more professional to use the correct anatomical terminology, but this only adds to the difficulty of communicating about sensitive issues if no-one understands what you are talking about! It may be better to use terms that are commonly understood, that you are happy to say yourself. If you are embarrassed you will convey that to clients, reducing the effectiveness of the interaction. Find alternative terms where necessary. Make sure you know what words and terms mean, by checking with others and, where there is confusion, clarify your understanding with clients who use them. Perhaps you could have a glossary of terms, with explanations, available in your ward, practice, unit or patch?

Another thing that may be helpful is to have anatomically correct diagrams available, to assist in clarifying what clients mean, or to improve explanations to clients. While nursing in a gynaecology setting, it became apparent to the author that very few women knew the term vulva, and therefore used vagina, a word they were more familiar with and which they perceived to be the proper term for any part of their genitalia. Diagrams of the vulva and the internal genitalia would have been extremely useful in that particular context.

Improving your knowledge base

It is important to identify where your knowledge deficits are. Sometimes it is difficult to know what we don't know, so it may be useful to look at some texts that outline the general issues.

If you need further guidance on the potential knowledge you require to promote sexual health and address sexual health-care needs, an excellent overview is available in the guidelines for good practice in sexual health education and training, produced by the English National Board for Nursing, Midwifery and Health Visiting (ENB 1994, pp. 18–19). Waterhouse (1996) also outlines the aspects of sexual health care that could be integrated into nursing practice.

Learning activity 10.6

Compile a list of the knowledge you feel would be beneficial to you, and your practice area, to enhance the sexual health care you provide. Prioritize the components of your list, and decide how best to improve your knowledge base.

It may be that you wish to share the responsibility for finding out more. Everyone could complete a literature search on a designated topic and share the findings with others, e.g. produce a summary and suggested reading list, present a seminar, or develop a resource file.

It is likely to be helpful to compare your thoughts with colleagues. If several of you identify the same knowledge deficits and you have prioritized them as important, perhaps your line manager, or a person responsible for staff training, could arrange appropriate education or training on a group basis. Formal courses may also be an option, and further details of local and national provision can be obtained from your local nursing library. If formal study is not an option, there are several pertinent open learning materials relevant to sexual health care. Good sources are your local library and health promotion departments, most of which have a designated sexual health worker, and learning materials you can borrow. Perhaps you could invite colleagues from other disciplines to unit or departmental meetings to increase your knowledge base. For example, the staff from an accident and emergency unit could ask the health adviser from the genitourinary medicine department to update them on managing and referring appropriately clients who present with sexually transmissible conditions.

Utilizing specialist resources

Although increasing knowledge does tend to increase confidence about dealing with sexual health-care problems, it may be helpful to know who is available locally with specialist knowledge and skills, and who can provide advice and support.

Learning activity 10.7

Produce a local directory of agencies, contacts, referral sources and services that provide sexual health-related care.

Many resources may already be listed in the local authorities' guide to voluntary agencies, or your local Citizens' Advice Bureau or sexual health promotion officer may be able to help. Perhaps some of the agencies will have publicity materials that you could use for clients and their families or friends. Making contact can be helpful, in that it gives you a better idea of where, and to whom, you are referring clients, and improves the likelihood of effective communication. It may also lead to the development of shared protocols which enhance care.

CONCLUSION

Implementation of any of these suggestions would be a useful and constructive coping strategy.

It would be helpful to reflect regularly upon not only your increasing knowledge and skills, but on how this has influenced your practice. Recognizing improvements in the care provided produces motivation to continue. Remember: using constructive coping strategies takes time and effort, but provides the only long-term solution to stress. If you are committed to improving your knowledge, skills and comfort with sensitive issues, you may have several things in your personal action plan still outstanding. Use the other chapters in this book to assist you, and continue to reflect upon your development and achievements. With a clearer understanding of your personal stressors, and how you may overcome them, you are more likely to succeed. Using constructive coping strategies also usually results in the stimulation of emotions which are best expressed in a safe environment. In order for this to occur, you may need to read further about eliciting personal and professional support.

ANNOTATED FURTHER READING

Donohoe G 1992 Sensitivity can break the taboo: female sexual problems and treatment approaches. Professional Nurse 2: 304–308

This article outlines common medical and surgical disorders, and drug therapy which has the potential to interfere with sexuality or sexual functioning.

Oojen E V, Charnock A 1994 Sexuality and patient care, a guide for nurses and teachers. Chapman & Hall, London

Chapters 3 and 7 may be helpful in developing your knowledge about the relevance of sexual health care to your practice.

Redfern S 1991 Sexuality and arthritis. Nursing 4 (44): 17–19

This article assists nurses to acknowledge and respond to the common effects and treatment side-effects of arthritic illness.

There are of course many more articles pertinent to specific areas of practice, or illnesses, which can be obtained via a keyword literature search.

Using reflective practice

Dewing J 1990 Reflective practice. Senior Nurse 10: 26–28

Powell J H 1989 The reflective practitioner in nursing. Journal of Advanced Nursing 14: 824–832

Smith A, Russell J 1991 Using critical learning incidents in nurse education. Nurse Education Today 11: 284–291

Developing interpersonal skills

Continuing Nurse Education Programme 1986 Interpersonal skills – open learning for nurses. Barnet and Central Manchester Open Tech Project, London and Manchester

This open learning text is not specific to sexual health, but is an extremely useful resource.

ENB 1994 Caring for people with sexually transmitted diseases, including HIV disease. ENB, London

This open learning package includes useful sections: see Section 6, part 2

Faulkner A 1992 Effective interaction with patients. Churchill Livingstone, Edinburgh

A pragmatic approach to developing interpersonal skills.

Groenman N H, Slevin O D'A, Buckenham M 1992 Social and behavioural sciences for nurses. Campion Press, Edinburgh

Module 5 of this text, sections 1–4, is helpful.

Oojen E V, Charnock A 1994 Sexuality and patient care, a guide for nurses and teachers. Chapman & Hall, London

Chapters 6 and 7 deal with interpersonal skills and their application in sexuality in ill health.

Ross M R, Channon-Little L D 1991 Discussing sexuality: a guide for health practitioners. MacLennan & Petty, Australia

This is an excellent, pragmatic text with application to various care contexts

Few C 1993 Safer Sex. Community Outlook, September

Developing a glossary of terms for promoting sexual health

REFERENCES

Annon J S 1976 The PLISSIT model: a proposed conceptual scheme for the behavioural treatment of sexual problems. Journal of Sex Education Therapy 2: 1–15

Briggs L M 1994 Sexual healing: caring for patients recovering from myocardial infarctions. British Journal of Nursing 3(16): 837–842

Brogan M 1996 The sexual needs of elderly people: addressing the issue. Nursing Standard 10(24): 42–45

ENB 1994 Sexual health education and training: guidelines for good practice in the teaching of nurses, midwives and health visitors. ENB, London

Freud S 1975 Beyond the pleasure principle. Hogarth Press, New York

Gamel C, Davis B D, Hengeveld M 1993 Nurses' provision of teaching and counselling on sexuality: review of the literature. Journal of Advanced Nursing 18(8): 1219–1227

Gordon D, Benner P 1984 Guidelines for recording critical incidents. In: Benner P From novice to expert. Addison Wesley, London, pp. 299–302

Holmes T H, Rahe R H 1967 The social readjustment scale. Journal of Psychosomatic Research 11: 213–218

Hott J R, Ryan-Merritt M 1982 National study of nursing research in human sexuality. Nursing Clinics of North America 17: 429–447

Jeffers S 1989 Feel the fear and do it anyway. Rider, London

Johnson M 1979 Anxiety/stress and the effects on disclosure between nurses and patients. Advances in Nursing Science 1(4): 1–20

Kautz D D, Dickey C A, Stevens M N 1990 Using research to identify why nurses do not meet established sexuality nursing care standards. Journal of Nursing Quality Assurance 4(3): 69–78

Lewis S, Bor R 1994 Nurses' knowledge of and attitudes towards sexuality and the relationship of these with nursing practice. Journal of Advanced Nursing 20: 251–259

MacLaren A 1995 Primary health care for women: comprehensive sexual health assessment. Journal of Nurse Midwifery 40: 104–119

McHaffie H 1993 Improving awareness. Nursing Times 89(18): 29–31

Ross M R, Channon-Little L D 1991 Discussing sexuality: a guide for health practitioners. MacLennan & Petty, Australia

Seligman M E P, Rosenhan D L 1984 Abnormal psychology. Norton, New York

Shuman N A, Bohanick P 1987 Nurses' attitudes towards sexual counselling. Dimensions of Critical Care Nursing 6: 75–80

Smith A, Russell J 1991 Using critical learning incidents in nurse education. Nurse Education Today 11: 284–291

Wall-Haas C L 1991 Nurses' attitudes toward sexuality in adolescent patients. Paediatric Nursing 17(6): 549–557

Waterhouse S 1996 Nursing practice related to sexuality: a review and recommendations. Nursing Times Research 1(6): 412–418

Young E W 1987 Sexual needs of psychiatric clients. Journal of Psychosocial Nursing and Mental Health Services 25(7): 30–32

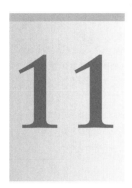

Sexual health, the process: primary care

David T. Evans

> '*Remember: Sex doesn't make you sick – diseases do.*'
> (Berkowitz & Callen 1983)

KEY ISSUES/CONCEPTS

◆ Identifying the audiences: primary care, associated care, and their clients

◆ Exploring the needs of clients and their professional caregivers

◆ Highlighting the atypical: looking for sexual health issues of people and situations not routinely covered

◆ Examining ways to learn from good practice

OVERVIEW

Chapter 11, *Sexual health the process: primary care*, explores sexual health from two main perspectives. The first is sexual health within the structures of primary health care, for example primary health-care teams. The second is from the primary, or first presenting, care needs of the client, irrespective of which professional service they avail themselves of. For many people the concepts of sexual health are still in their infancy, and is frequently reduced either to contraceptive advice such as family planning, cervical screening campaigns, or to the avoidance of sexually transmitted infections. This chapter attempts to widen this view, first by exploring the ways in which the primary health-care team and allied services can address the issues, and secondly by examining the sexual health-care responsibilities of other health and social care professionals. Such responsibilities emanate from the client's needs.

Given the limitations of length in this section, the main focus will frequently concentrate on services for people from non-traditional groups, i.e. those not usually considered as being in need of 'run of the mill' sexual health services.

INTRODUCTION

The world of health and social care is no stranger to the process of continuous change. One noticeable philosophical development to affect clients is the desire to move away from pathologizing their lives. In certain circumstances this is evident in the frequent change of title from 'patient' to the more empowering 'client' or consumerist 'service user'. With this change has come an added emphasis on first access to treatment, either when things go wrong or, preferably, by way of prevention and health promotion.

Many of these changes parallel the development of primary health-care teams (PHCTs), which usually operate in a general practice setting, including receptionists, GPs, practice nurses, and then, to varying degrees, a manager and other associated services (Fig. 11.1). From April 1999 there was another major development in England, with the reorganization of health and social care under the auspices of primary care groups (PCGs). Similar organizational structures will affect Scotland, Wales and Northern Ireland (Antrobus 1999).

With the focus of this book on sexual health, the approach to primary care may be twofold:

◆ primary health care in the form of PHCTs
◆ *primary* care, as in the first point of access for clients with sexual health needs.

Primary health care (PHC) refers to the first tier of health provision, provided in local community settings by generalists (Naidoo and Wills 1994). For many people access to primary health services is initiated by some particular health deficit or need. However,

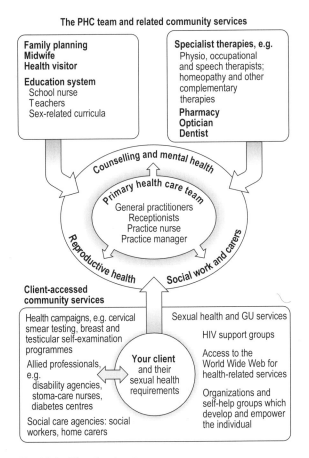

The PHC team and related community services

Family planning
Midwife
Health visitor

Education system
School nurse
Teachers
Sex-related curricula

Specialist therapies, e.g.
Physio, occupational
and speech therapists;
homeopathy and other
complementary
therapies

Pharmacy
Optician
Dentist

Counselling and mental health

Primary health care team
General practitioners
Receptionists
Practice nurse
Practice manager

Reproductive health

Social work and carers

**Client-accessed
community services**

Health campaigns, e.g. cervical
smear testing, breast and
testicular self-examination
programmes

Allied professionals,
e.g.
disability agencies,
stoma-care nurses,
diabetes centres

Social care agencies: social
workers, home carers

Your client
and their
sexual health
requirements

Sexual health and GU services

HIV support groups

Access to the
World Wide Web for
health-related services

Organizations and
self-help groups which
develop and empower
the individual

Fig. 11.1 The client's primary care resources.

there is an increasing emphasis on the benefits of proactive health promotion. As the ancient dictum states: prevention is better than cure. Generally, it also costs a lot less.

As far as sexual health is concerned the PHCT may not be the first team a client wishes to approach. Therefore, other services may provide the first point of contact, and either take on the complete management of care themselves, or treat and then refer certain clients back to their own PHCT. These other services include sexual health or genitourinary (GU) clinics; contraceptive and family planning services; and health, education and social care agencies whose members have a health promotion remit.

A television advertisement in vogue from late 1998 shows a young man going into a pharmacy to purchase some condoms. He is embarrassed, and tries to do this secretively. The young female assistant holds up a pack of condoms and shouts out to a colleague, asking the price. The young man is mortified!

Barriers, imaginary or real, to accessing services may occur when clients with sexual health needs consider approaching their PHCT. It is not too difficult to list some of these, with the first being embarrassment at revealing problems to the 'gatekeepers' of PHC: the receptionists, especially in a crowded waiting room. Then there is the concern of some clients in knowing their GP, especially if the GP has been the family doctor for many years. Finally, there are concerns of prejudice and discrimination, from the insurance and mortgage industries, frequently related to sexual disease issues and most particularly to non-heterosexual lifestyles. These relate to the legal requirements on a GP, and the GP's conditional approach to confidentiality regarding sexual health issues. For example, a GP may be asked for details concerning their patient's history of sexually transmitted diseases (STDs), hepatitis B virus (HBV) and the human immuno-deficiency virus (HIV). They may also be asked about sexual orientation and lifestyle. The law requires that they answer such questions honestly and completely.

Dealing with sexual issues in the health-care setting often requires the building up of a rapport with the client which indicates that the practitioner will refrain from prejudging and judging them, as well as from condemning them and discriminating against them, but such problems are frequently experienced by clients (McFarlane 1998). It also requires the health-care professional to try, as far as they can, to have a positive regard for each person. This may not always be easy, given the misconceptions and fears around the issues of sex. It is, however, vital if a genuine therapeutic encounter is to take place (Flaskerud and Ungvarski 1992). Foucault (1990) once urged society to ask why we burden ourselves today with so much guilt for having once made sex a sin.

This chapter will therefore explore some of the main issues concerning sexual health from the perspective of the PHCT, other primary care facilities, and the clients or service users themselves.

SEXUAL HEALTH AND PRIMARY CARE

The primary health-care team

It would be stating the obvious to point out that there are significantly more women working in health-care settings, and accessing health-care services, than men. This would seem to indicate a good relationship between the majority of service providers and users. However, where sexual health is concerned, nothing can be taken for granted. Nurses, both female and male, along with many other health-care professionals, frequently show suboptimal standards of care in relation to sexual health (McHaffie 1993). The levels of knowledge on sexual health-care matters, and the ability to communicate on such matters, often leaves much to be desired (Bor and Watts 1993). Superimposed upon this are the numerous ways in which individuals are discriminated against on the grounds of their sexual health needs, practices, orientation, age or physical and mental ability. For example, there is an abundance of studies showing just how homophobic health-care professionals can be (Rose 1994, James et al. 1994, Douglas et al. 1997, Polansky et al. 1997, McFarlane 1998). However, homophobia is just one problem. Reflect on the number of stereotypical media images – especially on the television – that use young, white, 'beautiful', able-bodied, financially solvent, heterosexual models to sell products. Now ask yourself how those products would be sold using alternative images, for example physically disabled people.

The concept of the PHCT has a great deal to offer clients regarding their sexual health and wellbeing. Unfortunately, many opportunities are missed or reduced to a minimum requirement of statistical obligations. For example, with quantitative research data looking at targets and statistics, 'the percentage of women over 16 being offered contraceptives' seems a fair starting point. However, contraception is far from being the only sexual health need of sexually active women. In this example, other missed opportunities include:

◆ not dealing with the health needs of sexually active under-16-year-olds
◆ failing to educate clients about preventing the spread of STDs (while at the same time giving advice leading to the uptake of non-barrier methods of contraception, such as the pill and the intrauterine contraceptive device (IUCD) or 'coil')
◆ failing to assess and advise on the self-empowering skills often needed to negotiate safer sex and condom use
◆ under-identifying the women to be screened and educated for cervical and breast cancers.

In the PHCT setting there are also opportunities to address sexual health issues through Well Woman and Well Man clinics. Among other services, Well Woman clinics offer advice and screening against cervical and breast cancers. They can also educate women on the need for regular breast self-examination. Three groups of women often missed – or *dis*-missed – for cervical screening include those presumed not to have sexual intercourse, such as lesbians, women with certain disabilities, and celibate women such as nuns (Weston 1994).

For men, advice on regular testicular self-examination (TSE) is sadly lacking. Coupled to this is the reluctance of many men to access health services until problems are well and truly present (see below). Given the annual rates of preventable testicular cancer, there are far too many men who are totally unaware of TSE and other sexual health matters.

With the current frequency of role and organizational change there is a possibility that nursing care may overlap (Jones 1998). This can offer added incentives for continuity of care, from GP practice through all branches of nursing service in primary care: the practice nurse, district nurse and, where appropriate, community midwife and health visitor. Unfortunately, there is another pitfall in that professionals often assume that somebody else is addressing sexual health issues, i.e. shifting the responsibility. Sexual health issues can thus easily slip through the net.

It is inappropriate for just one or two individuals to take on the mantle of sexual health care:

sexual health is tightly interwoven with total health (Savage 1998), as is the continuity of effective, holistic care. The changing roles of health and social care provision will give nurses an unparalleled opportunity to take an active part in the planning, provision and evaluation of services to clients in their local areas and primary care groups (Antrobus 1999). Consequently, the more proactive nurses, midwives and health visitors are on the sexual health front, the more such needs will be identified and provided for.

One final impact to consider on the changing role of the PHCT is the process currently gaining momentum of 'normalizing HIV'. In the early days of all new illnesses, the initial response and allocation of services is referred to as the period of 'exceptionalization' (Steffen 1998, Cattacin, 1998, Noël et al. 1998). After the new phenomenon has been brought under an acceptable level of control, the process changes to that of 'normalization'. This has certain effects on the PHCT, not least a shift in financial resources from specialist services to the budgets directly maintained in various primary health-care settings.

Recent practices, such as antenatal screening for HIV, and the guidelines from the British Medical Association and Department of Health, view ways of integrating HIV issues, especially testing and related counselling, into the mainstream of GP care. As with all issues there are many pros and cons.

In favour of this process is the normalizing of HIV disease, which may help destigmatize many of the issues and people for whom HIV has often meant a reason for hostility from others (Sontag 1991). Also in favour are the generally well advanced levels of sexual awareness, client empowerment and knowledge of treatment options found in some parts of this client group. Many of the ways in which HIV-positive clients have learned to improve their status can give very positive images to other (disempowered) client groups. Against this normalization is the lack of knowledge, the ignorance and prejudice, that still remains with many health-care professionals (O'Hanlan et al. 1997), as well as the risk, as mentioned above, of knowledge of sexual lifestyles being obtained by outside agencies, such as insur-ers and mortgage lenders, which is then used to penalize certain people.

Reflection point 11.1

Before moving on to the next section, take a few minutes to recall the sexual health services and materials (e.g. posters, leaflets, specialist clinics) available in your PHCT/GP centre.

Make a list of

◆ the sexual health services

◆ the sexual health resources.

When you have time, telephone or visit the practice and find out exactly what is on offer. You may wish to discuss your findings with a member of staff in the practice, by way of giving feedback as a service user. This would be especially important to those involved in service-related decision making.

Services allied to the PHCT

Figure 11.1 shows numerous other services and professionals allied to the PHCT. It is conceivable that these may be the first line of contact for numerous clients. Some of the professionals involved have an obvious role to play in sexual health, such as midwives, family planning services, and to some extent health visitors and school nurses. Nevertheless, studies have shown that just because a professional is expected to address sexual health does not mean that they feel comfortable in doing so (McHaffie 1993, Chalmers 1994, Evans 1997). Many may limit the focus to that which is directly relevant to their casework, and no more.

It does not always follow that because a person is a health-care professional they will automatically be able to deal with sexual health matters. Take the case of Dorothea (Case study 11.1). She had always thought that she was well placed and well equipped to deal with the sexual health needs of school pupils. Unfortunately, she held inaccurate and culturally specific beliefs that clouded her judgement and the subsequent 'advice' she gave. Coupled with this was the erroneous belief of the teaching staff that they could leave all the sexual matters to the nurse.

Like many school nurses, Dorothea increasingly finds herself having to give advice, or teach, on the subjects of sex, sexuality and sexual health. Sometimes this work is directly with pupils; at other times with the teachers. Working with teachers may be by way of offering support and professional or 'expert' (e.g. medical) opinion, or as a form of cascade learning, as in 'training the trainers'. In Dorothea's case, her contact was directly with young people, who looked to her as the 'professional' with all the right answers.

Case study 11.1

Dorothea was a school nurse who wished to advance her knowledge and expertise in sexual health matters, so she attended a relevant course. During the course, many of the learners seemed to be in awe at Dorothea's wealth of knowledge and experience. She kept reaffirming how she felt totally comfortable in dealing with all matters sexual. 'I've been round the block a few times!' was her way of explaining her breadth and depth of knowledge.

However, during a session on legal issues relating to sex and young people, the topic of the unequal ages of sexual consent was raised. This was explored from many different angles, but Dorothea insisted that she always warns 'young homosexuals' not to start having sex 'too soon'. Even if the law is changed, to reflect an equal age of consent at 16, Dorothea said that they ought to be dissuaded from having sex until as late as possible.

When she was questioned as to why this should be, she pinched her index finger and thumb together and screwed up her face as though to show the smallness of the finger and thumb image she was making. Then she said: 'Because at 16 the anus isn't fully developed!'.(See Learning activity 11.1.)

Many health-care professionals, such as the majority of mental health nurses, social workers and physiotherapists, do not have a specific sexual health remit. However, no profession that claims to offer holistic care can do so unless they are open to all aspects of life, including sexual health. A client with walking difficulties or disability may

Learning activity 11.1

From an anatomical point of view, how was Dorothea wrong?

Check out in Wellings et al. (1994) the percentages – and sexual orientations – of people who engage in anal intercourse in the UK.

List ways in which the impact of wrong sexual information can be detrimental to the health and development of young people.

Spend a few moments to think of erroneous messages about sex that you received in your school years. Who gave you those messages? How have you learned to correct them since?

spend hours each week working with a physiotherapist, and develop great levels of rapport and trust. This client may also conceivably have sexual health needs related to their physical mobility problems, such as people with spinal injuries. In an ideal world they may be able to engage in a therapeutic relationship that addresses their sexual health, as well as their physical health, but unfortunately this is not always the case.

Step 1 in addressing the sexual health aspects of life is therefore an acknowledgement that such needs actually exist. Next will be the opportunities to identify and explore the issues within the wider context of care. Many of the professionals allied to the PHCT may have a definite role to play in helping a client address those needs. However, as Savage (1998) says, much wider aspects need to be investigated too, and incorporated into the curricula of all health-care learners. These wider aspects include issues of sex and disability (sensory, physical and learning), the impact of illness on sexuality, drugs and sex (prescribed medication, recreational drugs and alcohol), and infections related to the sex organs. The latter should, of course, include all parts of the body used in sex, and the ways in which they may be involved in a disease process, such as the nipples, mouth and rectum.

The reason why so many of these issues are routinely neglected is because of a common tendency to view sex as both a private matter and something predominantly related to heterosexual couples and the ability to procreate (Ussher and Baker 1993). These views, often unwittingly taken on board by health-care professionals, express general beliefs in society at large (Grey 1993). Throughout the ages, in all parts of the world, there are examples of societies whose approach to sex, sexuality and sexual health has been less than positive and supportive. Obviously, such an approach can be reflected in the health-care systems of a given society.

In a multicultural nation such as the UK there are peoples from all different ethnic, religious and cultural backgrounds. Some of these people are health carers, some are clients, and some are, at one time or another, both. The personal and societal 'baggage' people bring with them can therefore affect their approach to the sex issues of health care. This is seen predominantly in the reluctance to communicate on these issues within the therapeutic encounter. Reasons include the following:

◆ many people see sex as pre-eminently for (married) couples and/or for having babies
◆ that too much sex is bad/leads to promiscuity, STDs and HIV
◆ penis + vagina is the only 'normal' form of sex, i.e. non-penetration, and oral or anal sex are somehow abnormal, wrong or perverted. In certain societies and cultures such practices are punishable by law. Likewise, in some cultures and religions, sex by oneself (e.g. masturbation) is frowned upon or thought 'selfish' (Howe 1995), as is non-procreative sex, e.g. using certain forms of contraception, sex between people of the same sex, or sex with postmenopausal women
◆ sex is for the good-looking – see the comment on media images above
◆ one partner for life/at a time (e.g. serial monogamy)
◆ sex before or outside marriage is wrong
◆ sex is only for the young and able-bodied.

Another point to be mentioned is that not all people wish to express their sexuality procre-atively. Such an idea can be alien to many societies, although many people would probably admit that not everyone has sex simply for making babies! The other side of this statement is that there are many people who *do* have sex to have children, but who, for one reason or another, are unable to. Cultural interpretations on this may reflect negatively on individuals who cannot have children of their own.

For some, impaired or reduced physical performance in sex can be perceived as a disgrace or stigma. Consider the early debates on the availability of the anti-impotence drug Viagra. Impotence, and the inability to have children, may affect people in different ways. Some men, for example, may feel a loss of their manhood or masculine identity, whereas women may have the added burden of having their sexuality constantly linked to children, i.e. 'women and children'.

Many health-care services and institutions use images of women and children together, e.g. the Women and Children's Directorate, or in the logo for hospital or Trust services. This would seem to totally negate a woman's sexual identity outside procreation. Just think of the different ways in which 'career women' are often spoken of, especially when they choose not to have children. There may be one approach to career women in the business and finance industries, but the approach to women in the caring professions may be very different. Assessing a woman from the point of view of whether she has had children or not has the potential to miss out on addressing many other aspects of her sexual health needs.

 Reflection point 11.2

Spend a few minutes considering how you may presume, or prejudge, the sexual needs of:

◆ a 10-year-old client
◆ a 15-year-old client (female)
◆ a 17-year-old client (male)
◆ a 43-year-old female client
◆ a 79-year-old male client

Feedback on Reflection point 11.2

Did you consider:

◆ 10-year-old client: many people do not consider that children or young people have sexual/sexual health needs (Grey 1993)

◆ 15-year-old female: the UK has one of the highest underage pregnancy rates in western Europe

◆ 17-year-old male: sex between males and females is legal at the age of 16; sex between males is currently 18. This affects various sexual health promotion initiatives and services

◆ 43-year-old female: many women experience psychological traumas at the thought and implications of the menopause. There are many myths and stereotypes attached to this point in life

◆ 79-year-old male: society generally perceives older people to have ceased sexual activities; the risk of prostate cancer increases with age

Addressing secondary sexual health issues

Sexual health may not be the primary reason for referral to a health-care professional. However, in the presence of a therapeutic environment which is both non-judgemental and receptive to exploring a client's holistic needs, sexual health issues may never be too far from being relevant. Case study 11.2 is an example.

Case study 11.2

Niamh is a 43-year-old woman seeking help from the community psychiatric services. She has numerous alcohol-related problems: personal, medical, relational and social. Niamh is alcohol dependent. Because of this she has been unable to find and/or keep regular employment. She has had three children, all taken into care by social services; her whole social network consists of other people with alcohol problems, and she has an abusive relationship with her husband.

Niamh's husband, also with alcohol dependency and associated problems, works as a labourer. They share a council flat together, and Niamh is concerned that if she and her husband separated she would be homeless and without adequate money. For these reasons she puts up with the abusive relationship. Sometimes, when the abuse is physical, Niamh will 'give him as good as I get'. She sometimes talks about going 'back home' to Ireland, but owing to lack of support this is not a viable option.

Niamh's husband regularly has sex outside his marriage, often with women he meets in pubs, when both are heavily intoxicated; sometimes he pays for sex. This makes Niamh feel unwanted and unloved. Her self-esteem appears exceptionally low, and she is prepared to do anything to keep her husband. Niamh says that she sometimes uses the pill as contraception, but sees no need to protect herself from sexually acquired infections, including HIV.

(Adapted from a personal communication with Matthew Wilding, RN/DipHE student (mental health branch), Wolfson Institute of Health Science, TVU, London. Biographical details changed to maintain client's confidentiality.)

 Learning activity 11.2

List some of Niamh's primary sexual health needs, which are:

◆ physical

◆ emotional

◆ relational.

How can these needs be met by a CPN?

What other services/professionals may be appropriate to help Niamh, and why?

How does the exploration of this case study make *you* feel? What issues does it evoke for you?

Make some notes in your reflective journal, and take the opportunity to discuss the issues with a confidant or mentor.

Feedback on Learning activity 11.2

Here are just a few possibilities you might have thought of:

1. Assessing the client's needs

Physical

◆ Niamh is at risk of sexually transmitted infections, from unprotected intercourse with her husband.

◆ Abuse from her husband has physical, as well as psychological, dangers. Each of these is dangerous in itself, but may also lead her further into a cycle of abuse, e.g. more heavy drinking, more 'Dutch courage' to physically fight back, and reduced inhibitions to taking more sexual risks.

◆ Unsatisfying sexual relationship, from all aspects: physical, emotional and relational.

Emotional

◆ Low self-esteem.

◆ Perpetuating risk-taking behaviours.

◆ Inability to be self-assertive and defend her own rights.

◆ Feels trapped to accept what she has, because it appears the most viable option.

Relational

◆ Failure to keep children with her (and the guilt and other feelings of inadequacy this brings).

◆ Feelings of guilt at not 'providing', or 'being adequate' to meet her husband's needs (i.e. he turns to others for sex, including paying for it).

2. The CPN's role in addressing these issues

◆ Clearly assess the needs, and discuss appropriate professionals who may help.

◆ Plan care which sees the interrelatedness of the problems in Niamh's life, not just the alcohol dependence.

◆ With the client, outline possible outcomes to therapeutic interventions, by both the CPN and other multiagency supports/treatments.

◆ Explore ways of empowering the client, so she can make positive health choices.

◆ Map out realistic and achievable goals, as well as a time for progression, review and achievement.

◆ Examine accurate ways of monitoring and supporting the client's progress and choices (even those which are not the CPN's own).

◆ Adequate support and supervision for the CPN, to deal with her/his own feelings and professional judgements and actions.

3. Services and other professionals to help

◆ Sexual health/Genitourinary clinic for sexual health check; session with health adviser re safer sex and related skills, and condoms, should the client so decide.

◆ Alcohol and/or women's support group.

◆ Social workers, for a 'safe house' or other accommodation and social supports, including financial.

◆ Counsellors/therapists: to combat low self-esteem, and addictive behaviours, and improve assertiveness skills.

◆ PHCT for medical services from GP, and contraceptive advice including barrier methods, e.g. from family planning services.

4. Reflecting on your own personal feelings on this case

◆ Examine your feelings and responses to this situation.

◆ Explore possible ways of informing/improving your practice in the light of this learning.

Shernoff (1991) highlighted how people who devalue themselves – indeed, sometimes even despise themselves – are likely to be filled with self-loathing and self-hate. In these circumstances, not only may a person be more vulnerable to taking risks, they may actively seek to do so. Such a person is of course also putting others at risk.

Learning activity 11.3

Identify sexual health issues with which a client may approach the different health-care professionals: for example, a person with a spinal injury and their physiotherapist; a person with incontinence and their continence adviser; a person with a colostomy and their stoma nurse; a person with HIV and their specialist clinic staff; the primary carer/partner of a person with dementia, and their key support worker (add others as relevant to your area and experience).

◆ Contact some of these professions (either locally or nationally) and ask for their printed materials on dealing with sexual health issues.

◆ Analyse what you perceive as clients' needs, and the service provision offered by the professions.

◆ Assess the impact on clients when their needs are not addressed/met.

◆ Contemplate ways of highlighting your findings to colleagues, peers and educators.

PRIMARY SEXUAL HEALTH CARE

Identifying the clients

Identifying both the clients and their sexual health needs will involve thinking beyond traditional areas of health care and promotion. This is because sexual health has frequently been reduced to set goals, such as cervical screening of a given percentage of a population; reducing teenage and unwanted pregnancies; reducing the new incidence of sexually transmitted diseases etc. (DoH 1992, 1993). Identifying the clients means going a lot further than that. If we consider that every human being is a sexual being, then it is not too hard to imagine that many may have sexual health

issues that can be addressed in the therapeutic encounter.

Take, for example, the case of Agnes, in case study 11.3. This profile shows how her needs were appropriately addressed by a health-care professional once they had been identified and accurately assessed.

Case study 11.3

Agnes is an 80-year-old woman whose husband died 2 weeks before this visit. Her husband had been cared for at home and this visit was part of her community bereavement follow-up.

As she welcomed me into her home, Agnes told me that she had a problem about which she felt embarrassed. Her embarrassment stemmed partly from the fact that I am a man, and many years younger than her. She was unaccustomed to talking of 'personal' matters, with either men or women. However, the rapport we had built up, on the few earlier occasions in which we had met, meant that she trusted me and my professional opinion/judgement in the matter. Ultimately, the gender difference did not prove a barrier to her care.

*Agnes explained how she had been cruelly abused as a child. The scars of this abuse were known fully only to her husband, her one and only partner, of 65 years. The abuse had left physical scars, which meant she dressed differently from most women of her generation, throughout her life. Agnes said that, after having a baby, her 'womb dropped'. 'My husband was always **good** to me': she winked, nodded and nudged me, to indicate that she was referring to their sexual relations. But 'it' always hurt. She suffered both sex and the pain from the prolapsed uterus for well over 50 years, and told nobody.*

*The week before this present visit, Agnes said that a new lady doctor had visited and she had told the doctor about her prolapsed uterus. The GP inserted a ring pessary to hold the uterus in place. 'Honestly', she said, 'I've been walking around with a smile on my face ever since. My husband was good to me, but **this**! Do you think it's a sin – should I have it out?'*

Learning activity 11.4

◆ Make a list of questions that arise from Case study 11.3 regarding the sexual health needs of people over 65 years of age.

◆ Explore where *you* stand in relation to the answers to these questions.

◆ Ask the same questions of colleagues from different health-care professional groups.

◆ Evaluate the answers and reflect on ways of informing and improving care to clients in this age group.

It's a woman's world!

Many aspects of daily life, from catching a bus, through shopping in the supermarkets, to accessing various health services, regularly give priority to women. In particular, many of the services are specifically developed to be suitable for women. Look a little closer and we see that in many circumstances it is not just women who are being targeted, but women and children.

This can have great benefits in society. It also means that, on the individual level, women with children are positively catered for. In the health-care world there are many examples of this, right down to the current government recruitment campaign to entice nurses back into the profession. In so doing, child-care needs are receiving unparalleled attention and resources.

Unfortunately, this is not all as positive as it sounds, first, because many women feel they are not treated as an individual in their own right, but only in relation to their capacity to produce offspring. Also, if the starting point is to focus attention and services on 'women and children', again this will miss all those women who do not have or want children.

It is true to say, too, that there are ways in which society's bent for procreation can send out the wrong messages. This is seen in individuals who are unable fully to address their own needs, but who at the same time feel compelled to have children. As Heller (1998) states: 'Life choices for young people growing up on the estate are severely limited. The young women often choose to have babies at a very early age and turn their energies to the next generation in the hope of finding meaning and fulfilment. Children being born to children.'

Many of the messages concerning sexual health, including safer sex and contraceptive advice, are frequently aimed at people with more readily accessible skills and means than those who are disempowered and disenfranchized. If the provision of services and resources appears hostile to women, the implications may go much further than the individual woman herself, as in Heller's case even to the next generation.

A concrete example can be found in safer sex leaflets and posters. The images and language used frequently depict lifestyles – and reading ability – that may be inaccessible to a large proportion of the population. Conversely, many of the more erotic images developed for use by the sections of the 'gay community' have been deemed by some to be too sexually explicit to learn from. And yet these images, once the moral condemnation has been removed, actually speak positively, to many people, in ways that are meaningful *for them*.

Many services appear to suggest that they are woman friendly, but it does not take too much imagination to see how they mean just certain women – especially those with children – and in ways that may totally exclude others. One simple example is to look at the name for many of the contraceptive service organizations: *Family* Planning, when most of their users are actively trying to avoid creating families!

Learning activity 11.5

Collect a sample of sexual health resources from a local PHCT, written specifically for women. Ask yourself some of the following questions:

Which groups of women are they directed towards?

◆ Age

◆ Family status

◆ Socioeconomic class

◆ Reading ability

◆ Sexual orientation/lifestyles/practices

◆ Ethnicity/language/culture.

Do the messages actively promote the benefits of sexual health, or are they reduced to disease prevention initiatives?

Which groups of people are present in the local population yet may feel excluded from accessing these materials/services?

'The trouble with men is . . .'

. . . threefold:

◆ Males are frequently treated stereotypically, as though 'all men are the same', with same needs, attitudes, behaviours and practices.

◆ Many men fail to make full use of the various self-help and health-promotion initiatives, which could maximize their health and wellbeing and prevent the development of disease.

◆ Many men leave health problems until it is too late; consequently, the treatment is either radical or unsuccessful.

Men's sexual health needs relate to gender, sexual orientation/identity and sexual practices. In the UK there are more men than women born each year, yet men have a shorter lifespan, consult their doctors less often, and have higher rates of admission to hospital, which is a widely accepted indicator of serious health problems (Lloyd 1996).

Gender-related sexual health problems may be linked to notions of sexual activity and performance, which include peer pressure and bullying from an early age (Douglas et al. 1997). As far as illnesses and disease are concerned, there is also a tendency among males, particularly young ones, to hold misinformed beliefs that 'nothing like that could *ever* happen to me'. Finally, many men are

generally assumed not to talk about health or their feelings and needs.

Notions of a machismo character, of competitive sexual prowess and fecundity (Bloor 1995) are compounded with related problems, such as fast cars and daredevil practices, which are ultimately indicative of risk perception and risk-taking activities. For example, young men form the highest group of people killed in road traffic accidents each year (Lloyd 1996). Alcohol, too, is a major contributor to the male persona. Men tend to consume more alcohol than women. In some this may boost their sexual bravado, giving them so-called 'Dutch courage', or, conversely, inhibit their libido and sexual performance. It may also lead to greater risk taking, as do certain recreational drugs.

There are significantly higher gender-related pathologies, too, such as cancers. It is estimated that in the UK some 70 000 men each year die of cancer (Lloyd 1996). The specifically sexual health-related tumours include:

◆ **testicular**: predominantly in the 20–34-year age group, with about 1400 new cases diagnosed each year

◆ **prostatic**: 9000 deaths recorded in 1994: six times higher than female deaths from cervical cancer

◆ **penis**: 400 new cases a year

◆ **bladder**

◆ **rectum**.

Another important factor for both men's and women's sexual health is that HIV infection is higher in men than in women, the current ratio being 7:1 (PHLS 1998). AIDS-related deaths are therefore also higher in men. HIV infection in the UK continues to affect gay, bisexual and other men who have sex with men disproportionately in relation to all other groups.

Added to this list would be cancers and other conditions that may indirectly affect sexual health, such as body-image pathologies and changes, physical disfigurement and performance-debilitating conditions, as well as their psychosocial implications. Some conditions that affect men's sexual health may also be related to the higher proportion of men injured in road traffic accidents, accidents at work, and traumas caused while on military service.

One aspect to affect men's psychological health in relation to sex has had media prominence since late 1998, owing to the availability of the anti-impotence drug Viagra. A service allied to the PHCT that has a definite role to play in impotence or sexual dysfunction, is the diabetic nurse and team. Nevertheless, we should not forget that there are other psychological issues that can be equally as traumatic as impotence, but which receive little serious attention from many men. These include the effects of low self-esteem, and victimization or bullying by other men.

In both sexes low self-esteem can perpetuate an unfulfilled craving for love, affection and attention (Grey 1993, King 1993, Evans 1997). In some, these feelings may increase their risk taking, especially in sexual practices, which may put them at risk from STDs, including HIV, or lead to ultimate despair and suicide. In young men, the latter increases annually. Anecdotal evidence also suggests that suicide among young people, in particular men, may be related to unhappiness about sexual orientation (for example when faced with societal pressure) (Davies and Neil 1997). There is definite evidence of a higher suicide rate in men who are HIV positive (Washer 1994).

Specific sexual health needs relating to sexual orientation may be affected by media representations of men. Whether in sitcoms such as the BBC's 'Men Behaving Badly', or in men's health magazines, the images are often directed to the under-40 heterosexual. Again, such a focus treats all males as an amorphous mass, with little individuality or alternative group identity, and with no real difference in potential health risks.

An examination of the sexual health focus of many PHC settings will reveal a lamentable lack of information readily available to men whose needs vary because of their sexual orientation, lifestyle, or physical and psychological abilities.

THE WAY AHEAD: LEARNING FROM MISTAKES

Throughout this chapter there has been an underlying emphasis on sexual health, clients' needs and service provision. First, this has included elements of needs analysis: the client's needs, as well as the need for adequately trained personnel and the provision of relevant health services and resources. From such an analysis it is possible to influence policy for education, service provision and resourcing. This is especially relevant with the ever-increasing role of the nurse, as in the PCGs and their new management structures.

Implementation may be by way of offering feedback on the quality and quantity of appropriate services; it may also include specifically targeted actions and resources to address the issues identified. Next comes reflection on the outcomes of service change or provision. This is one way of supporting the process of evaluation. Evaluation, as an ongoing reflective process, involves ensuring that the client's needs are appropriately assessed, met and regularly reviewed. Also, in this chapter there has been a focus on people who are frequently left out of the various 'general population' campaigns and services for sexual health (Field et al. 1997). It has been emphasized that there is no point in prejudging groups of people, such as 'women and children', 'men', 'the young', 'the old' etc., as this only leads to popular assumptions that everyone in the group will have identical needs. An example of a group which has been stereotyped is that of gay men.

Listening to the gay community

'One headline you won't see in the mass media:
"Safer sex works; gay men prove it".'
Canadian AIDS Society

Since the advent of HIV gay, bisexual and other men who have sex with men in numerous countries have taken the lead in sexual health promotion and disease prevention initiatives (Paglia 1990, Kippax et al. 1993), frequently against a background of hostility from governments, religions, the media, health professions and the general population (Sontag 1991, King 1993, Field et al. 1997). Yet despite this, the numerous resources mobilized to help gay men deal with this epidemic have shown that sexual health really does matter. The initiatives have also shown that we cannot address sexual health fully unless we take the 'sex' bit of it seriously.

Many of the printed materials on safer sex used by the various gay communities show a sexual explicitness not formerly seen in many health promotion campaigns. This has obviously led to a backlash from certain moral monopolists, who still believe theirs is the only way to educate people about sex. The lamentable state of affairs of teenage and unwanted pregnancies, and the numbers of preventable STDs and HIV in the UK, should be clear evidence against this. Yet there are two other significant outcomes of the use of erotica in safer sex messages. One is that it helps to depathologize the lives of people who are often discriminated against on the grounds of their sexual orientation and practices. It also sends the message that safer sex *is* a sexy alternative to risky behaviour.

Work carried out on social constructionist views of health education and promotion, as seen in Australia with Kippax et al. (1993) and in the UK with Project Sigma (King 1993), clearly shows how the whole sexual health movement and philosophy have a great deal to learn from elements of the gay community. To neglect or dismiss this learning will mean that the approach to sexual health in the UK will remain with the traditional behaviourist philosophies used to date. These are not always the most appropriate for client needs, carers' education or service provision.

Finally, there have been numerous examples of missed opportunities, or occasions where sexual health needs have not been adequately addressed. One final activity for this chapter includes a visit to a sexual health clinic. The aim of this is to explore the array of services that *may* be available locally. Many of the services in sexual health clinics can be relevant to the professionals identified in Figure 11.1, as collaboration between services is to receive increased emphasis in the future health of the nation.

Learning activity 11.6

Aim: to gather information and develop resources relevant to local client needs

Draw up a list of local services and resources, e.g. GU services, outreach facilities, voluntary and statutory organizations (you can do this by checking in the local telephone directories, the *National AIDS Manual* (often held in NHS Trusts and some public libraries) and/or some service user media, e.g. the weekly free gay papers, Well Woman clinic information sheets etc.

What are the different services offered by each organization? Which ones are unique? Which ones are duplicated or overlap?

How do they relate to your work and your clients?

Reflection point 11.3

In your journal, you may like to reflect on the following questions:

◆ How easy was it to find the services?

◆ If you were a service user, how accessible would they have been to you (conversely, what hindrances may prevent you from using them, e.g. distance, opening hours, level of appropriate privacy and confidentiality)?

◆ What sort of welcome and help were you given?

◆ What type of feelings might clients experience in accessing these services?

◆ As a professional enquirer (as opposed to a service user), how did your feelings differ from the ones you imagined clients may experience?

Many service users still find accessing some sexual health, GU or HIV services embarrassing and difficult to talk about. Try discussing your visits and personal reflections on them with a friend or colleague to whom you might not normally talk about such issues.

CONCLUSION

This chapter has explored aspects of sexual health which might not always be seen as the most usual topics in this area. The primary aim in this was to highlight the many people for whom, and the many ways in which, sexual health is not routinely addressed. Such failure means that the world of health care misses out on a significant part of a holistic therapeutic encounter.

The focus of this chapter is meant as a supplement to the many ways in which sexual health is regularly addressed in the primary care setting. Hopefully, it has encouraged the reader to explore the issues in more depth and breadth, and thus lead to a more holistic approach to the care and services they deliver.

RESOURCES AND ANNOTATED FURTHER READING

Education, Training and Consultancy in Sexual Health, 37 Kenilworth Gardens, Shooters Hill, London SE18 3JB. Tel: 020 8856 0234
e-mail: DTEvansSRN@aol.com

Project for Advice, Counselling and Education (PACE), 34 Hartham Road, London N7 9JL. Tel: 020 7700 1323
e-mail: pace@dircon.co.uk

The Terrence Higgins Trust, 52–54 Grays Inn Road, London WC1X 8JU.
Tel: 020 7831 0330

University of Hertfordshire (for diploma and degree courses in sexual health), Jon Whelan, Sexual Health Pathway Leader, Hatfield Campus, Hertfordshire AL10 9AB. Tel: 01707 285149
http://www.herts.ac.uk
e-mail:j.whelan@herts.ac.uk

Useful Internet sites: **http://www.**

Albert Kennedy Trust: akt.org.uk/
homeless, lesbian,
gay and bisexual
teenagers

AIDS Education and Trust Research	avert.org/
Black Liners: HIV charity/organization for black people	blink.org.uk/organ/ bliners.htm
Crusaid: HIV organization/charity	crusaid.org.uk
Deaf Queer: organization	deafqueer.org/
Gay and Lesbian Medical Association	glma.org/
Gay Men Fighting AIDS	gmfa.org.uk
Mental health and sexual health	mentalhelp.net/guide/
National AIDS Manual and British HIV Association, combined Website	aidsmap.com/index.htm
National AIDS Trust	nat.org.uk
National HIV Prevention Information Service (part of the UK's HEA)	hea.org.uk/nhpis
Outrage!: political lobby group	outrage.cygnet.co.uk /eqrights.htm
Sexual health/HIV Internet information service and resources	thebody.com/ index.html
Sexual health for teenage girls having heterosexual sex	open.gov.uk/ womens-uni/factsheet /2teen.htm
Pink Practice: gay, lesbian and bisexual counselling services and support	pinkpractice.co.uk /central.htm
Stonewall: gay, lesbian and bisexual people's political lobby group	stonewall.org.uk

The Terrence Higgins tht.org.uk
Trust, London

United Nations (AIDS) unaids.org/
organization

FURTHER READING

Bor R, Watts M 1993 Talking to patients about sexual matters. British Journal of Nursing 2(13): 657–661

This article effectively explores the reasons why the sex aspects of life ought to be addressed in the health-care setting. It also examines ways in which to go about it.

Caulfield H, Platzer H 1998 Next of kin. Nursing Standard 7(13): 47–49

Department of Health 1996 Guidelines for pre-test discussion on HIV testing. DoH, London

Department of Health 1998 Our healthier nation: a contract for health. Consultation paper. DoH, London

ENB (1994) Caring for people with sexually transmitted diseases, including HIV disease. English National Board, London

This pack is a distance learning resource which is contemporary and relevant. Each section has some 'offprints' related to the subject under study, as well as informative 'further reading' lists.

ENB (1994) Sexual health education and training – guidelines for good practice in the teaching of nurses, midwives and health visitors. English National Board, London

This booklet contains educationally sound principles for implementing learning, such as that gained from the ENB (1994 above), to a wider audience.

Few C, Hicken I, Butterworth T 1996 Partnerships in sexual health and sex education. University of Manchester, Manchester

Few C, Hicken I, Butterworth T 1996 Principles and practices of sexual health and sex education in schools. University of Manchester, Manchester

Grey, A 1993 Speaking of sex. The limits of language. Cassell, London.

This text will make the reader stop and question every utterance they make on sex! It shows ways in which sex and sexuality has been constructed by so-called 'pillars' of society. This reveals a societal approach to sex and sexuality which favours certain people, to the detriment of many others. The book looks at sex and law, politics, religion and health care. It also examines attitudes towards the sexuality of children, as well as challenging the reader to improve the status quo for the third millennium.

King E 1993 Safety in numbers: safer sex for gay men. Cassell, London

This book is for anyone interested in the ways institutionalized prejudices, especially homophobia, have led to gross failures in effective HIV prevention. It would profitably be 'compulsory reading' for anyone having to work with HIV-positive people, as well as for those teaching on the wider issues of sex, safer sex and sexuality.

Palmer H 1998 Exploring sexuality and sexual health in nursing. Professional Nurse 14(1): 15–20

REFERENCES

Antrobus S 1999 Community care services: the future framework. NT Learning Curve 2(11): 7–8

Berkowitz R, Callen M 1983 How to have sex in an epidemic: one approach. Cited in: King E 1993 Safety in numbers: safer sex for gay men. Cassell, London

Bor R, Watts M 1993 Talking to patients about sexual matters. British Journal of Nursing 2 (13): 657–661

Bloor M 1995 The sociology of HIV transmission. Sage Publications, London

Chalmers H A 1994 Nurse education – teaching about HIV infection and AIDS. AVERT (Aids Education and Research Trust), West Sussex

Cattacin S 1998 From risk to normalisation. Western European politics to fight HIV/AIDS. In: AIDS in Europe: Working Papers for Synthesis Sessions, 2nd European Conference on the Methods and Results of Social and Behavioural Research on AIDS, 12–15 January 1998, Paris

Davies D, Neal C (eds) 1997 Pink therapy – a guide for counsellors and therapists working with lesbian, gay and bisexual clients. Open University Press, Buckingham

Department of Health 1992 The health of the nation. DoH, London

Department of Health 1993 The health of the nation key area handbook: HIV/AIDS and sexual health. DoH, London

Douglas N, Warwick I, Kemp S, Whitty G 1997 Playing it safe: responses of secondary school teachers to lesbian, gay and bisexual pupils, bullying, HIV and AIDS education and Section 28. Institute of Education, University of London, London

Evans D T 1997 The psychic shadows of HIV and AIDS and the role of social representations in post-registration nurse education. MPhil Thesis (Unpublished), University of Wales

Field B, Wellings K, McVey D 1997 Promoting safer sex – a history of the Health Education Authority's mass media campaigns on HIV, AIDS and sexual health 1987–1996. HEA, London

Flaskerud J H, Ungvarski P J 1992 HIV/AIDS: a guide to nursing care, 2nd edn. W B Saunders, Philadelphia

Foucault M 1990 The history of sexuality – an introduction. Translated from the French by Robert Hurley. Penguin, London

Grey A 1993 Speaking of sex: the limits of language. Cassell, London

Heller T 1998 'Snowballs and acorns: medicine by impact'. In: Allott M, Robb M (eds) Understanding health and social care – an introductory reader. Sage Publications, London, pp 48–55

Howe J 1995 A natural remedy: giving patients permission to masturbate. Nursing Standard 9 (29): 46–47

James T, Harding I, Corbett K 1994 Biased Care? Lesbians and gay men. Nursing Times 90 (51): 29–31

Jones L J 1998 Evaluating market principles in health care. In: Allott M, Robb M (eds) Understanding health and social care – an introductory reader. Sage Publications, London, pp 295–301

King E 1993 Safety in numbers: safer sex for gay men. Cassell, London

Kippax S, Connell R W, Dowsett G W, Crawford J 1993 Social aspects of AIDS. Sustaining safer sex: gay communities respond to AIDS. Falmer Press, London

Lloyd T 1996 Men's health review. Royal College of Nursing, London

McFarlane L 1998 Diagnosis: homophobic – the experiences of lesbians, gay men and bisexuals in mental health services. PACE (Project for Advice, Counselling and Education), London

McHaffie H E 1993 The care of patients with HIV and AIDS: a survey of nurse education in the UK. Institute of Medical Ethics, University of Edinburgh, Edinburgh

Naidoo J, Wills J 1994 Health promotion: foundations for practice. Baillière Tindall, London

Noël G, McGarrigle C A, Donda N D, Sinka K 1998 UK HIV testing policy: results, changes, and challenges – will normalisation of HIV testing weaken, rather than strengthen, primary prevention? In: AIDS in Europe: Working Papers for Synthesis Sessions, 2nd European Conference on the Methods and Results of Social and Behavioural Research on AIDS, 12–15 January 1998, Paris

O'Hanlan K O, Cabaj R P, Schatz B, Lock J, Nemrow P 1997 A review of the medical consequences of homophobia with suggestions for resolution. Journal of the Gay and Lesbian Medical Association 1(1): 25–40

Paglia C 1990 Sexual personae: art and decadence from Nefertiti to Emily Dickinson. Yale University Press, New Haven

PHLS 1998 Communicable diseases report September 1998. Public Health Laboratory Service, London

Polansky J S, Karasic D H, Speier P L, Hastik K, Haller E 1997 Homophobia: therapeutic and training considerations for psychiatry. Journal of the Gay and Lesbian Medical Association 1 (1): 41–48

Rose L 1994 Homophobia among doctors. British Medical Journal 308: 586–587

Savage B 1998 Sex education for nurses. Professional Nurse 14(1): 5–6

Shernoff M 1991 Designing effective AIDS prevention workshops for gay and bisexual men. Cited in: King E 1993 Safety in numbers: safer sex for gay men. Cassell, London

Sontag S 1991 Illness as metaphor/AIDS as metaphor. Penguin, London

Steffen M 1998 The normalisation of AIDS policies in Europe: phases, levels, perspectives. In: AIDS in Europe: Working Papers for Synthesis Sessions, 2nd European Conference on the Methods and Results of Social and Behavioural Research on AIDS, 12–15 January 1998, Paris

Ussher J M, Baker C D (eds) 1993 Psychological perspectives on sexual problems. New directions in theory and practice. Routledge, London

Washer P 1994 Gay men, suicide and AIDS: autonomous choices at the end of life? MA Dissertation (unpublished), King's College, London

Wellings K, Field J, Johnson A M, Wadsworth J 1994 Sexual behaviour in Britain. The national survey of sexual attitudes and lifestyles. Penguin, London

Weston A 1994 'Sapphic sickness': A study of the health care experiences of women patients who disclose their sexual identity as lesbian. MSc dissertation (unpublished), Brunel University

The process: acute care

12

Sue McAndrew

'He questioned so calmly and easily about every aspect of my sexual development and my life that I gradually found myself talking with almost equal ease.' (Carl Rogers 1990 'Speaking Personally')

KEY ISSUES/CONCEPTS

◆ What is sexual health?

◆ The effects of acute illness and treatments on human sexuality

◆ Checking your own attitudes, values and beliefs with regard to sexuality and sexual health

◆ The process of taking a sexual history

◆ Planning and implementing appropriate interventions

◆ Assessing where you are as a practitioner with regard to sexual health

OVERVIEW

Chapter 12, *The process: acute care*, sets the scene by considering what currently happens with regard to a client's sexual health in an acute care setting, and why change should occur. It focuses on the practical aspects of sexual history taking before moving on to consider the range of options available.

INTRODUCTION

Acute illness and treatments often have a profound effect on a person's sexuality, which unfortunately health-care professionals may fail to recognize or even acknowledge. In order to address this particular deficit health-care professionals need to consider what sexual health is, what they know in relation to how acute illness and treatment affects a client's sexuality, and how their attitudes, values and beliefs on sexuality and sexual health affect the health care they provide.

The literature to date (Webb 1985, Savage 1995) demonstrates a reluctance on the part of health-care professionals to become involved in the process of taking a sexual history. For some this may be the result of not knowing how to introduce the topic of sexual health, not being sufficiently perceptive in picking up on cues that the client gives during the general assessment process, and avoiding pertinent areas for exploration. Avoiding taking a sexual health history, either deliberately or unintentionally, leads to missed opportunities for sexual health promotion, education and/or advice. The challenge facing the practitioner is to deal with any avoidance strategy in order to provide truly holistic care, of which sexual health is an integral part.

SEXUALITY AND ACUTE ILLNESS

Setting the scene

Health care at a very basic level concerns itself with wellbeing. When health is affected, resulting in ill health, it becomes the responsibility of health-care professionals to aid the person to return to a state of wellbeing. Unfortunately, when ill health occurs it is not as a rule compartmentalized to one specific part of the body; instead, it has a tendency towards the domino effect, causing other aspects of health to suffer, e.g. the common cold may cause tiredness and lethargy; appendicectomy may in the short term create a lack of confidence to do the things taken for granted before the operation; depression may lead to social isolation. If our responsibility as health-care professionals is to aid the process of recovery when ill health occurs, then, when assessing the effects of illness, account needs to be taken of the broader effects of the illness and how it is affecting the person's life.

It has been well documented (Hawton 1985, Bancroft 1989) that acute illness affects people's sexual health. However, it is often difficult to distinguish whether sexual health is disrupted by the physical illness, or whether it arises from the person's psychological reaction to the illness. An example of this could be a client who is admitted to hospital having had a myocardial infarction (MI). Several researchers (Wabrek and Burchell 1980, Sjorgen and Fugl-Meyer 1983) have noted a decrease in sexual activity following MI. This may be the result of circulatory problems and/or the prescription of diuretics and antihypertensive agents (both of which are known to cause impotence and ejaculatory problems in men). However, it may also be the result of fear, owing to the client's belief that the excitement resulting from sexual activity will cause a further MI or even death. If the client's partner shares this opinion then the belief will be reinforced. However if the partner does not share this belief, then a decrease in sexual activity may lead to frustration within the relationship.

Table 12.1 offers a brief synopsis of how some of the more common acute illnesses affect sexuality. It is also important to remember that not only illness, but also treatment, can impinge on sexual wellbeing, e.g. phenothiazines may cause retrograde ejaculation; radium therapy may cause body scarring, which may leave the person feeling unattractive; surgery may also create an undesirable body image and/or directly affect sexual ability (prostatectomy is a common cause of retrograde ejaculation).

Table 12.1 The effects of different types of acute illness on sexuality

Cardiovascular system	Circulatory problems, heart attack	Erectile dysfunction Fear may cause loss of interest in sex
Respiratory system	Bronchitis, asthma, pneumonia	Ability to participate in and enjoy sexual activity may be impaired
Endocrine system	Diabetes, Addison's disease, menopause	Erectile dysfunction, impaired or loss of sexual interest, vaginal dryness
Genitourinary system	Prostatitis, HIV, pelvic inflammatory disease	Painful ejaculation, painful intercourse Fear may cause suppression of sexuality
Surgery leading to altered body image	Colostomy, rectal resection, mastectomy, skin grafts	Embarrassment about engaging in sexual activity, erectile dysfunction
Musculoskeletal system	Arthritis	Impaired sexual activity and interest owing to pain and fatigue
Neurological	Brain lesions, strokes	May have impaired sexual interest, ejaculatory problems
Mental health	Depression, manic illness	Loss of interest, problems with sex, disinhibited sexual behaviour
Renal system	Renal failure, dialysis	Impaired sexual interest

Because of the complexity of sexual problems that arise through acute illness it is very important that health-care professionals should be vigilant during assessment and take account of both the physical and the psychological state of the person. It is very useful to establish at the earliest opportunity what feelings the client has about his or her illness, and, if they are in a relationship, what are their perceptions regarding their partner's feelings towards the illness.

Sexuality and sexual behaviour are not confined to the young and attractive, and therefore in terms of health care should be an integral part of care provision. It is also pertinent for practitioners to think wider than their own preferences (homosexuality, heterosexuality, celibacy), as it is easy to make assumptions based on one's own values and beliefs, and thus deny the client full understanding of the difficulties that face them. Unfortunately, research (Webb 1985, Waterhouse and Metcalf 1991) shows that health-care professionals are extremely poor at addressing clients' sexual health needs. The challenge is that their area of practice will almost certainly encompass clients whose illness and/or treatment will impinge on their sexual health needs.

THE PROCESS OF TAKING A SEXUAL HISTORY

In the beginning

In recent years nursing literature has promoted the notion of holism with regard to client care, but this will be achieved only if all aspects of the client's life are taken into account, including their sexuality. Much of the documentation used as part of a nursing model acknowledges sexuality, but practitioners employing the model often fail to use this part of the documentation effectively. For example, in areas where they use the Roper, Logan and Tierney model the box marked sexuality will often include comments such as: wears false teeth; wears make-up; married. This is a technique on the part of the practitioner to avoid asking about sensitive areas of the client's life, but without this knowledge truly holistic care cannot be offered.

Reflection point 12.1

- ◆ Consider for a moment any nursing model that you have used.
- ◆ Did it include sexuality and/or sexual health?
- ◆ What did you write in response to that?

Taking a sexual history should therefore be an integral part of the assessment process, as it will enable a clearer understanding of the client in the context of his or her current situation, and this will in turn facilitate accurate care planning that will meet the client's needs. Although sexuality is seen as fundamental to holism, obtaining knowledge about the client's sexual health is not easy as it requires a great deal of thought and sensitivity coupled with good use of interpersonal skills. Because sexuality is expressed through a whole spectrum of behaviours, and these will vary greatly from person to person, taking and interpreting a sexual history can be very complex. These complexities arise from two human beings (client and practitioner), both of whom bring their own values, attitudes and beliefs to the assessment, trying to find common ground and language for this neglected and unfamiliar area of health. Because of this, before reaching the point of taking a sexual history it is important for practitioners to have the opportunity to obtain a clearer understanding of what sexual health means to them personally. It is hoped that this will facilitate a better understanding of its relevance to client care. Learning activity 12.1 is designed to trigger this process.

Despite the move towards holistic care, literature (Hawton 1985, Gillan 1987) related to sexual health care does not offer a blueprint for taking a sexual history. The starting point for taking a sexual history might be considering why you need such information.

As previously suggested, if clients are to be offered holistic care then addressing sexual health needs is fundamental. Most illnesses and/or treatment will impinge on a person's sexual health,

Learning activity 12.1

Identify how clients' sexual health needs are currently recognized in the health-care setting in which you work. List the common words and phrases used in relation to clients' sexuality and their sexual health needs. This can now be put to one side.

Write down 8–12 words which you feel describe and are important to your own sexuality. If you are doing this exercise as part of a group you could now do 'rounds', each person in the group sharing one of their words or phrases at a time until everyone has shared all the words/phrases that they feel able to. These words can be listed as they are shared and then grouped accordingly, e.g. you may wish to group all the words related to appearance, all those related to relationships, and all those related to sexual activity.

The final part of the exercise involves comparing the two lists: the one used professionally for clients and the one used personally. Discuss the similarities and the differences, and explore why these occur.

Reflection point 12.2

Think of six people that you have looked after in the past 2 weeks and write down their diagnoses and treatments. For each one, brainstorm the areas of their lives in which the illness may have had a knock-on effect. Now try to assess how, in the wider context of that illness, their sexual health might have been affected.

and for that reason alone health-care professionals should be vigilant about giving clients the opportunity to express any concerns they might have.

Creating this opportunity by broaching the subject of sexual health, thereby demonstrating a willingness to discuss such important issues, is the first stage of taking a sexual history, but this will only be achieved if you feel confident about discussing such issues with the client. As research (Webb 1985, Savage 1995) demonstrates, a large proportion of nurses do not feel confident in asking questions related to a client's sexual health, and one of the major reasons for this is a lack of knowledge and understanding of how illness affects sexuality. Although this cannot be put right in one chapter of a book, the examples in Table 12.1 highlight how illness can affect a person's sexuality.

Many practitioners who lack confidence in this area will often rationalize their decision not to broach the subject by saying that if the client wishes to discuss it they will approach the practitioner. This is a myth. Because of the power imbalance implicit in the practitioner–client relationship – the practitioner being powerful whereas the client, in unfamiliar surroundings and in a state of vulnerability, is disempowered – waiting to see if the client mentions it sends out a covert message that the subject is not important and therefore not to be discussed in this situation.

In order to promote good practice health professionals need to be mindful of their power and to develop the skill of using it positively and effectively. With regard to sexual health this means acknowledging that it is their responsibility to open up communication that will facilitate a client's exploration of how their illness may impinge on their sexuality. However, this needs to be done sensitively, and before embarking on such a process the following points should be considered.

◆ All assessments that involve gathering personal information should be carried out in private. In this instance this means that the informant feels that they are in a safe environment, that any information given or received cannot be overheard, and that what is said is confidential. Whenever questions are being asked of clients it is a good idea to offer a rationale for why they are being asked, i.e. what relationship the questions have to their illness and/or their treatment.

◆ Timing is essential. During the initial interview, where personal issues are being discussed, it is important for the practitioner to raise the issue of sexual health. This gives the client the opportunity to ask any questions they might have and, perhaps more importantly, demonstrates that there is a willingness to talk about such issues. It is important to take note of the client's non-verbal communication, e.g. do they appear anxious? Do they respond verbally by saying that everything is fine but at the same time avoid eye contact? These cues may tell you that the person is not ready to discuss their sexual health at the present time, but as you have opened up these specific lines of communication it may well be appropriate to return to the subject at a later date.

◆ Be aware of your own verbal and non-verbal communication. Are you relaxed, giving eye contact, sitting at an appropriate distance, i.e. a distance at which the person can be heard without having to raise their voice, and presenting yourself in a non-threatening manner? Are you using the right tone of voice, and are your questions direct, understandable and open, thus allowing the client the opportunity to explore their own feelings? It is important to listen to what the client is saying so that you can gain a good understanding of their situation. It is also important to use the right language, i.e. words and phrases the client will understand and with which you will feel comfortable.

◆ Know your limitations and do not be frightened of telling the client what they are. Remember, if you are going to establish a trusting relationship there must be honesty between you and the client from the outset.

What this initial process is seeking to achieve is to open up lines of communication between yourself and the client, which will give clarity and understanding to your relationship and which in turn will enable you to give holistic care. With these points in mind it might be useful now to move on and give some thought to how you would introduce the topic of sexual health to the client.

Learning activity 12.2

Give some thought to ways in which you would feel comfortable introducing the topic of sexual health to a client.

Write out what you might say, e.g. I would now like to ask you some questions about your sexual health, as having an operation/medical problem/treatment often causes people to worry about how they will look/feel/perform, and how we look/feel/perform is very important to our sexual wellbeing. What are your thoughts about this?

In this example a statement has been made which has enabled communication specifically related to sexual health to be opened up; it demonstrates to the client that the practitioner is willing to discuss any concerns they have; it offers a rationale with regard to the importance of sexual health needs in relation to the rest of their health; and it leaves the client free to think about and hopefully explore the implications of either their illness and/or their treatment on their sexual health.

Once you have written out your introduction to the topic say it out loud to yourself a few times until you have found the words you feel comfortable with. These may need further refining when you are face to face with different clients, as both people and situations vary greatly. Once you feel comfortable with what you have written, find a colleague or a number of colleagues and ask them if you can try your introduction out on them; all you want in return is their honest feedback regarding:

◆ What were you actually asking? (Does their answer match up with what you thought you were asking?)

◆ Why were you asking the question? (Was your rationale clear?)

◆ What psychological message did your statement convey?

◆ Would they have been inclined to respond? What is the reason for this answer?

◆ How intrusive did it feel? (As well as asking this question, you might like to ask your colleague to rate the level of intrusiveness on a 0–10 scale, 0 being not intrusive at all and 10 being extremely intrusive.)

After obtaining their feedback you might wish to further modify what you had written.

EXPLORING ATTITUDES, VALUES AND BELIEFS

When those working in acute care settings are asked why they fail to address sexuality with clients a variety of reasons are presented: 'The client is not in hospital long enough'; 'It would be too embarrassing for the client'; 'Most people do not believe it to be important when they are acutely ill'; 'The doctors deal with that sort of thing'.

Reflection point 12.3

Challenge yourself by asking the following questions:

◆ Why have you or do you avoid asking clients about their sexuality?

◆ What is your level of embarrassment if and when faced with raising the issue of sexual health?

◆ How many times have you asked a client to prioritize issues related to their sexual health when they are acutely ill?

◆ Identify occasions when you have found it easier to pass the buck.

◆ What have you discussed with medical staff as regards addressing the sexual health needs of clients?

In answering these questions honestly, you may open up a way of exploring your own attitudes, values and beliefs in relation to sexuality.

Learning activity 12.3

This is a group exercise which would benefit from being facilitated. Set up a short debate, which may make use of literature but which will also be very dependent on 'gut' reactions.

Motion: This house believes that it is the practitioner's responsibility to concern him or herself with meeting the client's sexual health needs in the acute care setting.

The group should be split into two equal halves, one speaking for the motion, one against.

Preparation time of 10 minutes should be given, followed by 5 minutes for the first group to present their arguments and 5 minutes for the second group to present their opposing views.

Questions from one group to the other may then be raised and discussed; this should go on for no longer than 10 minutes. The debate can then be drawn to a close by the facilitator asking if anyone had changed their view as a result of what they had heard.

The facilitator could chair the debate and, during the process, note down the main points raised. These could then form the basis of a post-debate discussion exploring the attitudes, values and beliefs of those participating.

PICKING UP ON CUES

Talking about sexuality and sexual health problems can be difficult and embarrassing for both the client and the practitioner. It is hoped that as the practitioner gains knowledge and understanding as to the importance of sexual health in relation to being able to offer holistic care, and as he or she becomes more skilled in taking a sexual history, much of their embarrassment will be alleviated. However, the client may never have had this channel of communication opened up to them before, and may initially succumb to their embarrassment and try to avoid the topic. It is because of this that the practitioner needs to become skilled at picking up on both the verbal and non-verbal cues. It is these, plus the general history taken from the client, that will enable the practitioner to enhance the level of communication and understanding between themselves and the client.

Case study 12.1

Consider the following scenario and then try and answer the questions as fully as you are able.

Anne is a 46-year-old woman who has been admitted for a lumpectomy. Anne was divorced 4 years ago but has been living with her present partner for the past 2 years. Her partner John is 42 years old and runs a successful small business. Prior to meeting John Anne worked quite successfully as an independent finance adviser, but chose to give up her career when she moved away from her home to live with John. Anne has no children but enjoys a good relationship with John's 17-year-old daughter from a previous relationship, who spends most weekends with them. During the assessment process you notice that Anne appears anxious and admits to feeling somewhat worried about the operation. When you explore this further you discover that her main worries concern the fact that she is having a 'wedge cut out of her breast', and the prospect of having a 'general anaesthetic'. When you move on in your assessment to ask Anne about her sexual health there is an initial few seconds' silence; she then turns her head away and she just laughs, saying 'Chance would be a fine thing!' and 'There is plenty of time to worry about that later'. Anne then asks when she will be going to theatre and will John be allowed to come in and see her before she is properly awake from the anaesthetic?

What, from Anne's general history, might you pick up on when trying to establish how her illness may impinge on her sexuality?

How would you interpret Anne's willingness to discuss her sexual health?

Would you have pursued the subject of her sexual health at this point?

What is your rationale for your answer to the above question?

Would you pursue the subject of Anne's sexual health at any other time?

If your answer to the above question is yes, when would you pursue it and what questions do you feel would be important to ask?

If your answer was no, state your reasons for not pursuing it, both in relation to Anne and in relation to yourself as a practitioner.

Again, this exercise would be useful if carried out by a group, as the answers could form the basis for discussion and self-exploration.

THE ACTUAL HISTORY TAKING

As previously stated, there is no blueprint for taking a sexual history. There is, however, a range of questionnaires/assessment protocols available that can be used to aid the process. These range from collecting very broad, limited and superficial information to those that provide very detailed, in-depth and focused information.

If a specific sexual health problem is identified then there are models of sexual history taking that have a specific focus (Hawton 1985, Rust and Golombek 1986, Rust et al. 1986). Although these are used primarily in clinics where people are referred specifically for sexual and/or relationship problems, it may be useful to consider some of the questions asked and areas covered as a means of informing your preliminary enquiries. The following should be used only as a guide.

◆ What does the client feel about their illness?
◆ If the client is in a relationship, what perceptions do they have regarding how their partner feels about their illness?
◆ How would they describe their general relationship with their partner?
◆ How would they describe their sexual relationship with their partner?
◆ How does the client see him or herself in terms of attractiveness?
◆ Does the client have any other physical or mental health problems that affect their sexual health?
◆ How important is their sexuality to them? And to their relationship?
◆ What are the client's cultural beliefs?
◆ What are the client's religious beliefs?

◆ What prescribed and non-prescribed drugs does the client take?
◆ What is the client's usual alcohol intake?

Perhaps one of the most useful and simplistic frameworks for taking a sexual history is that identified by Hawton (1985), that is, looking at the precipitants, maintaining factors and predisposing factors.

To ascertain the precipitants the question that needs to be asked is, when exactly did this problem start? For example, why was sex OK in June but not in July? What happened in the client's life during that time? It is useful to pursue this question of precipitating factors as it is not always the obvious that has initiated the problem. My own experience in working with clients has been that precipitants can include such life occurrences as redundancy, retirement, childbirth, bereavement and short-term hospitalization of a partner, child or parent.

When possible causal factors have been identified, consideration then needs to be given to what has contributed to the problem continuing? What stopped it from being resolved? It might be that the client has been afraid to talk to a partner about the problem; they may feel resentment towards someone; or they could be grieving for a significant loss.

Lastly, the predisposing factors need to be considered. Why has it affected this particular person in this particular way? e.g. why has Mr Brown stopped having sexual intercourse following his heart operation when Mr Smith has continued with his sexual relationship? What are Mr Brown's beliefs about heart operations? What are his beliefs relating to sexuality and his age? What meaning has his illness in spiritual terms? How open, honest and trusting is his relationship with his partner?

Learning activity 12.4

Think of two or three friends, colleagues and/or clients who have been in a similar predicament. Try to identify the precipitating factors, the maintaining factors and the predisposing factors.

When a person's sexual health is affected it is important to remember that there is a strong likelihood that not only will it affect them physically, it will also affect them psychologically, and as a practitioner offering holistic care you must address both. Taking a sexual history can act as a screening process, i.e. during this process you may detect a previously undetected physical problem, such as diabetes. In order to take a sexual history effectively, it is important to develop the necessary skills.

Skill development

'It ain't what you do, it's the way that you do it', and sexual history taking is no exception. In previous chapters your awareness was drawn to the importance of good interpersonal skills when asking people about their sexual health. The skills that have particular relevance when initiating the process of taking a sexual history include:

◆ building a trusting relationship which offers the client a feeling of safety
◆ being able to demonstrate sensitivity
◆ responding appropriately
◆ listening to the client and being able to put into context what has been said
◆ the use of open and closed questions
◆ sharing a common language with which both you and the client feel comfortable
◆ observing for congruent and/or incongruent verbal and non-verbal communication
◆ knowing yourself, i.e. having an awareness of your own sexuality.

Case study 12.2

The following will enable you to explore a person's sexual history using your interpersonal skills and taking account of your attitudes, values and beliefs.

Dan Baker is 46 years old and was recently admitted for coronary heart disease. He is currently being treated on a number of drugs, which include an antihypertensive. Dan has been on a similar drug regimen for the past 2 years but 'never felt happy at having to take them'. Since starting on the medication 2 years ago Dan has had difficulty in achieving and maintaining an erection, but has not told anyone about this. As Dan's named nurse, how would you start asking him about his sexual health?

When you ask Dan if he is in a relationship he tells you that he has been married for 25 years: he then looks down at the ground as he tells you, in a low voice, that his marriage is OK. How would you explore this further?

Dan goes on to say that he and his wife have very separate lives these days: both have jobs that involve shiftwork, and they have no interests in common. He says that since the youngest of their two daughters left home to go to college last year, their relationship seems to have become more distant. When you go on to explore what Dan means by 'distant', he says that they are not together much, although he does confess to their having a very busy social life together at the weekends.

How might you use this information to challenge Dan further?

It now becomes apparent that what Dan really means by 'distant' is that for the past 18 months his wife has showed no interest in their sexual relationship, and for 2 years before that they had sexual intercourse only on a very irregular basis (less than once a week).

What might you explore with Dan at this point?

Stop now and consider:

♦ *What was your immediate response to reading this last statement?*
♦ *Where has that response come from?*
♦ *What are your own beliefs regarding sex on a regular basis?*
♦ *Is there a disparity in your beliefs about regularity of sex for yourself and for Dan?*
♦ *If so, what influences that?*
♦ *How might you respond to this statement if you had (a) responded immediately; (b) responded after doing this brief self-exploration?*

Dan eventually admits that 20 months ago he had the 'full works' with a prostitute, which he describes, in a very quiet voice, as enjoyable. Dan says that he does feel a bit guilty about

this, and jokes that perhaps being on these tablets for the rest of his life is his punishment!

What is your gut reaction to the last piece of information?

How has it affected your perception of Dan's problem?

What other information might be useful if you are to offer Dan some constructive help?

Planning and implementation of sexual health care

If during the assessment process it becomes apparent that a client does have concerns about their sexual health, the practitioner needs to clarify what help, if any, they would like. You should avoid assuming that, because a client has discussed and/or identified a problem, they will automatically wish for help to resolve it: speaking about it may be all they wish to do. However, they may need help in one of the following ways.

More time to explore the problem

This might be with yourself, given that the client may feel that they can trust you and may be relieved that you have given them the opportunity to talk about their sexual health. Time in acute care settings can be limited, and even if this is not the reality clients often believe that they do not have the right to monopolize the practitioner's time. Practitioners themselves may have a sense of being seen by colleagues as 'just talking to clients', rather than doing the 'important work'. Being mindful of these pressures, it may well be beneficial to both client and practitioner to arrange a time when you can explore the problem further. However, it is important to remember that if such an arrangement is made it should be carried through.

After raising the issue of sexual health with the client it might become obvious during your conversation that you do not have sufficient knowledge to help. If this is the case then you should explain your limitations to the client, at the same time offering the option of more time with someone who does have the right level of knowledge and who would be willing to give them quality time.

Reassurance from a significant person

The client may simply be looking for reassurance from a significant person, e.g. a nurse, doctor or partner. The practitioner should in this instance clarify exactly who the client wants reassurance from. If it is the practitioner, then the practitioner must be able to give the appropriate reassurance, i.e. they must have the appropriate knowledge and understanding. There is very little value in telling a woman who has had a lumpectomy that 'lots of women feel the way she feels' and that 'in a couple of months she will be back to normal and her partner will not even notice the scar'. These are platitudes, not reassurances! It would be more reassuring to offer an honest description of what her breast may look like, and what is available to enhance its appearance postoperatively.

If, however, the client is seeking reassurance from a partner then the practitioner may need to work with the client to enable them to meet this need. Often clients want reassurance from a partner but are frightened to seek it. This needs to be dealt with sensitively and the practitioner should be mindful that partner reassurance should only be sought when the client feels ready and able to do so. Do not set yourself up as an intermediary by volunteering to speak to the partner yourself, as you might not like what they say and you are then left with the dilemma of how to explain it to the client. Equally, no matter how much you think that discussion with the partner will relieve some of the client's tension, you have no right to force the matter: always respect that the client knows him or herself best.

Education: what effects and long-term consequences will the illness have?

Again this needs to be undertaken by someone who has the appropriate knowledge and understanding of both the illness and/or treatment and its effects on the client's sexual health. It is also important to remember that both the physical and the psychological effects need to be taken into account. For example, if a client is diagnosed as having arthritis the physical aspects of stiff joints and pain need to be considered, as do the psychological effects of pain, such as fatigue and low self-esteem. The client may need educating about different positions which are more appropriate for sexual activity if joints are stiff and painful, and they may need advice about which times of the day sexual activity would be more acceptable, given that they may be tired at certain times. Such advice may enable the person to continue to enjoy being sexually active, and thereby raise their self-esteem.

If this level of education is difficult in your area of work then remember that there are a lot of good books on the market which are directed at the client. Having books available in your area of practice might be useful. If recommending books it is important that prior to choosing them someone who has knowledge and understanding of sexual health should critically review them. It is also important to remember that clients may still wish to check out what they have read.

Professional advice, e.g. where to go for more expert help

It might be that as a practitioner who has personal/professional and/or external limitations, what you can most appropriately do is act as a resource person for the client, directing them to the right sort of support and help.

Sex therapy/brief counselling

This should only be offered by those who are appropriately educated and trained. Sex therapy is normally based on behavioural techniques, and although the details are widely published in books and magazines it is often the presence of a skilled therapist that enables the clients (often if people are in a relationship then both are encouraged to attend) to use the therapy appropriately. The therapy also often involves brief counselling, which may be the added vital dimension to its success.

Reflection point 12.4

Think about yourself as a practitioner having a responsibility to meet the sexual health needs of your clients in the acute care setting. Carry out a SWOT (strengths, weaknesses, opportunities and threats) analysis based on your thoughts. From this, develop an action plan for yourself which clearly identifies your own needs with regard to improving your practice. Try to establish how your needs might be met both within and outside the organization you work for. Try to write specific objectives for yourself, and put a time limit on when you would like to achieve each of them.

CONCLUSION

Sexual history taking is a challenging but essential contribution to holistic health care. Without it clients experience a reduced service and nurses do not fulfil their professional role. Opportunities for sexual health promotion can be enhanced by appropriate interview and examination skills, and can provide the high-quality service clients deserve.

While acknowledging that it is not easy for nurses to engage in this activity, the more knowledge and experience they can gain in practice will contribute to the development of clinical competence and confidence.

In the same way that nurses can pick up the cues given out by clients, it is important to remember that clients can also pick up cues from health-care professionals and avoid presenting their prime health concerns. To complete the circle of care, clients deserve caring, competent and confident practitioners who can assess their needs and implement appropriate care strategies.

RESOURCES AND ANNOTATED FURTHER READING

Association of Marital and Sex Therapists, PO Box 62, Sheffield S10 3TS

Run courses in dealing with marital and psycho-sexual difficulties. Also keep up-to-date list of therapists.

English National Board for Health Visiting, Midwifery and Nursing, ENB Careers, P O Box 2EN, London W1A 2EN
Sexual Health Courses: N87, N90

Skrine R L (ed) 1989 Introduction to psychosexual medicine. Montana Press, Carllisla

Describes one method of helping patients overcome sexual problems. It is readable and offers an attitude towards patients which is necessary if therapy is to be effective.

Bancroft J 1989. Human sexuality and its problems. Churchill Livingstone, Edinburgh

An excellent classic text that provides information on the physiology, anatomy, psychology and sociology of sexuality. It offers a whole chapter on the assessment of sexual problems and takes account of newer investigative methods and up-to-date developments.

Yaffe M, Fenwick E 1986 Sexual happiness for men. Dorling Kindersley, London

An easy book to read, with much of the text being supported by diagrams. Useful for both clients and practitioners.

Zilbergeld B 1980 Men and sex. Fontana, London
Raises and discusses many problems men may encounter through their sexual lives.

Dickson A 1985 The mirror within. Quartet, London
Gives a good understanding of women's sexuality. Useful for both practitioners and clients.

REFERENCES

Bancroft J 1989 Human sexuality and its problems. Churchill Livingstone, Edinburgh

Gillan P 1987 Sex therapy manual. Blackwell Scientific Publications, Oxford

Hawton K 1985 Sex therapy. A practical guide. Oxford Medical Press, Oxford

Rust J, Golombek S 1986 Golombek–Rust inventory of sexual satisfaction. NFER Nelson, Windsor

Rust J, Bennum I, Crowe M, Golombek S 1986 Golombek–Rust inventory of marital state (GRIMS) test and handbook. NFER Nelson, Windsor

Savage J 1995 Nursing intimacy, an ethnographic approach to nurse–patient interaction. Scutari Press, London

Sjorgen K, Fugl-Meyer A 1983 Some factors influencing quality of sexual life after myocardial infarction. International Rehabilitation Medicine 5: 197–201

Wabrek A J, Burchell R C 1980 Male sexual dysfunction associated with coronary heart disease. Archives of Sexual Behaviour 9: 69–75

Waterhouse J, Metcalf M 1991 Attitudes towards nurses discussing sexual concerns with patients. Journal of Advanced Nursing 16: 1048–1054

Webb C 1985 Sexuality, nursing and health. Wiley, Chichester

13

Sexual health in the continuing care setting

Steve Jamieson   Sue McAndrew   Heather Wilson

> *'We British, and especially we English, are a bad case of "Sex in the head".'* (D. H. Lawrence)

KEY ISSUES/CONCEPTS

- ◆ Sexual health in the context of the continuing care setting
- ◆ Stigmatization
- ◆ Barriers to exploring sexual health needs
- ◆ Meeting the challenge
- ◆ Sexual health promotion and education

OVERVIEW

Chapter 13, *Sexual health in the continuing care setting*, explores the attitudes, values and beliefs of health-care professionals in relation to clients who are reliant upon long-term care. It challenges current practice and discusses some of the ethical dilemmas facing those who work in the continuing care setting. The final part of the chapter looks at health promotion strategies that health-care professionals may adopt to enable them to meet the sexual health needs of their clients.

INTRODUCTION

The positive and attractive aspects of sex and sexuality too often fall under the shadow of preoccupation with their problematic aspects. Such problems must not overshadow the joys of healthy sex: this is the reason for promoting sexual health in a positive sense. We must not be ensnared by religion or other ideologies into seeing sexuality as a problem. There will always be obstacles to sexual health and expressions of sexuality; however, solutions to the problems of HIV infection and other STDs must be founded on a basic belief in sexuality as a positive force, and the right to sexual health along the lines of the right to health in general.

Sexuality and gender are an important part of being human and are often seen as keystones in development (Burns 1986). Rowan (1988) argues that sexuality and the sexual act are inextricably linked with an individual's state of being: their intrapersonal domain. The humanistic concept of developing self-awareness is, it has been argued (Rogers 1951) essential to the effective functioning of individuals within interpersonal relationships. Those who work with individuals in continuing care settings rely on effective interpersonal relationships in order to function meaningfully, and therefore need to heighten their self-awareness in a way that can be translated into effective and therapeutic relationships with clients.

Talking with clients about their sexual behaviour is an important part of the caring process when working within a 'harm reduction framework'. Integrating sexual health with behavioural issues in the care setting is paramount. In order successfully to achieve such integration, it is imperative that health-care professionals examine their own attitudes in the hope that prejudices will be modified. This should then pave the way for more open communication with clients about their sexual health needs.

'ON SCENE' – THE NEED IN CONTINUING CARE SETTINGS

The sexual needs of people in continuing care settings are all too often ignored, or are classified as behaviour that is either asexual or hypersexed. To see clients as asexual is to devalue them, or not to consider them holistic beings. Perceiving clients as hypersexed is often justified by blaming their sexual behaviour on 'mental illness' or 'antisocial behaviour', rather than individual preference.

The sexuality of clients who identify as being lesbian, gay or bisexual may be considered by some practitioners as a cause or result of mental health difficulties, rather than as an alternative lifestyle. This is to some degree affirmed within our social authority: for example, in the case of clients who wish to undergo gender reassignment surgery, mental health assessment is a prerequisite. Thus the sex life of residents in continuing care settings, such as older people, those in rehabilitation units, hostels, homes for young people and psychiatric institutions, becomes invisible. Research suggests that although this may be a reality for the staff, it is not the reality for the clients living in these settings. Pratt (1986) found that sexual activity among psychiatric inpatients in long-stay units is fairly common. Open acknowledgement of sexual relationships in institutions has posed a dilemma for authorities. In general, access to sexual health resources – for example condoms, sexual information and privacy to engage in sexual activity – has been frowned upon. Therefore, relationships which do develop are, because they are covert, likely to include unprotected and perhaps unsatisfying sexual activity.

Apart from denial on the part of professionals that residents in continuing care settings are not sexual beings, another common response is to devalue sexuality and sexual activity by placing it towards the bottom of a 'hierarchy of needs'. A common belief and/or assumption among mental health nurses is that clients who have been diag-nosed as suffering from schizophrenia are 'too ill' or have 'too many other problems' to worry about their sexual health. The reality is that this particular client group is willing and able to talk about their feelings and needs, and the reason most frequently given for limiting their sexual activity was separation from their partner by hospitalization (Bell et al. 1993). Separation applies to a great number of people in continuing care settings. Nurses and other health professionals do not adequately address clients' sexual health needs, and yet clients are willing to discuss those needs (Wilson 1987). In particular, illness, hospitalization and medication often affect sexual functioning: this could lead to longer-term sexual problems and the discontinuation of treatment by some clients (Jacobs 1991).

Learning activity 13.1

Think of a client you have worked with in a continuing care setting. How did you address the sexual health needs of that client? Considering the client's circumstances, draw up a care plan demonstrating how you would now address their sexual health needs.

Nature/Nurture

It is easy to fall into thinking that all aspects of sexuality are 'natural' and that people do not need to learn how to behave appropriately. Most of us learn from our peer group about how to be attractive to potential partners, and how to function in safe sexual relationships. However, some people find themselves excluded from such information and informal education, and are therefore in need of more structured, individualized programmes to help them to make sense of their bodies and feelings. This is most evident in continuing care settings, where the environment isolates people from the usual social norms.

Sexual health and mental health

Sexual health and mental health are inextricably woven together. It is clear that many factors affecting a person's sexual health – such as sexual abuse, infection with an STD, or altered body image – may precipitate problems requiring help from a mental health professional. Similarly, a person's mental health problems may impinge on their sexual health, either because of the nature of the mental illness or as a result of the treatment.

Bhui and Puffett (1994) believe that among people with mental health problems,

> *'The side-effects of prescribed medication are too often named as the cause of sexual problems, and less attention is directed to other factors which may be amenable to psychological intervention.'*

This applies equally across other health-care situations and is an important point as it can be all too easy for health-care professionals to pass off sexual problems among clients as being inevitable or secondary to treatment. This may be a form of avoidance, given the evidence detailing the difficulties nurses and other professionals have in addressing this issue. Before reading the rest of this chapter it might be useful to consider your own views by filling in the questionnaire in Learning activity 13.2.

Learning activity 13.2

Questionnaire

1. Do you think clients have a right to form sexual relationships while in hospital?

Yes

No

Perhaps

Give reasons for your response.

If you have answered 'yes' or 'perhaps', please continue.

2. What difficulties might face clients who wish to have consenting sex in hospital?

3. In what circumstances do you think consenting sex between clients is acceptable?

4. Are there any circumstances in which you think consenting sex between clients is unacceptable?

5. Do you think clients should have more privacy for sexual expression?

Yes

No

Maybe

If you have answered 'no' or 'maybe', please give your reasons.

6. Where do you think clients should have the opportunity to have consenting sex?

7. Would it make a difference to you if the clients involved were of the same sex?

Yes

No

Maybe

If you answered 'yes' or maybe', please give your reasons.

KNOWLEDGE AND SEXUAL HEALTH

Knowledge is needed about sexual behaviour, not just physiology. We need to know the make-up of sexual identity and sexuality. We need to know about legislation and moral philosophy related to sex. Attitudes must be recognized and questioned. It is not difficult to learn about sexually transmitted diseases, their symptoms, transmission, treatment and local services available: it is much more demanding to understand safer sex (Few 1994). In order to promote sexual health effectively we need to examine how a range of factors can influence our approach to sexual health-care issues. Knowledge of different cultures is essential to ensure effective health care that addresses cultural needs and values. Fear of stigmatization must not be used as an excuse for inaction in relation to sexual health programmes and activities directed towards members of minority groups.

Learning activity 13.3

List the different ethnic groups included in the main cultural elements of British society. Although many people will have spent most of their life in Britain they will have experienced certain family behaviours, beliefs and languages. Looking at your list, write down what you already know about each different group (male and female), their values, attitudes and beliefs with regard to sexuality and sexual health.

Where does your knowledge and understanding of different ethnic groups come from?

How do you know that your assumptions or knowledge are correct?

Have you identified deficits in your knowledge?

What sources of information are available to you to find out more about them?

Education and learning

Education is one key to change, but there is also a need for change within nurse education. The whole ethos requires a move from propagating conformity and similarity of thinking (Burnard 1989) to 'promoting individuality, autonomous thinking and critical self- and social awareness'.

Savage (1987) states:

> 'In reality it is only through struggling to incorporate sexuality amid all our doubts and feelings of inadequacy that we will begin to learn about ourselves and our clients and grow in confidence. Whether it is possible to attain a state of grace and ever come to deal with sexuality in a dispassionate way seems doubtful. I do not even know that this is a worthy goal. After all, if we become glib about sexuality, can we still empathise with most clients' unease?'

Human sexuality is a complex attribute of every person, involving deep needs for identity, relationships, love and immorality. It is more than biological and physiological processes, gender or modes of behaviour: it involves one's self-concept and one's self-esteem. Sexuality involves masculine and feminine self-image, the expression of emotional states of being, the communication of feelings for others, and encompasses everything that the individual is, thinks, feels or does during their entire lifespan. Sexual behaviour is ultimately related to emotional wellbeing, yet is often misunderstood, feared and misused.

> 'Before embarking upon entering into the world of another, the "right" to do so must be earned by looking into your own world first.'
> Dexter and Wash (1986)

Much the same message comes over in a WHO report:

> 'People have the right and the duty to participate, individually and collectively, in the planning and implementation of their health care. Consequently, community involvement in shaping its own health and socioeconomic future, including mass involvement of women, men and youth, is a key factor in the strategy.'

STIGMATIZATION

What is stigma?

Human beings will distance themselves both emotionally and physically because of abhorrence, lack of awareness and understanding, and issues that challenge their belief systems; the consequence is stigmatization. For those who become stigmatized, that is, those who are viewed as offenders of social order, the consequences are likely to involve victimization.

Stigmatization and nursing

Stigmatization is a broad and complex issue when related to sexual health and it evokes many internal feelings, especially when applied to a nurse as a professional, who is often at the front line and expected to behave appropriately and act as a role model in society.

In a continuing care setting it could be argued that the professional relationship with the client is different from that in an acute setting, by virtue of the duration of the client's stay. However, despite the length of the professional relationship there seems to be little evidence to indicate that stigmatization is decreased in any significant way. This may be due to professionals making assumptions about the sexual health-care needs of this client group. The very nature of institutionalized settings brings about changes in client behaviour, and what is assumed to be their 'normal' behaviour in this setting may be very different from their 'normal' behaviour at home.

Attitudes of health-care professionals

Kelly (1988), in two separate studies of nurses and physicians, found a negative bias and attribution towards clients who have sexual health concerns (including HIV/AIDS). The findings ranged from an unwillingness to engage in even casual interaction to viewing clients with AIDS as more responsible for their illness and less deserving of sympathy than other clients. This indicates the severity of negativity in attitude and the stigmatizing of sexual health. It appears that this is particularly pertinent to those who suffer HIV/AIDS, as this is well known publicly to affect mainly homosexuals and intravenous drug users. These particular groups of people raise moral and ethical issues, and negative responses can range from individuals vocalizing their beliefs or to ignoring and distancing themselves from clients.

An example of this is given by Sontag (1989):

> 'The unsafe behaviour that produces HIV disease is judged to be more than just weakness, it is indulgence, delinquency – addictions to chemicals that are illegal and to sex regarded as deviant'.

This strongly indicates that these people have been judged for what they practise rather than for who they are as individuals. This has led to HIV and sexual health acquiring negative labels and creating a negative attitude in nurses, leading to conflict on several levels. There is a personal issue, i.e their own belief and value system; a cultural issue, which deems these people to be unclean; and a professional issue.

Currently those diagnosed with HIV disease or AIDS can now receive treatment that prolongs life. This client group may well therefore become in need of long-term care. Considering the research evidence health-care professionals are challenged to become more proactive and to consider how they will pre-empt stigma and address the sexual health needs of those with HIV/AIDS in the continuing care settings of tomorrow.

BARRIERS TO MEETING SEXUAL HEALTH-CARE NEEDS

For most of us sex is an absorbing topic. We chatter endlessly about it, but despite this tidal wave of sex talk, current attitudes still leave a lot to be desired. The advances in academic and specialist knowledge about the physical and psychological aspects of sexuality have not been matched by similar progress in personal, social, religious, legal and public attitudes.

Now that we find ourselves in the era of HIV, when precise descriptions of which sexual acts are safe and which are not is literally a matter of life or death, language and medical inhibition is not merely idiotic, it is lethal. During the past decade, governments have shrunk from funding educational programmes that use 'frank sex talk', pitched at a level the target audience will readily understand.

A common belief is that workers should 'examine their own attitudes' and 'modify their prejudices' to enable them to talk with clients about sex. This is a facile argument, as it does not acknowledge the skills and training required to undertake sexual counselling, but rather enables the worker to intellectualize the issues and thus protect themselves from fear and ignorance: 'If I am broadminded about matters sexual, then I am a good counsellor about sex'. Grey (1993) states:

'We have to be honest with ourselves about our own sexual desires and needs to feel comfortable about them before we can hope to be good news sexually to other people'.

Prejudice in the matter of sex is a barrier towards effective communications in the client/staff relationship. According to the *Concise Oxford Dictionary*, prejudice is a preconceived (i.e. based) opinion. Ambrose Bierce, in his *Devil's Dictionary*, defines prejudice as 'a vagrant opinion without visible means of support'. Prejudice is, as Bierce dryly makes clear, 'intellectually disreputable', yet this does not prevent its proliferation in the sexual sphere, and one is bound to wonder why. Part of the answer, Grey (1993) believes, is to be found in so many people's anxiety about sexuality (not only their own, but other people's), which leads them to experience a need for sexual control, again not only for themselves but also of other people, so that they can feel safe.

Assailed by constant media images and discussion of sexual matters, they seek to limit, if not to ban, sexual items from the public arena. Because of prejudice they believe that sex is obscene, and label it 'offensive'.

Reflection point 13.1

Brainstorm a list of all the sexual activities that you have heard about through the media. Identify from your list those behaviours that (a) you would participate in, (b) you would find acceptable, and (c) you would find abhorrent. How does your personal point of view influence the therapeutic relationship with clients in relation to activities you find abhorrent?

Tackling the issues

It is not enough to intervene when a crisis has arisen. Health-care staff can no longer remain 'inactive' and feel that their responsibilities end with completing an incident form when clients have been found engaging in sexual activity.

Sometimes there will be dilemmas that cannot be resolved, and the service will have to support the individual in their right to sexual expression.

'There is a growing body of knowledge that relates to prevention programmes with the chronic mentally ill. Programmes are effective if they are simple, brief, amoral, accommodate questions and are prepared for pathological response.' (Graham and Cates 1992).

To equip staff to respond to clients' needs with regard to sexual matters, suitable educational programmes will need to be made available. Numerous courses surrounding topics of sex and sexuality, HIV awareness, condom use, sexually transmitted diseases and sexual counselling are provided nationwide, but there remains a lack of enthusiasm which needs to be explored.

Needing to meet the challenge

The challenge of sexual health, and especially HIV disease, has presented the health-care profession with the need to equip itself not only with the basic knowledge of aetiology and methods of transmission of HIV, but also an understanding of the psychosocial effects of HIV and AIDS. Both nationally and internationally, nurses have been faced with a condition that forces them to examine and evaluate attitudes to the plethora of social taboos. Sexuality, loss, bereavement, drug use and abuse and individual lifestyles are just a few of the complex issues that our society has for too long chosen to disregard (Szasz 1972).

Practitioners are facing increasing pressure to develop their role in meeting the sexual health needs of their clients, and are well placed to be effective educators. Consumers expect to receive health care from informed and humane professionals whose diagnostic, treatment and human relations skills have been developed by systematic and thoughtful preparation. Such preparation confronts the very nature of a person's beliefs and practices, and should facilitate better understanding of self as well as an appreciation of a more holistic approach to the consumer in need of sexual health care. The concept of sexual health has generated a great deal of discussion. Many professionals have had difficulty in agreeing a definition that encompasses all the essential components of human sexuality in the context of health and illness. Most individuals tend to believe that sex and sexuality are 'natural' and 'inevitable', the result of instinctive animal urges (Argyle 1983). This is a powerful way of addressing the issues surrounding sex in relation to one's lifestyle, but taking cognisance of the history and cultural variations around the world leads us to question such assumptions. Sexual preferences and patterns of sexual behaviour vary a great deal over time and between cultures. However, it is becoming increasingly difficult to define sexual health in a society where cultural and social boundaries and expectations change very rapidly (ENB 1994).

Powerful social forces in politics, religion, and even in medicine encourage the distinction between acceptable and unacceptable sexual acts or behaviours. Human sexuality is thought about, fantasized about, talked about, written about and scripted into action. It is enmeshed in the dialogues of theology, philosophy, medicine, literature, law, morality, psychiatry and the sciences.

'Sex and gender are interrelated in complex ways. Sex permeates our symbolism and much of our art. In many languages, inanimate objects are endowed with gender.' (Bancroft 1989)

One issue that has become increasingly apparent is the fact that sexual health is not just about sexually transmitted diseases. The World Health Organization (1986) defined sexual health using key elements: the advantage of this approach is the acknowledgement that sexuality is related to sexual activity in health, disability and illness, and that it changes and evolves over time.

One of the implications of the key concepts approach is that individuals need to acknowledge the importance of sexuality within their own lives in order to be sensitive to the needs of others. A recognition of the importance of sexual health is an essential part of the concept of holistic care. Education and training in sexual health have to take into account that within this area of care there is a deli-

cate interface between 'professional' and 'personal' (ENB 1994). It has been acknowledged by the World Health Organization that education of health professionals is crucial.

It is important that relationships between client and practitioner are open and supportive if work on sex and sexual health is to be undertaken. The practitioner should be totally comfortable with the whole issue of sexual health as it can be counterproductive if the client picks up a sense of anxiety. Learning about sexual health is not only the responsibility of the client: professionals also need to regularly examine their own attitudes and actions.

The needs of students undertaking education and training in sexual health will vary depending on their previous experiences, cultural beliefs and values, motivation and abilities. The aim is to facilitate the development of mature learners with a greater insight and understanding in relation to sexual health issues. Human sexuality encompasses a far wider range of behaviours and identities than is sometimes acknowledged (Aggleton et al. 1989).

Reflection point 13.2

What would be the challenges for you when addressing clients' sexual health-care needs in a continuing care setting?

ETHICAL DILEMMAS

In relation to mental health nurses, Thomas (1989) acknowledges that historically psychiatric nurses have only addressed sexuality when it was perceived as a problem, such as a client masturbating in a public area. This tendency is not unique to mental health nursing.

Case study 13.1

Paul is a 24-year-old client who, following a road traffic accident, has been admitted for rehabilitation to your ward, where it is anticipated that he will spend the next 6–12 months.

He often displays overt sexual behaviour, particularly with younger female staff, attempting to touch their breasts, fondling his penis, and asking staff to get into bed with him. He had a girlfriend before his accident, but she ended the relationship shortly after he was admitted to hospital.

In what ways could you ensure that Paul is able to deal with his sexual needs?

What are the issues you would have to discuss?

Who would need to be involved in the discussion?

How would you go about arranging the environment to ensure his privacy and dignity were being maintained?

When clients have been discovered engaging in sexual activity the traditional response has been to try to control it. Thus, most local policies state that sexual relationships between clients are not permitted, and that staff should intervene to stop any overt expressions of sexuality. Such policies tend to give vague or impractical guidance on how to control sexual expression. To date the authors are not aware of the development of any clear policies which offer guidance to staff on how to intervene in such situations.

Despite this tendency to avoid sexuality, there is a growing body of research-based evidence that people with mental health problems who are sexually active:

◆ experience sexual problems (Bhui and Puffett 1994)
◆ engage in unprotected sex, which carries the risk of sexually transmitted disease and unplanned pregnancies (Kelly et al. 1992)
◆ have significant gaps in their knowledge regarding safer sex (Goisman et al. 1991)
◆ are vulnerable to exploitation and abuse (Cournos et al. 1994).

One concern in continuing care settings is that of the risk behaviour individuals adopt when engaging in sexual activity. Some of the more common risk behaviours are:

◆ Sex in exchange for money, drugs or a place to stay

◆ Being pressurized into unwanted sex
◆ Unprotected sex after using alcohol or drugs
◆ Being amenable to anal intercourse
◆ Having unprotected sex with an infected drug user.

Bor and Watts (1993) suggest that talking to clients about sexual matters is as difficult as addressing death and dying. They quote USA research which suggests that the main factors accounting for nurses' reluctance to take a sexual history are embarrassment, a belief that it is not relevant to the client's care, and a feeling of being inadequately trained for the task.

Reflection point 13.3

List your excuses for not addressing clients' sexual health-care needs in the continuing care setting.

There is clear evidence that clients do engage in sexual activity which places them at risk of STDs and unplanned pregnancy, along with evidence that a significant number engage in sex in return for money or scarce goods, all of which only raises concerns about exploitation. The alarming evidence that homeless people with mental health problems may engage in more sexual risk behaviours causes major concern for health-care providers, especially in view of the lack of condoms and information available to this group.

A number of studies have shown that people with mental health problems have significant gaps in their knowledge regarding the risk of sexual activity and the use of condoms, and limited access to resources such as condoms and genito-urinary/sexual health clinics or family planning services. There is also a lack of training courses on sexual health promotion in mental health and an absence of any distance learning or teaching packs to help staff develop their skills and practice in this area, although these exist for other client groups, such as people with learning difficulties.

Health-care professionals frequently express concern about the harmful effects of appearing to encourage or condone sexual expression, in whatever form. Among the reasons staff have given for this response is that it is a potential cause of conflict in the ward if clients are seen to be physically attracted to each other; that such activity detracts from their treatment and recovery; and that staff are concerned about vulnerability and exploitation. Although some of these may be genuine concerns, it does not seem to fit with an ethos of individualized care which recognizes sexual expression as a contributing factor to wellbeing to have a blanket ban on such activities. Clearly, there needs to be some criteria for staff to assess each individual situation and relationship before deciding on the best course of action.

People who are vulnerable, such as those with mental health problems, may be more at risk of STDs and sexual abuse for a number of reasons:

◆ Cognitive deficits may affect their ability to take in new information (Goisman et al. 1991).
◆ They may have reduced ability to refuse sexual advances and negotiate the type of sex they engage in (Kelly and St Lawrence 1987).

Learning activity 13.4

The following exercise is a productive and enjoyable way for practitioners to openly discuss sexual health issues in their area of work.

The group is divided into two and each subgroup is asked to be for or against the following motion:

This house believes that clients with mental health problems should not be permitted to have consensual relationships while undergoing inpatient treatment

Twenty minutes should be allowed for preparation of the debate and then 30 minutes for the actual debate.

This will stimulate a lot of discussion and will allow participants to express their views, concerns and fears in a safe, yet productive way.

◆ Lack of access to resources such as condoms and lack of appropriate written information (Firn 1994).

It is well recognized that health promotion initiatives need to be targeted at at-risk groups and presented in ways which are accessible and meaningful to their lifestyles and experiences. It is therefore very important that resources are developed and that sensitive and effective training and education are implemented that address knowledge deficits and empower clients to negotiate safe and comfortable forms of sexual expression.

The practice of making condoms available in continuing care settings is fraught with ethical concerns. Often staff say they don't know how to actually go about making the condoms available,

Learning activity 13.5

How would you answer the following in relation to a continuing care setting?

◆ Should condoms be freely available in dispensers in care areas, or should staff have some control about how many are given out and to whom?

◆ Should condoms be provided free, or should clients have to pay for them? Is the use of vending machines a part of normalization philosophy in continuing care services, and does this override the need for open access?

◆ Should condoms be kept in the care area, or is it sufficient and less controversial to have information about how and where to obtain them, such as a local GUM clinic, GP or commercial outlet?

◆ If condoms are not available in each care area, are machines in visitors' toilets, outpatient departments or the hospital social club appropriate?

◆ Where the continuing care setting is within a hospital, should condoms be sold in the hospital shop? How will the concerns and possible objections of clients and staff be taken into account and dealt with?

and see it as a 'hot potato' and are concerned about legal issues.

Clearly, access to condoms is not a complete solution to sexual risk behaviour. There is evidence that people with mental health problems have similar negative views towards condoms as the general population, including perceiving them as messy, likely to reduce pleasure, and an unwelcome interruption to foreplay – which reduces usage. These issues need to be addressed by further research and during education sessions with clients.

Recognizing and accepting that clients engage in sexual activities makes it imperative for staff to have clear guidelines so that they can respond sensitively and sympathetically, not denying the clients' right to be sexual but also ensuring that there is no harm to any client in the unit.

Whenever clients are known or thought to be engaging in sexual relationships, management and care decisions need to be based upon an individual assessment of the specific circumstances. The nurse's principal role is to assess whether both parties consent to the sexual relationship. For clients with mental health problems an important consideration will be whether either partner is detained under a section of the Mental Health Act (1983), as this may indicate that they are unable to make informed judgements.

Some people have raised the concern that hospital setting must be viewed as a public place. Therefore, it could be argued, men having sex with men would be illegal, and sex between men and women would fall foul of the public decency laws. However, it is by no means clear that a bedroom in a psychiatric hospital, for example, is a public place within the particular laws governing sexual activity. A draft report by the Special Hospital Services Authority (SHSA 1993) took legal advice which suggested that under European law it is probably illegal to prevent two consenting adults detained in a special hospital from engaging in sexual intercourse.

Many nurses will have come across clients masturbating in view of staff, residents and visitors. Many would agree that, even if the door cannot be locked from inside, the client's bedroom might be an acceptable place for them to masturbate, as long as they cannot be seen from outside.

Consideration must be given to the issue of sexual activity between a client in a psychiatric hospital and a partner who is not a client. Some organizations have called for the provision of 'safe private spaces for service users to engage in consensual, intimate activities' (RCN 1996), particularly if the client is likely to have a prolonged stay in hospital and has limited opportunities for leave. In such a scenario the nurse would still need to be sure the client was able to consent freely to sexual relations, even with an established partner. This may be particularly difficult if the client is unable to articulate their sexual health needs, for example those suffering from dementia or aphasia.

SEXUAL HEALTH PROMOTION AND EDUCATION

The concept of the nurse as health educator is implicit. The UK 'Project 2000' curricula identify the importance of learners achieving competencies to a stated level, to acquire and develop skills to identify the health needs of patients and clients, families and friends, and to participate in health promotion activities.

Social cognitive theory and the health belief model

Today, in the age of HIV/AIDS, 'the role of the nurse in primary, secondary and tertiary prevention is paramount' (Pratt 1991). To assist in this process there are various models of health education, all having relevance and uses with different individuals, cultures and situations. Social cognitive theory, originally described by Bandura (1986), states that behaviour is determined by the interaction between an individual's beliefs, opinions and expectations and the incentives associated with a particular behaviour.

The health belief model (Rosenstock et al. 1988) states that in order to change their behaviour individuals must have sufficient concern about health issues and believe that they are susceptible, that the condition is serious, and that the recommended action is going to work and does not involve significant cost. Rosenstock, Stretcher and

Becker (1988) argue that, in combination, the social cognitive theory and the health belief model provide the best available account of health-related behaviour, and hence are the best guide for effective behavioural interventions.

According to these models, to change behaviour the individual must perceive a risk and the behaviour change must be attractive at minimal cost. The theory underlying the self-empowerment approach is based on liberal principles of education, where individuals are free to make their own decisions. Self-empowerment is described by Hopson and Scally (1981) as

'a process by which one increasingly takes greater charge of oneself and one's life, self-empowerment means believing that there is always an alternative we can choose, and having the ability to identify the alternatives in any situation, and to choose on the basis of one's values, priorities and commitments'.

The underlying principle of the self-empowerment approach is that each individual has the power and motivation to adopt a healthier lifestyle. One criticism of this approach is that, at its extreme, the individual may make behaviour choices regardless of the consequences for others.

The collective action approach

The collective action or radical political approach aims to improve health by acting on the environment. Unlike policy development within existing structures, collective action seeks change from the grassroots up. This is achieved by motivating individuals or community groups to act in their own interests. There are similarities between this approach and self-empowerment, as both require well informed, assertive individuals to act to improve their health (Aggleton and Homans 1987).

The collective action approach is concerned with the physical, social and political environment, which is seen as a key determinant of health where the emphasis of self-empowerment is the individual, who is perceived as being of prime importance. Although no single model of health education is ideal in the variety of situations found in clinical practice, probably the most useful for nurses is an eclectic 'educational model'. This is based on the belief that health behaviour is a product of prior learning, and can be changed by the educational process. This is often referred to as teaching for health. A belief that health promotion will reduce health-care costs has led many to see health promotion as a way of saving money, but this is not the primary objective: health promotion professes to be centrally concerned with the social policy process. Building a healthy public policy is one of the five means of health promotion action to achieve Health for All by the Year 2000. Healthy public policy, which is fundamental to

Learning activity 13.6

Devise an education package to use with a client in a continuing care setting which addresses the issues of safer sex.

health promotion, is emerging as a discrete area of study (Bunton and Macdonald 1992). The study of social policy contributes greatly to key areas of study within healthy public policy.

Widespread ignorance and prejudice in relation to HIV/AIDS and sexual health in general have been reported among health professionals. Instances of this ignorance and inhumane or insensitive treatment abound (McHaffie 1993). The development of healthy attitudes and values, as well as professional skills, may be encouraged by education. Motivation, however, is an essential factor, in addition to the ability; responsibility rests with the individual as well as the nurse educators.

One of The Health of the Nation's key target areas was HIV/AIDS and sexual health: this highlights the importance of educating the nurses of tomorrow, as their function may involve dispensing information and offering guidance to individuals in the sphere of sexual health. If health-care professionals are to achieve this, not only do they need to develop their knowledge, they also need to examine attitudes and develop skills. Sexuality workshops should be incorporated within the curricula to enable client needs to be met in both health and illness. The overall aim would be to facilitate group members to begin to explore and internalize some of the issues surrounding the concept of sexuality, developing an awareness of the influence of care delivery to individuals who encounter sexual health problems.

FUTURE PRACTICE

In order to address the sexual health-care needs of clients in continuing care settings, examples of good practice should include the following:

◆ A named nurse to act as a coordinator for sexual health programmes within the care setting
◆ Provision of condoms and sexual health education to all clients
◆ Provision of safer sex literature in appropriate and accessible areas
◆ Sexual health training for staff
◆ Liaison with other areas, such as GU clinics, HIV/AIDS prevention services, substance misuse service
◆ Updating and access to latest information for staff
◆ Development and implementation of policies that address sexual health needs of clients in the continuing care setting
◆ Resource pack for wards and departments
◆ Setting up user forums/groups
◆ Access to HIV counselling and testing
◆ Hepatitis B vaccine available for clients.

CONCLUSION

In this chapter a number of challenges for health-care professionals have been raised in relation to meeting the sexual health-care needs of their clients. It is essential that professionals working in the continuing care environment gain sufficient knowledge and understanding of sexual health issues to be able to question their own values, attitudes and beliefs, as well as being able to develop their skills and sensitivity

in meeting client needs. The ethical dilemmas that have been outlined draw attention to areas of practice that are difficult but which none the less require thought and discussion, to enable professionals to take a more proactive stance to ensure that clients in continuing care settings will be in an environment that takes account of their total wellbeing. Lastly, models of health promotion and education were explored. It is hoped that these will provide a framework for health-care professionals who wish to improve their practice in meeting the sexual health-care needs of their clients.

REFERENCES

Aggleton P 1989 Evaluating health education about AIDS. In: Aggleton P, Davies P, Hart G (eds) AIDS: sexual representations, social practice. Falmer Press, Lewes

Aggleton P, Homans H 1987 Educating about AIDS. NHS Training Authority, London

Argyle M 1983 The psychology of interpersonal behaviour. Penguin, Harmondsworth

Bancroft J 1989 Human sexuality and its problems. Churchill Livingstone, Edinburgh

Bandura A 1986 Social foundations of thought and action: a social cognitive theory. Prentice Hall, Englewood Cliffs

Bell C E, Wringer P H, Davidhizer R, Samuels M C 1993 Self-reported sexual behaviour of schizophrenic clients and non-institutionalised adults. Perspectives in Psychiatric Care 29(2): 30–36

Bhui K, Puffett A 1994 Sexual problems in the psychiatric and mentally handicapped populations. British Journal of Hospital Medicine, 51(9): 459–464

Bor R, Watts M 1993 Talking to patients about sexual matters. British Journal of Nursing 2(13): 657–661

Bunton R, MacDonald G (eds) 1992 Health promotion: disciplines and diversity. Routledge, London

Burnard P 1989 Fads and fashions. Nursing Times 85: 69–71

Burns R B 1986 Child development: a text for the caring professions. Croom Helm, London

Cournos F, Guido J R, Coomaraswamy S 1994 Sexual acts and risks of HIV infection among patients with schizophrenia. American Journal of Psychiatry 151(2): 228–232

Dexter G, Wash M 1986 Psychiatric nursing skills: patient centred approach. Croom Helm, London

English National Board for Health Visiting, Midwifery and Nursing 1994 Sexual health education and training. ENB, London

Few C 1994 Promoting sexual health. Community Outlook 4(2): 29–31

Firn S 1994 No sex please: patients in psychiatric hospitals. Nursing Times 90(14): 57

Graham L L, Cates J A 1992 How to reduce the risk of HIV infection for the severe mentally ill. Journal of Psychosocial Nursing and Mental Health Services 30(6): 9–13, 34–35

Grey A 1993 Speaking of sex. The limits of language. Cassell, London

Hopson B, Scally M 1981 Lifeskills teaching. McGraw–Hill, London

Jacobs M 1991 Insight and experience.

A manual of training in the technique and theory of psychodynamic counselling. Open University Press, Milton Keynes

Kelly J A 1988 Nurses' attitudes towards AIDS. Journal of Continuing Education in Nursing 19(2): 78–83

Kelly J A, Lawrance J S 1987 Caution about condoms in prevention of AIDS. (Letter) Lancet 1(8528): 323

Kelly J A, Murphy D A, Bahr G R et al. 1992 AIDS/HIV Risk behavior among the chronic mentally ill. American Journal of Psychiatry 149(7): 886–889

McHaffie H 1993 The care of patients with HIV and AIDS: a survey of nurse education in the UK. A report. Institute of Medical Ethics, University of Edinburgh, Edinburgh

Mental Health Act 1983. HMSO, London

Pratt R J 1986 AIDS: a strategy for nursing care. Edward Arnold, London

Pratt R J 1991 AIDS: a strategy for nursing care. Edward Arnold, London

Rogers C 1951 Client centred therapy. Constable, London

Rosenstock I M, Strecher V J, Becker M H 1988 Social learning theory and the health belief model. Health Education Quarterly 15(2): 175–183

Rowan J 1988 Ordinary ecstasy. Humanistic psychology in action, 2nd edn. Routledge, London

Royal College of Nursing 1996 Sexual health. Key issues within mental health services. RCN, London

Savage J 1987 Nurses, gender and sexuality.

Nursing Today Series. Heinemann Nursing, London

Sontag S 1989 AIDS and its metaphors. Allen Lane, London

Szasz T 1972 Manufacture of madness: a comparative study of the inquisition and the mental health movement. Routledge and Keegan, London

Thomas B 1989 HIV and encephalopathy. Nursing Times 3(46): 4–7

Wilson G D 1987 Variant sexuality research and theory. Croom Helm, London

World Health Organization 1986 Concepts of Sexual Health. EUR/ICP/MCH 521. WHO, Copenhagen

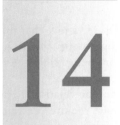

14

Sexual health: support and supervision

Hugh Palmer Sam Samociuk

'It was then that I realized the world's greatest truth: one bum vibe leads to another.' (Neil, 'The Young Ones' (BBC TV, 1984))

KEY ISSUES/CONCEPTS

◆ Reflective practice

◆ Defining support and supervision

◆ Formal supportive relationships

◆ Clinical supervision

◆ Types, structures and models of clinical supervision

◆ Qualities and skills of a supervisor

◆ Training to be a supervisee and a supervisor

OVERVIEW

Chapter 14, *Support and supervision*, focuses on the support needs you may have in relation to sexual health-related practice. It explores ways of identifying appropriate support mechanisms and offers ways of establishing and offering support to others. It emphasizes the importance of reflecting on practice, particularly as issues of a sexual nature can have a powerful personal impact.

INTRODUCTION

Working in sexual health may present challenges and will sometimes raise issues you may find difficult. It is important to consider what support you will need as you develop greater awareness and experience working in the sexual health arena. Support and supervision is an essential process through which you can use reflection to explore and develop greater self-awareness and sensitivity.

There are particular types of support (not all of which may be immediately available to you), the nature of which may vary considerably.

This chapter will offer you ways to think about support and supervision; your task will be to consider which would be best for you and your situation in relation to working in the sexual health arena.

To help you to do this, Kath, Keith and Sarah will be introduced as case studies. As you work through the chapter, you will be asked to consider their unique support needs and decide which strategies would be most appropriate for each of them.

Case study 14.1

Kath was working on an acute psychiatric ward when she discovered that a client who was due to be admitted had a history of sexual offences, including child sexual abuse. Kath felt that she would be unable to work with this client under any circumstances, and was considering taking time off sick rather than be on the ward at the same time as this person.

Keith was a staff nurse on an orthopaedic ward. A young man who was recovering from a head injury, currently being nursed in a bay with four beds, had begun to masturbate regularly in public. This caused embarrassment for staff, clients and visitors. Keith felt that, as the only male nurse on the team, it was his responsibility to deal with the issue, but did not know what to do.

Sarah had been working on a respiratory disease ward for some time. When Emma, a young client, was admitted with asthma, Sarah felt an immediate attraction towards her. This was not something Sarah had experienced before at work; she felt confused, embarrassed and flustered when attending to Emma, but nevertheless found that she was spending progressively more of her time with this client. She had never experienced these feelings towards another woman.

The above examples illustrate situations that may occur in clinical practice, where practitioners require some form of support or supervision in order to be able to carry out their job. All have a sexual issue at their core, whether related to the sexuality of the client, the practitioner or both. However, the support required by Kath, Keith and Sarah will be different, and as no one method of support can meet everybody's needs, it may be that more than one type will be needed.

WHAT IS REFLECTIVE PRACTICE?

In 1983 Donald Schön published a book entitled *The reflective practitioner: how professionals think in action*. This had an enormous impact on many professions. In his book, Schön highlighted how changes occurring in society were affecting professionals, who were not adequately prepared for the range and scope of change by their traditional 'scientific' training programmes. Schön proposed that one means of adapting to these changes was what he called reflective practice. Despite having specialized knowledge and technical ability obtained through traditional education, the reflective practitioner is not an 'expert' who knows 'everything', in contrast to clients who know little. The reflective practitioner's skill lies in the ability to utilize skills and knowledge flexibly in the unique context of each client. The implication is

that both practitioner and client recognize that the other brings an understanding to the situation, and that the process of communicating these understandings is of paramount importance. In order to facilitate this manner of relating to a client the reflective practitioner requires certain skills, notably those of reflection-in-action and reflection-on-action (Schön 1983). Conway (1994) provides a useful description of reflection-in-action as the ability to 'think on your feet' through devising and testing hypotheses in order to find a solution.

As this happens during a situation, the process seems to be unconscious: the solution to a problem just seems to 'pop up'. Schön argues that, in addition to using the practitioner's traditional knowledge base, these situations also demonstrate artistry. In contrast, reflection-on-action takes place after the situation, or during a pause within the situation. As reflection-on-action can be a conscious process, it can be done intentionally and given a structure. To reflect-on-action requires that you have a knowledge base, but you will also need to consciously reflect on the experience in the light of your past experience.

Reflection can be defined in several ways, but two useful definitions are given below:

'Reflective learning is the process of internally examining and exploring an issue of concern, triggered by an experience, which creates and clarifies meaning in terms of self, and which results in a changed conceptual perspective.'
(Boyd and Fales 1983)

'Reflection in the context of learning is a generic term for those intellectual and affective activities in which individuals engage to explore their experiences in order to lead to new understandings and appreciations.'
(Boud et al. 1985)

Both these definitions indicate that the authors' understanding of reflection is of an activity that takes place following an incident, in other words, these are definitions of reflection-on-action. Both illustrate that the effect of reflection is a change, either in perspective or in understanding.

Reflection point 14.1

Consider the ways in which reflection helps you to develop your work in sexual health-related practice. Think of some examples from your work, both positive and negative. What did you learn from these situations? How did you use the reflective process? Was it happening 'in action' or was it a reflection 'on action'? Do you use your reflective diary from previous events to demonstrate to yourself what you have been learning in practice?

Structured reflection

Johns (1995) offers a model of structured reflection that you may find useful in conjunction with support and supervision processes. It will give you a framework to think about situations you encounter, and help you select material to bring to a supervision session or use in the support process. Johns has integrated the four ways of knowing described by Carper (1978) into his model, which is well worth using. Some explanation of Carper's ways of knowing will be necessary before going on to consider Johns' model.

Carper's ways of knowing

Carper (1978), following a review of nursing literature, established that there are four patterns of knowing used by nurses which are aesthetic, personal, ethical and empirical. These patterns are also used by other caring professions.

◆ **Aesthetic knowing** Aesthetics is about the artistry exhibited by someone who is able to grasp a situation and deal with it effectively without appearing even to consciously think about it. This is the previously mentioned artistry seen in the professional who reflects-in-action, as described by Schön (1983). As Chinn and Kramer (1991) point out, the aesthetic way of knowing is expressed directly in the situation and will be unique to that particular experience.

◆ **Personal knowing** The personal way of knowing is about the process of becoming increasingly aware of your inner self. Johns (1995) describes three interrelated factors in the knowing of self: the perception of your feelings and prejudices within a situation; the management of those feelings and prejudices in order to respond appropriately; and managing anxiety and sustaining the self. It is not possible to suspend all prejudices and feelings, let alone even to be aware of them at times; hence becoming aware of these feelings is an essential first step in managing them.

◆ **Ethical knowing** The ethical way of knowing relates to what is right or wrong in a situation and your understanding of what is your moral obligation under the circumstances. This does not simply mean that you have the knowledge base of ethics to work from, but that you also have the ability to make judgements about what is right or wrong in the situation and to make 'on the spot judgements' (Chinn and Kramer 1991). There may be times when you feel uncomfortable about a situation, for example when you may have behaved in a way that was incongruent with your beliefs.

◆ **Empirical knowing** Empirical knowledge equates to the traditional scientific knowledge that you must have in relation to your practice. Again, you will see a parallel with Schön's (1983) writing, in that essential, empirical or scientific knowledge alone is not sufficient to make an effective practitioner. However, it is vital that you continue to maintain and develop your understanding of the science that relates to your practice.

Johns' model of structured reflection may help you to frame your thoughts on a situation before a support or supervision session. It may be that you and your supervisor or support person negotiate to use this framework to structure the process of the sessions too. Although the model is largely self-explanatory, you are best advised to read the original article to appreciate it more fully.

Learning activity 14.1

Identify a specific situation or incident related to sexual health. Consider Carper's four ways of knowing. Under each heading, write down how each one related to your practice.

Feedback on Learning activity 14.1

Did you come up with some of the following:

Aesthetic

Was it a situation where you seemed to know just what to do, without having to consciously think about it? When you recall this sort of situation, could you identify all the elements of the process? Why did you know what to do and how to behave? What was it about the situation, the client, the environment, the timing, that enabled this to happen? Were there any other contributory factors? Was it an activity you have been involved in before? How high were your personal confidence levels in this situation? How relaxed or comfortable did you feel?

Personal

This may involve reflecting on your self-awareness of your own sexuality, and how you relate to clients' expressions of sexuality. Do you feel comfortable with your sexuality and communicating with people who have differing personal views from yours?

Ethical

This could involve reflecting on what you consider to be right or wrong in relation to your sexual health practice. How did your views, values and beliefs affect the situation? Did you demonstrate an awareness of the client's rights in relation to their sexual health? Was the context in which the intervention took place appropriate?

Empirical

What theories underpinned your practice? Did you apply theories of human sexuality?

Learning activity 14.2

Using your example from Learning activity 14.1, work through the following using Johns' model of structured reflection (10th version). Write a description of the experience.

Cue questions:

Aesthetic

What was I trying to achieve?

Why did I respond as I did?

What were the consequences of that for:

◆ the client?

◆ others?

◆ myself?

How was this person (or these persons) feeling?

How did I know this?

Personal

How did I feel in this situation?

What internal factors were influencing me?

Ethical

How did my actions match with beliefs?

What factors made me act in incongruent ways?

Empirical

What knowledge did or should have informed me?

Reflexivity

How does this connect with previous experiences?

Could I handle this better in similar situations?

What would be the consequences of alternative actions for:

◆ the client?

◆ others?

◆ myself?

How do I *now* feel about this experience?

Can I support myself and others better as a consequence?

Has this changed my ways of knowing?

DEFINING SUPPORT AND SUPERVISION

What is support?

Having explored the concept of reflection it will now be useful to go on to investigate and describe support. The concept of support is frequently used in health care, whether in terms of clients or staff, yet support can have many different facets. Many people support a charity or a football team: others need the physical support of a walking frame or the psychological (but double-edged) support of alcohol or tobacco. Support can relate to any of the dimensions of a person: physical, emotional, social, spiritual and intellectual (Landrum et al. 1993), and a few examples are given below.

You will be able to think of other types of support in these dimensions too. Physical support could include things such as a plaster cast for a broken arm, a walking aid or a 'fireman's lift'. Emotional support could be anything from formal counselling to a sympathetic ear or shoulder to cry on. Social support could be financial, and spiritual support could be through participation in religious activities. Finally, intellectual support could range from reading this chapter to remedial classes intended for people with learning difficulties.

Another useful way of thinking about support related to your clinical work is to use categories called formative, normative and restorative. Proctor (1988) coined these terms and originally referred to them as functions of supervision; however, they are useful categories to consider in your general support needs.

◆ **Formative** Formative needs are those that relate to education; the things you need to know or learn in relation to your work. This would include developing skills, knowledge and understanding in relation to your sexual health practice.

◆ **Normative** Normative needs are those that relate to providing the good, quality service that is demanded by your employer and professional bodies. An example of this would be working in a non-discriminatory way with your clients.

◆ **Restorative** Your restorative needs are those that relate to the emotional issues arising from your work. Dealing with other people's pain and distress can create an emotional burden and it is important to deal with these issues before the practitioner's formative and normative needs can be effectively met.

Reflection point 14.2

Do you remember Kath, Keith and Sarah from the beginning of the chapter? What do you think their formative, normative and restorative needs might be?

You may consider that Kath's needs are normative: should she try to avoid caring for her client? Alternatively, you may believe that her needs are mainly restorative, owing largely to her needing help with the distress caused to her by this client's past activities. It could be that a range of supportive interventions are needed by Kath, including addressing very painful personal issues.

Keith's needs seem to be mainly formative, relating to skill development. He also needs to challenge his assumption that, as a male, he should be the one to deal with the situation. However, he may have restorative needs in relation to the difficulties in dealing with sexual health-related situations generally.

Sarah's needs are also complex, and although at first glance there may be concern about her confused feelings, it is important to ensure that normative support enables her to maintain a professional relationship with Emma.

Formal and informal support

There are two broad types of support: formal and informal. Formal support mechanisms usually have a structure, and may even have a cost implication for you or your employer. Types of formal support include clinical supervision, mentorship, preceptorship and appraisal methods, such as individual performance review. Personal therapy and counselling would also constitute formal support, although they are not necessarily available via your employer. These forms of support are usually structured and may have an impact on your practice. Informal support is not usually structured and does not normally cost anything (except your time), and can range from a coffee break chat with colleagues to talking about your concerns to friends or family.

Informal support

This is probably the form of support with which you are most familiar. Unstructured and often ad hoc, informal support usually is helpful in meeting practitioners' restorative needs, although it can be potentially damaging if it is used merely as a forum for complaining about clients, colleagues or management, without any constructive benefits.

Formative aspects of informal support are common in the workplace, for example informally asking a colleague about a procedure. Informal support has the advantage of immediacy: informal debriefing with colleagues after a critical incident can take place relatively soon after the incident, and the events will be fresh in your mind, thus making recollections more accurate.

Formal support

Formal support methods usually require planning, and have requirements for both the supporter and the supported. Such requirements may include knowledge and skill in relation to the process being used, and also limitations as to the nature of the material brought to the process by the person seeking support. Discussion of different support methods will include exploration of the areas of practice for which they are best suited.

Case study 14.2

Michael was a student nurse on a placement caring for older people with psychiatric illness. During the first few weeks he had grown very fond of Mabel, who had Alzheimer's disease, and used to enjoy caring for her. Despite her illness she had a good sense of humour and was always keen to chat. However, one evening, as he was helping her to undress for bed, Mabel said that she felt lonely and asked if he would get into bed with her. Michael found this extremely embarrassing and did not know how to respond. He mumbled something about needing to help another client and quickly left. Michael was not sure what to say to the other staff, as he thought that they would laugh at him, and wondered if he ought to say nothing at all. On the way home he met another student from his group, and mentioned what had happened. The other student said that something similar had happened to her and she had told the ward staff, who were surprisingly sympathetic. In addition to reassuring her, they had looked at improving the situation on their ward in relation to clients' needs for intimacy and comfort.

Following this conversation Michael decided to approach his mentor to discuss his feelings and to explore strategies for dealing with future situations.

The above example is not unusual. It can be difficult dealing with situations where sexual issues arise, and Michael's initial reaction is not uncommon. The need for support and supervision is clear in this example: Mabel's need for intimacy was not met and Michael was left feeling embarrassed and confused. However, with appropriate skills Michael could have been more able to react in a helpful way, even if only by acknowledging her feelings. Through formal support such as clinical supervision, Michael may be able to explore his feelings in relation to this type of situation, and to develop relevant skills. Although Michael did make use of informal support, which in this case reassured him and encouraged him to approach his mentor, his fellow student might not have reacted in such a positive way.

Learning activity 14.3

List all the sources of support to which you have access.

Starting with yourself in the centre, draw a diagrammatical representation that shows your current sources of support. Include formal and informal support both at work and outside. Use space to indicate how accessible each of your support systems is: the most accessible should be closest to you in the centre.

Are you getting the support you need?

Does this support help you to challenge and evaluate your practice?

What are the strengths and weaknesses of your current support?

What are the advantages and disadvantages of formal and informal support mechanisms?

Supervision

As you may have gathered from the previous section, support is a broad term that encompasses both formal and informal mechanisms. Supervision would fall into the formal category, and is commonly thought of as a means of inspection and control by one person over another, especially as supervision is considered a management role.

However, through the development of counselling supervision, many people would now regard supervision as a means of supporting a practitioner in the development of their practice, without the connotations of a manager overseeing a subordinate. This type of supervision can be carried out by someone with expertise in the type of practice the supervisee is engaged in, without necessarily being in a senior position. Clinical supervision is in a sense a logical development of counselling supervision, where the supervisee, with the support of the supervisor, is able to focus on and develop issues related to clinical practice. Clinical supervision will be explored in greater depth later.

FORMAL SUPPORT RELATIONSHIPS

Reading this section will enable you to begin to consider various formal methods of support and supervision that may be available to you or that you may wish to experience. As it is possible only to give a brief outline of some of these methods, it is recommended that you seek further information and make careful consideration before engaging in what could be a costly exercise. The types of formal support that you may consider in relation to your sexual health-related practice are: counselling, psychotherapy, mentorship, preceptorship, appraisal, individual performance review and clinical supervision. Clinical supervision will be dealt with in more depth than the others, as this is a broader type of support and, as will be seen, may be more flexible in meeting your needs.

Counselling and psychotherapy

Both counselling and psychotherapy are formal and deal with specific personal problems or distress. As they are very specific interventions, this chapter cannot offer any more detail. For further details look in the library or on the Internet.

Mentorship

A mentor is described by Morton-Cooper and Palmer (1993) as:

> '*Someone who provides an enabling relationship that facilitates another's personal growth and development. The relationship is dynamic, reciprocal, and can be emotionally intense. Within such a relationship the mentor assists with career development and guides the mentoree through the organizational, social and political networks.*'

As you will have noticed, the focus of mentoring is clearly on career development and is seen as an intense relationship. Some current thinking links mentorship with the role of a qualified practitioner supporting the development of someone undergoing professional training or education. This is a popular interpretation in current nursing literature: Butterworth and Faugier (1992) adopt this view in their model of clinical supervision and mentorship. The history of mentoring is a long one, and it should be borne in mind that how it is interpreted may change again. Morton-Cooper and Palmer (1993) point out that the term comes from the classics: in Homer's *Odyssey*, Mentor was a character nominated by Ulysses as tutor-adviser to his son Telemachus, and guardian of his estates. Morton-Cooper and Palmer (1993) add that mentoring was quite a common arrangement in ancient Greece, where young men were assigned older, wiser men to act as role models.

It should be appreciated that there should be an amount of freedom for both mentor and mentoree in choosing each other, to ensure this sort of intense relationship and, if you are a student in a clinical environment, you may need to assertively exercise your right to that choice. In the example of Michael given earlier, the support of his mentor would have been of value in helping him to develop his skills and feel more confident about his abilities.

Preceptorship

Preceptorship is generally interpreted in the UK as the support given to a newly qualified professional, or one who is returning to work after a break of 5 or more years in their career. The United Kingdom Central Council for Nursing, Midwifery and Health Visiting (UKCC 1993) recommends that this period of support should be for a duration of 4 months, and it is one of the requirements outlined in their *Preparation for Professional Practice* (PREP) document. The purpose of preceptorship is to meet the support needs of a newly qualified or returning practitioner in relation to developing the skills and attitude required of a responsible, accountable professional. The preceptor should be a first-level practitioner who has been working in a relevant clinical area for at least 12 months, who will be able to support the practitioner in relating knowledge to clinical practice. In effect, a preceptor acts as a role model, demonstrating clinical skills and

assisting the practitioner's transition into a confident and competent caring professional.

Appraisal and individual performance review

The aim of appraisal is to improve managerial control by improving the self-direction of all workers (Riseborough and Walters 1988), and individual performance review is simply an appraisal method. Some appraisal methods focus on the developmental needs of workers, whereas others focus on their past performance. Grohar and DiCroce (1992) state that the goals of performance appraisal are to:

◆ evaluate performance
◆ identify staff development and training needs
◆ identify unrecognized talent and ability
◆ influence motivation
◆ assign rewards
◆ take disciplinary action
◆ encourage career goal planning.

Generally, appraisal and individual performance review methods are designed to meet the organization's requirements that your progress and development be monitored, while enabling you to plan your development within the organization's objectives.

Your employer may not recognize that you have developmental needs in relation to sexual health practice, and using an appraisal system to highlight these needs may be useful. If you establish objectives to work to in this area you may find that your manager will support you, for example in applying to take a course on sexual health care.

CLINICAL SUPERVISION

Clinical supervision has been the subject of much recent discussion within the nursing profession, largely in recognition of the benefits already demonstrated by supervision processes in other health and social care professions (examples are social work, psychology, youth work, counselling and psychotherapy).

The Department of Health's document *A vision for the future* (1993) identifies the exploration and development of clinical supervision as one of 12 targets for the professions of nursing, midwifery and health visiting, stating that:

'The concept of clinical supervision should be explored and developed. Discussions should be held at a local and national level on a range and appropriateness of models of clinical supervision and a report made available to the professions.'

The UKCC, in its position papers (1995, 1996), is explicit in its support of the development of clinical supervision for all qualified practitioners in all fields of nursing.

Defining clinical supervision

There are diverse, often conflicting definitions and models of clinical supervision, probably related to its two roots: supervisory management and counselling. At this point it is essential to draw a distinction between professional/personal supervision and clinical supervision. Hawkins (1982) drew a map of the territory of supervision, symbolized by three equal overlapping circles, one representing the organization, one the client and one the practitioner. These three areas encapsulate the totality of the practitioner's professional 'work world'.

When the practitioner wishes to have formal support for the whole of this territory, they are acknowledging the need for professional/personal support and development to enrich their overall professional wellbeing. This type of supervision would give the practitioner the scope to discuss their place in their organization, interprofessional issues and concerns, and the impact of changing policies on them and their client group, as well as their direct clinical work and the inter- and intrapersonal effects of this. This type of supervision is very close to mentoring in its breadth and flexibility.

As a result of this type of supervision the practitioner is restored to optimum working potential; hence the overall quality of their professional performance is enhanced in each sphere of their professional territory.

Clinical supervision, in its purest form, is concerned solely with the practitioner's direct clinical work. This, and this alone, poses the greatest challenge to nursing. Clinical supervision requires the serious consideration of the intrinsic nature of nursing. If nursing still centres predominantly on tasks and procedures carried out mechanistically without true 'engagement' in the activity, then maybe a traditional supervisory management style of supervision is all that nursing deserves.

If nursing has moved away from the medicalization of the person and truly embraces the theories of holism, seeing itself as engaging with the individual in a therapeutic, caring relationship, then a more complex activity is called for. There has to be a range of tools that can be employed to support the practitioner effectively so that they are freer to become more creative, to engage in positive risk-taking and thus enrich the experience of carer and those cared for.

Butterworth and Faugier (1992) describe clinical supervision as: '. . . an exchange between practising professionals to enable the development of professional skills'. The British Association of Counselling (BAC) (1990) defines counselling supervision as: 'A formal arrangement which enables counsellors to discuss their counselling regularly with one or more people who have an understanding of counselling and counselling supervision or consultative support. Its purpose is to ensure the efficacy of the counsellor/client relationship. It is a confidential relationship'.

These definitions describe clinical supervision as an enabling and developmental process. The BAC states clearly that it is a 'formal' activity which is confidential: these aspects should not be lost when establishing systems of supervision. Other writers (Burnard 1991, Kaberry 1992, Wilkin 1992, Davies 1993) support these definitions by emphasizing the developmental and supportive elements of clinical supervision.

Bishop (1994a), who worked on *A vision for the future*, gives the Butterworth/Faugier definition of clinical supervision and goes on to state its aims as: '. . . to support the delivery of optimum care by safeguarding standards and by developing professional expertise'.

Clinical supervision itself may be divided into two distinct forms, managerial and consultative, with a third, educational, being a hybrid of the two. All three forms are still focused on the practitioner's direct clinical work and although there are great similarities between them, it is important to be clear about the differences and how these may affect the supervisory arrangements and relationship.

TYPES, STRUCTURES AND MODELS OF SUPERVISION

Managerial

There is a managerial aspect to all forms of clinical supervision in that minimum standards of professional competence and conduct are maintained, but it is not normally a line-management function, although someone who has a managerial role may carry it out. The key issue here is that the supervisor is likely to have direct responsibility for the practitioners' client group, and may also have other overall responsibilities, including the coordination of the clinical team and management of the therapeutic milieu.

Platt-Koch (1986) commented that clinical supervision is often taken to mean observation by an administrative superior who inspects, directs, controls and evaluates the nurse's work. This managerial model may fit with issues of audit and quality assurance, and would overlap with appraisal or individual performance review, which do have a distinct employee–line manager relationship. It would be in contrast to managerial *clinical* supervision, as this is a collaborative relationship which aims to explore the practitioner's clinical work, with the intention of increasing their insight and understanding and thus improving their clinical effectiveness.

There may be negative connotations of managerial clinical supervision for many nurses because of the perceived conflict of interests between the practitioner and the manager. In the instance of Kath, it may prove very difficult for her to discuss her true feelings about the client

who has been a sex offender, with her line manager. She may, however, feel able to discuss them with someone of the same managerial grade who works in another clinical area.

Where nurses feel that they are being judged or assessed by a senior colleague, which may result in disciplinary action or impaired promotion prospects or, at the very least, censure, they are less likely to be open about all aspects of their work, which will limit the depth of clinical review.

> '*It is practically impossible to wear the "halo" of disciplinarian one day and the "cap" of an empathic, flexible facilitator the next.*'
> (Long and Chambers 1996)

These negative feelings may be behind the extremely low response rate (0.2%) to a questionnaire on clinical supervision in a previous edition of the *Nursing Times* (Bishop 1994b).

Systems of clinical supervision may be implemented by the managers of organizations, albeit with the best intentions, but if they fail to take account of how they will be perceived by the practitioners, they are in danger of creating resentment, hostility and non-compliance.

When managerial clinical supervision is seen as the only practicable option, then clarification of the supervisors' and supervisees' roles and associated professional boundaries is essential at the contracting stage. (Contracting will be discussed in more depth later).

Consultative (or non-managerial) clinical supervision

This form of clinical supervision will be conducted with someone who has no direct clinical responsibility for either the practitioner's client group or their workplace. Consequently, the supervisor would generally be located outside the practitioner's immediate work environment.

The reasons for opting for consultative supervision are that it removes the immediate conflict of interest associated with managerial supervision, and will usually involve someone who has greater clinical expertise, impartiality, and a desire to work in depth with the practitioners' clinical case load.

True holistic practice must have 'true' clinical supervision interwoven through it. It is a recognition that nursing is not a mechanistic formulaic activity but a complex, multilevel relationship between three key people: the client, the practitioner and the supervisor. Nursing practice should not be given credence until all three of these key people's needs are addressed by having appropriate systems of clinical supervision to support and inform the supervisee's practice.

Educational clinical supervision

This form of supervision is undertaken as part of an educational programme of study that leads to a professional practice qualification (e.g. in nursing, social work or therapy). The practitioner may be required to have supervision as part of the course requirements. Some courses stipulate who the supervisor will be, and others allow students to negotiate their own consultancy arrangements. The role of the supervisor is to assist the neophyte practitioner to integrate the particular disciplines, philosophy, values, knowledge and skills into their practice. In this instance the supervisor will have links with the educational institution and be required to maintain course requirements (e.g. reports) and monitor minimum standards of the professions' codes of competence and conduct.

This form of clinical supervision must not be confused with other forms of educational support, such as tutorials, study skills and academic supervision of assignments, where the focus is academic rather than clinical competence.

Proctor (1988) describes the functions of supervision by concentrating on the tasks of the supervisor, which are described as *formative*, *restorative* and *normative*.

Formative tasks are related to teaching and learning, the focus being on the educative processes of reflection and skills development in the supervisee. This function is the primary focus of educational clinical supervision, with normative and restorative being in the background. Restorative tasks are related to enabling the supervisee to deal with the emotional labour of caring: coping with stress and ventilating feelings. As a specific function this would be addressed by

regular personal supervision, but would not be excluded from clinical supervision. Normative tasks are related to the management of the supervisee, ensuring that organizational and professional standards are kept and monitored. This relates most closely to managerial clinical supervision, but again would be in the background of other types and forms of supervision.

Clinical supervisory structures

Clinical supervision can be provided by a variety of individuals, depending on the developmental needs of the practitioner. Houston (1990) has presented some useful methods of supervision which are eminently suitable for consideration by nurses:

- ◆ Regular one-to-one sessions with a supervisor from the same profession or discipline
- ◆ Regular supervision from a member of a different profession or discipline
- ◆ One-to-one peer supervision
- ◆ Group supervision with members of the profession/discipline
- ◆ Peer group supervision
- ◆ Network supervision, where individuals who do similar work but do not necessarily work in the same place, share elements of their supervisory practice with more experienced supervisors. Hawkins and Shohet (1989) have envisaged this method as potentially providing an interdisciplinary safety net for complex multiagency work.

 Learning activity 14.4

Undertake a small-scale informal survey among your colleagues (try to include a minimum of 20 people). Establish exactly what type of clinical supervision is operating in practice. How was this implemented? How is it practised and evaluated? What benefit does it offer for staff and clients? Compare your findings with the recommendations of *Vision for the future* (1993) and Butterworth and Faugier's *Clinical supervision: a position paper* (1994). Draw up a plan for improving and/or extending the current provision of clinical supervision in your area.

Reflection point 14.3

Review the above possibilities and locate yourself, in terms of either your current or proposed arrangements, and consider the advantages and disadvantages of the methods.

What would get in the way of your having the method you would prefer?

Are the constraints personal, e.g. the risk of approaching someone from another discipline; organizational, e.g. release from 'normal' duties to receive supervision; or practical, geographical isolation?

Models of clinical supervision and their application to sexual health practice

The supervisory requirements of practitioners who care for people with sexual health needs are diverse. They can range from inadequate knowledge through to personal attitudinal issues related to assumptions and prejudices about the clients. Clinical supervision has great potential. If used creatively, it can provide a generative model to meet these needs and enhance the effectiveness of the practitioner. This will be particularly pertinent if the supervisor can promote reflection on practice, act as a resource, facilitate self-exploration in relation to the client, and act as a catalyst for the supervisee to express feelings and emotions about their work.

Proctor's (1988) model would seem eminently suitable for adaptation by nurses working in sexual health. The formative aspect could help to address the knowledge deficits of practitioners. The restorative aspect could help to alleviate some of the stresses practitioners find themselves faced with, including embarrassment, lack of experience, and religious or moral dilemmas. The normative aspect could help to ensure that professional and organizational standards are being met, for example when working with transgendered or transvestite clients by ensuring that their privacy and dignity are respected. By encouraging reflec-

tion on practice, the sexual health practitioner is able to reinterpret his or her past experiences in the light of reflection, the outcome of which will inform future action (Schön 1983).

The critical analysis of feelings combined with knowledge leads to the development of new perspectives (Atkins and Murphy 1993), and this suggests that sensitive, informed clinical supervision, which is essential in sexual health practice, may be instrumental in achieving the attitudinal shifts vital to the provision of non-judgemental care, which is so important in the sexual health arena.

Applying models of clinical supervision in sexual health care

A great deal of attention has been focused on the need for clinical supervision (Platt-Koch 1986) and the benefits to the practitioner (Butterworth and Faugier 1994), thus affirming that it is a 'good thing'. The challenge now is for those working in sexual health care to become familiar with and skilled in the use of appropriate models of supervision.

Two models are useful as guides to understanding the overall processes and foci for supervision. Page and Woskett's (1994) 'cyclical model of counsellor supervision' and Hawkins and Shohet's (1989) 'modes of clinical supervision' provide principles that may be adapted and applied irrespective of the practitioner's discipline. The former has five stages:

- ◆ Contracting
- ◆ Focus
- ◆ Space
- ◆ Bridge
- ◆ Review.

Although the authors encourage the 'flexible and pragmatic' use of the model, they do identify the contract as an essential first stage. Contracting 'performs a vital function in underpinning the entire process and relationship' (Page and Woskett 1994, p. 34), not least by making a formal agreement as opposed to an 'ad hoc' arrangement.

Bordin (1983) espouses a supervisory working alliance whereby both parties agree and understand the goals, tasks and bonds of the relationship.

Learning activity 14.5

Think about a recent sexual health-care episode that could have been enhanced by clinical supervision. List the essential areas that could have been discussed.

In relation to your work area, what would you have liked to have seen in the basic contract?

What would you expect from your supervisor?

What do you think your supervisor would have expected from you?

What are the benefits and/or drawbacks to a formal written contract signed by both parties?

Feedback to Learning activity 14.5

A contract should explicitly address the following:

◆ Type and form of supervision

◆ Expectations of the roles and responsibilities of both parties

◆ Length of sessions, frequency, venue, time frame (open/limited)

◆ Boundaries of confidentiality

◆ Boundaries of associated personal and professional roles

◆ Methods of bringing material to sessions (verbal/written/audio/visual)

◆ Ongoing evaluation and review of the supervision (recontracting)

◆ Relationship with and requirements of employing organization (record of contact/contract/audit)

◆ Relationship with course tutors and requirements, where supervision is stipulated (reports)

◆ Provision for non-attendance (sickness, holidays)

◆ Fees, when applicable

It seems that whenever contracting is discussed there is an assumption that both parties have chosen the right person first time. It may be useful to consider a precontracting phase, when the supervisee has the opportunity to contact potential supervisors and check their compatibility in the light of expectations and needs, and then make a choice; at this point a clear and specific contract may be negotiated.

Returning to Page and Woskett's model, the second stage is the **Focus**. This refers to what the supervisee brings to supervision to explore and discuss. It is important to note here that the focus is determined by the supervisee, not the supervisor; this helps to distinguish the supervision from a general management activity. The supervisor's role here is to pay attention to whether the issue is appropriate to what has been agreed in the contracting phase.

The third stage is **Space**. The supervisor needs to create the right therapeutic climate for the supervisee to feel able to explore their issues, without being rushed into early, convenient resolutions. Houston (1990) says that to be supervised is to be

'Held, listened to, encouraged; Challenged, confronted, stimulated;
Disciplined, informed, answerable.'

Here the supervisor provides a 'containment' field for the supervisee's fears, uncertainties, triumphs and tribulations whilst on the quest for greater understanding of the complex issues associated with engaging in helping another person.

Stage four is the **Bridge**. This is about the impact that the understandings gained from supervision will have on the supervisee's actual practice. This may be at an awareness or attitudinal level, which may have a direct bearing on the practitioner's future behaviour.

The fifth stage is **Review**. Although it is likely that there is an internal ongoing monitoring of the supervision by both parties, it is essential that the relationship is kept healthy by regular explicit reviews. A good starting point may be the original contract, to check out how satisfied both parties are with the overall supervisory process, and whether the supervisee's needs are being met. A revision of the contract may help to refocus both on their respective needs, or to move the relationship onto another level.

Hawkins and Shohet (1989) show a way into the specific aspects of clinical work on which one may need to focus to open up what Ekstein (1969) referred to as practitioners' 'deaf', 'dumb' and 'blind' spots. These are particularly relevant for sexual health and are called **modes**. The six modes of clinical supervision are there for supervisors to use as reference points when assisting the supervisee to look at their practice concerns and issues.

In **mode I** the supervisor asks the supervisee to pay particular attention to the client, who they are, and how they present the content of their problems.

In **mode II** the supervisee is asked to focus on the actual approach and skills used with specific clients, so that they may consider what has worked well or not so well, and what they may try as alternative strategies and interventions. Evidence of practice may be useful here in the form of audio visual or written recordings.

In **mode III** the supervisor would question, explore and possibly challenge the supervisee's perception of how the client viewed their therapeutic relationship. In the example of Sarah, she would be encouraged to explore how she thought the new client saw her.

Mode IV is concerned with the relationship from the practitioner's perspective. Again using Sarah as an example, she would be encouraged to explore her attraction to the new client, to discover for herself what was prompting this reaction.

One may quickly see how difficult this would be if Sarah felt that what she talked about would be open to use by someone in a direct hierarchical position. The value of exploring her feelings in a safe environment is that she may then be able to use her insights to improve the care she offers in future.

In **mode V** the existence of a particular phenomenon is assumed and often referred to as the 'parallel process'. Difficulties experienced by the practitioner in their clinical work are played out in the practitioner–supervisor relationship (Ekstein and Wallerstein 1972). Unconsciously, the practitioner is 'doing to' the supervisor what their client has 'done to' them. For example, the supervisee adopts gestures and language that would cause discomfort to the supervisor. The supervisor would need to challenge and/or confront the supervisee with their discomfort by asking them to talk about their discomfort with the language and gestures used by the client.

Mode VI is an opportunity for the supervisor to share their responses to the material presented, in the form of impressions, metaphors or images. This is not an excuse for the supervisor to be a 'sage-like' dispenser of the 'truth' about the case material presented, but rather another means by which the supervisee may gain a different perspective on their problems.

QUALITIES AND SKILLS OF A SUPERVISOR

There is no 'blueprint' for the ideal supervisor; however, it is useful to consider exactly what you would be looking for in a potential supervisor in order to get the most out of the arrangement.

TRAINING TO BE A SUPERVISEE AND A SUPERVISOR

Practitioners will be supervisees, and supervisors will also need to be supervised. It therefore follows that all parties should receive some training and education for the roles they are to undertake. Supervision is being addressed in some preregistration courses, which is essential to foster the culture of clinical supervision as an intrinsic partner to professional practice. Many Trusts and clinical units are addressing this by ensuring that all staff have one or two study days to explore the nature of supervision and the structures endorsed by the employing organization. There are longer training events available, usually modules, which are CAT, rated at level two or three, and some carry the ENB RO1 Award. The advantage of these is that there is usually the opportunity to digest the concepts over a period of time, as well as having the

Learning activity 14.6

◆ What qualities and abilities would you expect your supervisor to have?

Make a two-column list; highlight words or phrases from each list that you deem to be essential.

◆ How would you know if a potential supervisor had these qualities and abilities?

Feedback on Learning activity 14.6

The following are some of the essential criteria highlighted by participants on a clinical supervision course:

◆ Primary importance is the relationship

◆ Approachable, trusting, respected, available, willing, reliable

◆ Skilled, able to challenge 'blind spots' and give honest constructive feedback

◆ Maintains boundaries of confidentiality

◆ Being able to say whatever you want without 'blowing the supervisor's mind'

◆ Knowing the supervisor won't crumble

◆ Maintaining boundaries of the relationship in all settings

◆ Being supported and encouraged to explore work issues

◆ Having clinical and academic credibility

◆ A role model, with the equivalent or more experience, and knowledge of your area of work

◆ Someone from a related discipline, so able to be on the same 'wavelength'

◆ Allows 'control' of session by supervisee.

opportunity to experience being supervised and practice the skills of supervising.

In establishing systems of supervision for sexual health-care workers it is important to acknowledge the complexity of their work, particularly its difficult emotional and psychological aspects. Practitioners need a safe environment to explore all of these to maintain their effectiveness and to provide the highest possible quality service to their clients.

ACKNOWLEDGEMENTS

We would like to thank Christopher Johns, University of Luton, for his encouragement and allowing us to use his guided model of reflection in this chapter. We would also like to acknowledge past work with Derek Lawton (a friend, colleague and humanistic practitioner in the Leeds CMHT) in unravelling and putting together key concepts regarding supervision and consultancy.

RESOURCES AND ANNOTATED FURTHER READING

Bond T 1992 HIV Counselling, 2nd edn. British Association for Counselling/Department of Health, Rugby

A good book which utilizes Proctor's model of supervision. This would be a useful resource for any practitioners working in sexual health, despite the focus on HIV.

English National Board for Nursing, Midwifery and Health Visiting 1994 Caring for people with sexually transmitted diseases, including HIV. ENB, London

This is a well thought-out package designed to enable practitioners to learn about caring for clients with sexual health-related issues. It comprises of several workbooks and, importantly, recognizes support and supervision as areas for practitioners to develop.

Lawton D, Samociuk G A 1997 The pocket guide to clinical supervision. Leeds Community and Mental Health Trust, Leeds

This concise booklet is available from the Leeds CMHT and has a useful question and answer section on supervision issues.

NHS Executive 1995 Clinical supervision – a resource pack. DoH, London

An excellent package full of resources related to clinical supervision.

Palmer H 1995 Clinical supervision for nurses working with people with HIV/AIDS. Professional Nurse 11(1): 20–22

Overview of the benefits of clinical supervision in relation to nurses working in the field of HIV/AIDS, particularly in meeting developmental and support needs.

Courses

The University of Manchester School of Nursing, Midwifery and Health Visiting Division of Continuing Education offers the ENB RO1 'Clinical Supervision Skills for Supervisors' with 40 level 2 credits.

The University of Leeds School of Healthcare Studies also offers modules at level 2 (Clinical Supervision Skills of Professional Practice) and level 3 (Clinical Supervision Skills for Supervisors). Contact the authors for the latest details on these modules.

Check with your local institution offering health-care education to see what they offer.

REFERENCES

Atkin S, Murphy K 1993 Reflection: a review of the literature. Journal of Advanced Nursing 18: 1188–1192

Bishop V 1994a Clinical supervision for an accountable profession. Nursing Times 90(39): 35–37

Bishop V 1994b Clinical supervision questionnaire results. Nursing Times 90(48): 40–42

Bordin, E S 1983 A working alliance based model of supervision. Counselling Psychologist 11(1): 35–42

Boud D, Keogh R, Walker D 1985 Reflection: turning experience into learning. Kogan Page, London

Boyd E M, Fales A W 1983 Reflective learning: key to learning from experience. Journal of Humanistic Psychology 23(2): 99–117

British Association of Counselling 1990 Code of ethics and practice for counsellors. BAC, Rugby

Burnard P 1991 Coping with stress in the health professions. Chapman & Hall, London

Butterworth C A 1994 Preparing to take on clinical supervision. Nursing Standard 8(52): 32–34

Butterworth C A, Faugier J 1992 Clinical supervision and mentorship in nursing. Chapman & Hall, London

Butterworth C A, Faugier J 1994 Clinical supervision: a position paper. University of Manchester School of Nursing Studies, Manchester

Carper B A 1978 Fundamental patterns of knowing in nursing. In: Nicoll L H (ed) Perspectives on nursing theory. Little Brown, Boston

Chinn P L, Kramer M K 1991 Theory and nursing: A systematic approach, 3rd edn. Mosby, St. Louis

Conway J 1994 Reflection, the art and science of nursing and the theory–practice gap. British Journal of Nursing 3(3): 114–118

Davies P 1993 Value yourself. Nursing Times 89 (4): 52

Department of Health 1993 A vision for the future. The nursing, midwifery and health visiting contribution to health and health care. Report of the Chief Nursing Officer. HMSO, London

Ekstein R 1969 Concerning the teaching and learning of psychoanalysis. Journal of the American Psychoanalytic Association (USA) 17(2): 312–332

Ekstein R, Wallerstein R W 1972 The teaching and learning of psychotherapy. International Universities Press, New York

English National Board for Nursing, Midwifery and Health Visiting 1994 Caring for people with sexually transmitted diseases, including HIV. ENB, London

Grohar M E, DiCroce H R 1992 Leadership and management in nursing. Appleton & Lange, East Norwalk

Hawkins P 1982 Mapping it out. Community Care, 22 July: 17–19

Hawkins P, Shohet R 1989 Supervision in the helping professions. Open University Press, Milton Keynes

Houston G 1990 Supervision and counselling. Rochester Foundation, London

Johns C C 1995 Framing learning through reflection within Carper's fundamental ways of knowing in nursing. Journal of Advanced Nursing 22: 226–234

Kaberry S 1992 Supervision – support for nurses? Senior Nurse 12(5): 38–40

Landrum P A, Beck C M, Rawlins R P, Williams S R 1993 The person as a client. In: Rawlins R P, Williams S R, Beck C M, (eds) Mental health – psychiatric nursing: a holistic life cycle approach. Mosby-Year Book, St. Louis, pp 17–39

Long A, Chambers M 1996 Supervision in counselling: a channel for personal and professional change. Counselling Journal, February, pp 50–54

Morton-Cooper A, Palmer A 1993 Mentoring and preceptorship: a guide to support roles in clinical practice. Blackwell, Oxford

Page S, Woskett V 1994 Supervising the counsellor: a cyclical model. Routledge, London

Platt-Koch L M 1986 Clinical supervision for psychiatric nurses. Journal of Psychosocial Nursing 26(1): 7–15

Proctor B 1988 Supervision: a co-operative exercise in accountability. In: Marken M, Rayne M (eds) Enabling and ensuring: supervision and practice. National Youth Bureau, Leicester, pp 21–34

Riseborough P, Walters M 1988 Management in health care. Wright, London

Schön D 1983 The reflective practitioner. Basic Books, New York

UKCC 1993 Registrar's letter: The council's position concerning a period of support and preceptorship: implementation of the post registration, education and practice project proposals. United Kingdom Central Council, London

UKCC 1995 Position statement on clinical supervision for nursing and health visiting: Annexe 1 to Registrar's Letter 4/1995. United Kingdom Central Council for Nursing, Midwifery and Health Visiting, London

UKCC 1996 Position statement on clinical supervision for nursing and health visiting. United Kingdom Central Council for Nursing, Midwifery and Health Visiting, London

Wilkin P 1992 Clinical supervision in community psychiatric nursing. In: Butterworth T, Faugier J (eds) Clinical supervision and mentorship in nursing. Chapman & Hall, London, pp 185–199

Index

Page numbers in **bold** type indicate figures and tables